Understanding
Autism

To Sharyn

Whose strength and courage was an inspiration
and who taught me never to give up.

You raise me up, so I can stand on mountains
You raise me up, to walk on stormy seas
I am strong, when I am on your shoulders
You raise me up, to more than I can be.

(Brendan Graham/Rolf Lovland)

Understanding
Autism

SUSAN DODD

ELSEVIER

Sydney Edinburgh London New York Philadelphia St Louis Toronto

ELSEVIER

Elsevier Australia
(a division of Reed International Books Australia Pty Ltd)
30–52 Smidmore Street, Marrickville, NSW 2204
ACN 001 002 357

The publisher acknowledges the kind assistance of Berri Limited and the Sanitarium
Health Food Company for their kind permission to reproduce images of their products
as visual supports.

National Library of Australia Cataloguing-in-Publication Data

Dodd, Susan M.
Understanding Autism.

Includes index.
ISBN-13: 978-1-875897-80-3
ISBN-10: 1-875897-80-1

1. Autism. I. Title.

616.85882

Publishing director: Vaughn Curtis
Publishing services manager: Helena Klijn
Project coordinator: Emma Hutchinson
Editor, project manager and proofreader: Persimmon Press
Designer and typesetter: Wing Ping Tong
Illustrators: Greg Gaul Graphics and Shelly Communications Pty Ltd
Indexers: Glenda Browne and Jon Jermey
Printed and bound in Australia by Ligare Pty Ltd

Contents

Acknowledgments

This work would not have been completed without the assistance and support of a number of people.

Firstly, my thanks go to Jordan for his many hours of 'at call' technical support and his absolute commitment to completing this manuscript.

Thank you to Clare for her unwavering support and determination that I would complete this manuscript and for the incisive comments and feedback provided on the numerous drafts that she read without complaint.

I wish to thank the following people who provided valuable comments on an earlier draft: Dr Tony Attwood, Michele Carson, Michele Whitehouse and Chris Kilham.

Photographic credits are owed to Linda Roberts. Linda took the photographs used in the visual supports in the book.

I am indebted and grateful to the hundreds of parents and individuals with autism I have been fortunate to work with over the past 20 years. Their courage, resilience and compassion is remarkable.

Finally, I have been privileged to work with so many outstanding professionals. My journey through autism, which is reflected in this book, has been enriched and enhanced by the interactions and stimulus of working alongside dedicated and genuinely interested colleagues.

Introduction

Understanding Autism is written for parents and professionals who live with, and work with, individuals with autism. The book reflects my accumulated knowledge gained from many years of working professionally with parents and individuals with autism. It attempts to answer many of the most commonly asked questions about autism and also to provide information about the latest research findings and teaching techniques. The ultimate goal is to leave the reader with a better understanding of autism and what autism means for those individuals who have the disorder.

Over the past twenty years in particular, there have been remarkable developments in our knowledge of what autism is, why it happens, and how it should be treated. We have a better understanding of how autism affects individuals and the impact that having a child with autism has on families and the communities in which they live. The developments have come from a variety of sources — from medical, psychological and educational research; from statistical analysis of sociological data; from accumulated experience of numerous teaching approaches and methods; and from individuals who have willingly shared their experiences of living with autism.

Autism is a developmental disorder and it is important to recognise that individuals with autism are different — they think differently, they learn differently and their needs and interests are different. They also have some incredible strengths and abilities that should be recognised and acknowledged and harnessed to assist them to manage their lives and move towards independence.

Children with classic autism are usually diagnosed between the ages of 2 and 4. However, children and adults with atypical autism, high functioning autism or Asperger's syndrome may not be diagnosed until much later, sometimes not until adulthood. Some parents are aware that something is wrong with their young child and spend months and years searching for answers. Other parents have no idea that there is a problem and a diagnosis of autism comes as a real shock. Some individuals grow up knowing they are different — struggling at school, constantly frustrated and anxious. They are not given the support and understanding they need to help them cope in a world that does not recognise their needs and, indeed, their unique potential contributions. For these parents, and the individuals with autism, the diagnosis leaves them floundering and asking 'What does it mean?' and 'What do I do now?'.

Many professionals are first introduced to autism when faced with a young child requiring therapy, a client requiring assessment, a new student in the classroom with high support needs or a young adult requiring help to cope with severe stress and anxiety. If they are not familiar with autism they may also be asking 'How do I help this person?', 'What therapies and approaches work best?', 'How does this person learn?'.

Understanding Autism addresses these questions and provides information about the triad of impairments of autism as well as practical strategies for parents and professionals to help individuals with autism to maximise their potential.

This book is not meant to be a catalogue of the latest research findings but rather a readable summary of the latest trends. It is a practical guide that offers insight into the needs and strengths of people with autism. It offers practical suggestions and strategies that are useful for parents, teachers, health professionals and individuals with autism. The strategies introduced throughout the book may be individualised and adapted to different situations.

The first section of *Understanding Autism* is designed to provide essential background information about the disorder and addresses topics such as what autism is, possible causes, diagnosis, incidence, current trends in research and treatment, controversies such as MMR (measles, mumps, rubella) vaccinations, and alternative treatments such as secretin, specific diets and vitamin therapy.

The next section addresses the triad of impairments in autism that consist of:

- impairments in communication;
- impairments in social interaction; and
- patterns of behaviour, interests and/or activities that are restricted, repetitive, or stereotypic.

In addition, the section also addresses the sensory impairments that are so prevalent among individuals with autism and impact on their ability to cope and live independently.

Having covered the theoretical background in the first sections, the book moves on to provide information about diagnostic and assessment procedures. Asperger's syndrome is explained in the context of the unique thinking and learning styles of individuals with autism; for example, their weak auditory processing skills as opposed to their ability to process information presented visually. Practical examples of visual supports that are used to augment communication are provided.

The next section considers behavioural issues and the problems associated with emotions, stress and anxiety. It outlines the use of positive behaviour supports to address these issues.

The final section of *Understanding Autism* offers practical suggestions that may be beneficial to parents and professionals involved with individuals with autism. It explains the importance of teaching young children with autism how to play socially and provides examples of play programs and suggestions on how to set up practical play sessions. Dealing with change is a major issue for individuals with autism and it is important to plan ahead for changes to routines. General teaching strategies and programming ideas to assist with behaviours such as aggression, problems at mealtimes and rest times, as well as skills such as toileting, are discussed.

Individuals with autism have great strengths and can make valuable contributions without having to conform to unrealistic social standards. The aim of *Understanding Autism* is to offer hope to parents and to individuals with autism — hope that each individual with autism can reach his or her potential and live a full and rich life by being him- or herself.

CHAPTER

1

What is Autism?

Autism may be defined as a pervasive developmental disorder, characterised by impairments in communication and social interaction, and restricted, repetitive and stereotypic patterns of behaviour, interests and activities.

Diagnostic and Statistical Manual of Mental Disorders 1994 (DSM-IV) (American Psychiatric Association)

Leo Kanner, in 1943, wrote the first accepted clinical paper describing the psychological features of a number of children he labeled as 'autistic'. The word autism, from the Greek words 'aut' meaning self and 'ism' implying orientation or state, suggested that these children were unusually absorbed in themselves and showed little interest in others.

Kanner's original conclusion was that the autistic child was born with an '... innate inability to form the usual biologically provided affective contact with people' (Kanner 1943, p 42–3). He perceived autism to be a biological disorder of affective functioning, listing the main characteristics as:

- an inability to establish social relatedness;
- a failure to use language normally for the purpose of communication;
- an obsessive desire for the maintenance of sameness;
- a fascination for objects; and
- good cognitive potentialities.

Furthermore, these characteristics were present in children before the age of 30 months.

Since Kanner's original description, many researchers have advanced different theories and provided alternative views on what constitutes a diagnosis of autism and what causes the disorder. Educational practices follow the lead of research and scientific theories, so that the teaching of these children has also varied over the years, in line with the scientific theories about cause.

During the 1950s and 1960s, treatments for autism were based on theories that prescribed an emotional aetiology (Bettelheim 1967). In 1956, Bettelheim claimed that autism consisted of 'a disturbance of the ability to reach out to the world' due to a lack of parental emotional warmth, introducing the term 'refrigerator parent' to describe the mothers of children with autism. It was not until some years later that these theories were entirely discredited.

As the hope of 'emotional recovery' faded, a new approach was developed in the 1970s that described autism as a cognitive and linguistic impairment (Rutter 1978; Wing 1976). Theories eventually moved toward a behavioural approach (Lovaas 1977) that emphasised structured teaching and initially paid only brief attention to the social and emotional growth of the children. Wing and Gould (1979) first introduced the term 'triad of impairments', to describe children with autism. They studied a group of children under the age of 15 with learning and behavioural difficulties and concluded from their findings that there was a marked social nature to the difficulties of their subjects. They identified an 'autism triad' of impairments:

- an impairment of social interaction;
- an impairment of social communication; and
- an impairment of social imagination.

Wing and Gould identified a number of children with 'Kanner's Syndrome' and a number of other children with similar behaviours but not quite meeting Kanner's original criteria. In 1988, Wing introduced a broader term, 'autistic continuum', to describe children with the triad of impairments and then revised the term to 'autistic spectrum' in 1996. Autism is now referred to as a spectrum disorder because the specific characteristics may be present in a variety of combinations and may range along a continuum from mild to severe.

The term spectrum allows a broader definition of autism based on the triad of impairments and forms the basis for a specific range of treatment and educational approaches for children and adults who are diagnosed within the autistic spectrum.

What is the triad of impairments?

Autistic disorders affect a person's abilities in the following areas:

- Communication — this includes all aspects of communication including the comprehension and use of verbal and non-verbal communication to interact and communicate with others.
- Social relating — means how a person relates and interacts with other people, objects and events and includes skills such as sharing, turn taking and attending to tasks.
- Restricted interests and repetitive behaviours — are likely to be the product of cognition (thinking) characteristics of autism and are shown as a lack of imagination, poor abstract reasoning, limited play skills, concrete thinking and a strong desire for consistency.

These three areas are known as the core features of autism or the triad of impairments (Wing and Gould 1979).

Since the early 1990s, research has extended beyond describing observable behaviours associated with a triad of impairments. Today, emphasis is placed on looking more at the particular thinking and learning styles of children and adults with autism and developing interventions to match these. In general, teaching approaches today focus on child and family-centred practices that assess individual needs, accommodate individual learning styles and teach functional skills in real-life situations. Emphasis is also placed on the importance of social context in teaching individuals with autism.

A major goal of any intervention program is to enhance communication and socialisation abilities by supporting the integration of people with autism with adults and peers in regular services, school, work and community settings. It is no longer seen as necessary to try to fit individuals with autism into normal learning patterns (rather like trying to fit a square peg into a round hole). People with autism think and learn differently and it has taken until the last few years for us to acknowledge this and to understand, accept and work with these differences.

Liane Holliday Willey is a Doctor of Education who has Asperger's syndrome, a form of autism. She has written extensively about her life while pretending to be normal, and her realisation that she is who she is and does not have to try to fit into any social mould. She has a wonderful understanding of the triad of impairments and what it means to be 'on the utistic spectrum' (Willey 1999, p 107):

> On any given day, I can be just like everyone else seems to be.
> Until I remember I do not have to be.
> The me that I am has finally made friends with the
> differences I no longer try to hide.
> With effervescence in my heart I now find it easy, natural, right to harvest
> what I will and what I need from the places I visit and the people I meet.
> And with joy in my soul I am content to hope I have left something
> worthwhile, something safe and sound, behind me.

What is the current focus in autism?

Over the past decade, a number of related features also associated with autism have received increased understanding and attention. These include:

- sensory sensitivities;
- cognitive aspects including the visual learning style, attention problems and information processing characteristics; and
- empathy impairment including emotional problems, joint attention, theory of mind and difficulties interpreting moods and behaviour in other people.

Figure 1.1 outlines the major differences in how autism has been perceived over the past three decades. The move today is away from looking simply at the overt behaviours of individuals and towards determining the underlying causes of these behaviours and questioning why they occur in children and adults with autism.

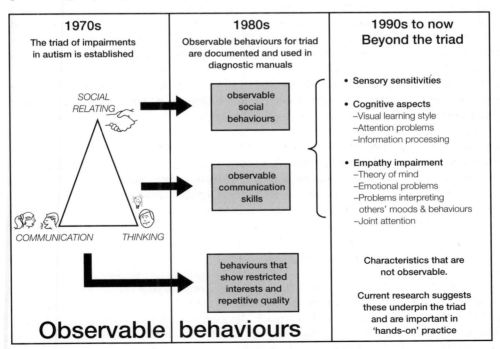

Figure 1.1 *A visual representation of how the picture of autism has changed over the past few decades. Developed by Jacqueline Roberts and Louise Ulliana, Autism Spectrum Australia (Aspect), 2000*

Unusual sensory responses and sensory sensitivities have been recognised in people with autism for a number of years. Among the current list of publications written by, or about, individuals with autism is a wealth of information about the sensory deficits that impact on their day-to-day existence and cause them problems throughout life. Over the past few years, an increasing focus on the importance of sensory integration and desensitisation programs for individuals with autism has proved successful in managing specific sensory problems.

It is also becoming more and more obvious that, in order to understand the disability and then to develop successful intervention strategies, we need to understand the particular thinking and learning styles of individuals with autism. Individuals with autism are different from their peers in several crucial ways: they tend to learn more effectively if information is presented visually; they have difficulty focusing and maintaining attention; and they have unique ways of obtaining and processing information from the environment.

Over the past decade, Kanner's original description of autism as the consequence of a complex disorder of brain development affecting many functions (Dawson 1989; Frith 1989) has once again been recognised and widely accepted.

Attention has also moved away from the linguistic difficulties associated with autism. The current focus on the social nature of the core difficulties has led to an interest in the research into impaired theory of mind functioning in autism and also research into the difficulties associated with shared attention (Baron-Cohen 1995). According to Baron-Cohen, the ability to engage in shared attention is the prerequisite for theory of mind to develop. Since this ability is impaired in autism and the child is unable to engage in shared attention, theory of mind fails to develop.

What is theory of mind?

Theory of mind research, represented by the work of Baron-Cohen, Leslie and Frith (1985) originated from research on social cognition. Bruner, in 1975, established the importance of communication in social exchanges and relationships and the findings of a number of studies concerning theory of mind deficits in autism put the spotlight on social cognition as a possible primary deficit in autism (Baron-Cohen 1991).

The concept of a 'theory of mind' in individuals was introduced by Wellman (1992) to explain the process of understanding the mental states of oneself and others. The term was coined on the basis that mental states are not visible and, therefore, have to be hypothesised. Baron-Cohen completed the original work in this area in 1985 with his false belief test, also known as the Sally/Anne Test.

The Sally/Anne Test was designed to show whether children understand the implications of a false belief. Before the ages of three or four, children do not appreciate the difference between their own belief and someone else's belief, and that there can be different beliefs about the same event. After that age, children realise that other people have different beliefs than they do and this helps their ability to understand and relate to others in the ordinary way. It has been hypothesised that children with autism do not develop a theory of mind and are therefore unable to understand that other people have different thoughts and beliefs.

Baron-Cohen, Leslie & Frith conducted the original research in this area in 1985 to test the hypothesis that children with autism fail to take account of beliefs (one type of mental state). They tested autistic, normal and developmentally delayed Down's syndrome children with a mental age above three years (see Appendix 1).

Tager-Flusberg (1996) concluded that young children with autism develop communicative functions that affect the behaviour of others, such as requesting; but that they do not develop communicative functions that affect other's mental states, such as commenting. Baron-Cohen

(1989) also found that toddlers with autism develop pointing to request, but fail to develop pointing to comment or to share information.

Frith (1989) found that the fundamental difficulty for people with autism is understanding their own and others' mental states. It is not merely that they are unable to understand what other people are thinking and feeling, but rather that they cannot understand that people do think and feel (that is, that people have minds).

Theory of mind involves the understanding that other people have thoughts, wishes and desires that are different from our own. It is based on the fact that individuals with autism are impaired in their ability to 'mind-read'. Children on the autism spectrum are 'mind blind'; they think that other people think and feel exactly as they do. They do not understand that other people they come in contact with — parents, teachers and peers — may not have exactly the same feelings and point of view as they do. They do not recognise that people vary in their thoughts, beliefs and desires that impact on their behaviour. Theory of mind proposes that people with autism do not develop the ability to think about others' thoughts so that they are impaired in some social, communicative and imaginative skills (Happe 1994).

Theory of mind can also be described as a mental state that exists apart from the reality of a particular situation. According to Baron-Cohen, the prerequisite for theory of mind to develop is the child's ability to engage in joint sharing of attention. It is known that this ability is impaired in children with autism and so theory of mind fails to develop.

How is autism classified?

In addition to an increasing interest in the core deficits, especially the social deficits of autism, there has been widespread confusion and conflict over diagnostic criteria. Children with autism are now typically classified according to either the World Health Organisation's International Classification of Diseases (ICD-10, WHO 1992) or the American Psychiatric Association's Diagnostic and Statistical Manual (DSM-IV, APA 1994). Both classification approaches incorporate the notion of a triad of impairments (Wing & Gould 1979) to describe autistic individuals. These impairments impact upon a person's ability to relate socially to others, to communicate effectively and to learn and think like other people.

In very young children, the problems appear as poor eye contact, limited social awareness, no joint sharing of attention or interaction with others, sensitivity to certain sounds and lack of anticipation of others' social approaches. In addition, vocalisations such as babbling are minimal or nonexistent and imitation of gestures and sounds and responsiveness to social overtures are absent or limited (Freeman & Ritvo 1984). Some children also display repetitive behaviours, such as rocking or hand flapping, obsessions with certain objects or routines, an inability to cope with change to normal routines, poor play skills and little interest in conventional toys.

In older children, adolescents and adults, the same problems exist but may be obvious in different ways. For example, language may be present but still appear disordered by echolalia, repetitive questioning, perseveration on certain topics of interest, literal thinking and poor verbal processing skills. Socially, children and adults with autism may have difficulty initiating social contact and also responding appropriately to others' attempts to interact. Most adults with autism may be described as social 'loners' with a marked preference for their own company and a lack of awareness of the thoughts and feelings of others. In addition, the need for sameness, the inability to attend to more than one stimuli at a time, or to 'read' the environment, continue to cause many difficulties as individuals with autism endeavour to 'fit' into society.

Although the primary characteristics of autism have been well documented over the past twenty years and classification systems are now in place, there is still a general feeling of reluctance on the part of doctors to define autism and to diagnose the disorder. This could be in part due to the fact that there is no single medical test that will definitively confirm the presence of the disorder. Many parents struggle for a number of years to obtain a diagnosis or for someone to confirm that their child has autism. Once the diagnosis is given, parents are then often left wondering what to do as they are provided with little information about what the term autism actually means.

What is a definition of autism?

Autism refers to a number of neuro-developmental disorders that affect some parts of the central nervous system (i.e. the brain and nervous system), particularly the way that both verbal and non-verbal information is processed. Autism affects how people understand their world and what is happening around them. Autism is seen as a lifelong disability because there is no known cure. However, children and adults with autism continue to change and grow and many show dramatic improvements in a range of skills throughout their lives.

The core features of autism vary in terms of severity. There is considerable variability in the levels of cognitive ability within the autism group, ranging from high-functioning individuals of normal or superior intelligence to those with a severe/profound intellectual disability. The triad of impairments in autism may also present in a single person quite differently at different ages. Currently, the idea of a spectrum of autism is widely accepted. This spectrum is referred to in the literature as either an autism spectrum disorder (ASD) or a pervasive developmental disorder (PDD).

The term pervasive developmental disorder was originally adopted to provide a formal diagnosis for individuals who shared many of the characteristics of people with autism but were unable to meet the full criteria for a diagnosis. The term PDD implies the global nature of the impairments that are associated with the disorders, while still differentiating autism from more general cognitive disabilities such as global developmental delay. A breakdown of the types of pervasive developmental disorders is illustrated in Figure 1.2.

The blanket term pervasive developmental disorder includes autism or autistic disorder, Asperger's syndrome, and atypical autism (or pervasive developmental disorder not otherwise specified (PDD-NOS) as well as Rett's syndrome, and childhood disintegrative disorder). The term autism spectrum disorders includes Asperger's syndrome, autistic disorder (also known

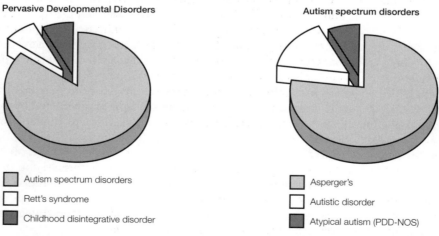

Pervasive Developmental Disorders

- Autism spectrum disorders
- Rett's syndrome
- Childhood disintegrative disorder

Autism spectrum disorders

- Asperger's
- Autistic disorder
- Atypical autism (PDD-NOS)

Figure 1.2 *A breakdown of sub-categories of pervasive developmental disorders*

Figure 1.3 *A breakdown of the sub-categories of autism spectrum disorders*

as infantile autism or Kanner's syndrome) and atypical autism (also known as PDD-NOS). Autism spectrum disorders are illustrated in Figure 1.3.

What is Asperger's syndrome?

Asperger's syndrome was first identified nearly sixty years ago by Hans Asperger, when he described a consistent pattern of abilities and behaviour in a group of young children made up predominantly of boys. 'The pattern included a lack of empathy, little ability to form friendships, one-sided conversations, intense absorption in a special interest and clumsy movements' (Attwood 1998). Asperger's syndrome is characterised by impaired ability to utilise social cues such as body language, irony, or other subtext of communication; restricted eye contact and socialisation; limited range of interests; perseverative, odd behaviours; didactic, verbose, monotone voice; concrete thinking; over-sensitivity to certain stimuli; and unusual movements.

What is Rett's syndrome

Rett's syndrome is a complex neurological disorder that mainly affects girls. It is present at birth but becomes more evident during the second year of life. Particularly noticeable is the loss of purposeful hand movements that are replaced by stereotypic movements including hand wringing or clapping. People with Rett's syndrome are profoundly and multiply disabled and require intense support throughout life. At least one in every 10,000 females born has Rett's syndrome. It is believed to be one of the most common causes of severe and profound learning disability in girls. Most individuals with Rett's syndrome have a mutation on the MECP2 gene on the X-chromosome and are diagnosed through a process of genetic screening.

What is childhood disintegrative disorder?

Childhood disintegrative disorder is characterised by a period of normal development for the first two to three years and then loss of previously acquired skills by the age of ten, especially in the areas of language, social, cognitive or motor skills.

What is pervasive developmental disorder not otherwise specified (PDD-NOS)?

Pervasive developmental disorder not otherwise specified (PDD-NOS) is often shown as atypical autism and refers to people who exhibit impairments in social, communication and stereotypic behaviours but do not meet full criteria for a diagnosis of autism.

Controversy remains over which disorders should be included in the spectrum and also how broadly the spectrum extends (Mahoney et al 1998), but there is almost universal agreement that there is a spectrum that best describes the range of 'autistic' behaviour. Autism may be differentiated from other PDDs in a number of ways. According to Lord & Risi (2000), factors that differentiate autism from other major pervasive developmental disorders include age of onset, presence of cognitive or language delays, severity of the disorder and presence of co-morbid factors. These factors are illustrated in Table 1.1.

How common is autism?

Autism affects as many as 19 cases for every 10,000 people in the population. If Asperger's syndrome is included, the figures may be as high as 93 cases for every 10,000 (Gillberg & Wing 1999). Autism may occur in isolation or in association with other conditions such as epilepsy, intellectual impairment, Down's syndrome, ADHD (attention deficit hyperactivity disorder), cerebral palsy and other specific genetic and developmental disorders.

There is disagreement in the literature about the prevalence of autism spectrum disorders. Trevarthen et al (1996) stated that autism affects approximately one person in every 400. Due

Table 1.1 *Factors that differentiate autism from other pervasive developmental disorders (PDDs). From Lord & Risi (2000)*

Disorder	Onset/course	Delay	Severity	Domain affected
Autism	Prior to 3 years	May or may not be associated with general delays	Exceeds standard thresholds of number of features	Social, communication, repetitive behaviours
Childhood disintegrative disorder	Typical development up to 2 years; loss of speech and at least one other skill	Usually associated with mental retardation requiring extensive supports	Thresholds not specified but appear same as autism	Abnormalities in two of three domains of autism
Asperger's syndrome	Onset may be before or after 3 years	No general delay in cognition or language	Must exceed threshold in social area	Social and circumscribed interests
Atypical autism (ICD-10)/ pervasive developmental disorder-not otherwise specified (DSM-IV)	May fail to meet autism onset criteria	May or may not be associated with developmental delays	May fall below threshold in one or more areas	Social and either communication or repetitive behaviours or both

to various factors — increased awareness by both the public and professionals, a widening of the spectrum, improved diagnostic techniques and different methodologies in research that have included related disorders such as Asperger's syndrome, Rett's syndrome and milder forms of autism — this estimate has increased over the past few years. Whether these factors are sufficient to account for the marked increase in the prevalence of autism, or whether there has been an actual increase in the number of people affected, is yet to be clarified.

According to Gillberg & Wing (1999) the ratio is closer to 1:100 (93 cases for every 10,000 people) of the general population, with approximately 60 in every 10,000 people diagnosed with Asperger's syndrome.

There is a higher incidence of autism among males. The ratio varies according to the definition but is commonly cited as 4:1 males to females for autism and rising to approximately 9:1 males to females when Asperger's syndrome is included (Attwood 1998; Gillberg 2002). Typically, when females are diagnosed with autism, they are more severely affected and have a significant degree of mental retardation.

Approximately 70% of people with an autistic disorder have intellectual disabilities ranging from mild through to severe. There is also considerable overlap between different subtypes and other related disorders such as severe intellectual disability, attention/hyperactivity disorder and obsessive/compulsive disorder.

What causes autism?

In most cases, it is not known what causes autism although it is now recognised as a biological/neurological problem affecting certain parts of the brain. It is generally accepted that autism is caused by abnormalities in brain structures or functions. Considerable research has been and continues to be conducted into possible causes. Using a variety of research tools to study human and animal brain growth, scientists are discovering more about normal development and how abnormalities occur. It seems clear that autism is caused by something that either damages the brain before, during or after birth, or prevents the brain from developing normally.

Different parts of the brain have a variety of functions:

- the hippocampus makes it possible to recall recent experience and new information;
- the amygdala directs emotional responses;
- the frontal lobes of the cerebrum help with problem solving, planning ahead, understanding the behaviour of others and restraining impulses;
- the parietal areas control hearing, speech and language;
- the cerebellum regulates balance, body movements, coordination and the muscles used in speaking; and
- the corpus callossum passes information from one side of the brain to the other.

These parts are shown in Figure 1.4.

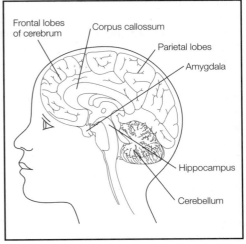

Figure 1.4 *Cross-section of the human brain*

Recent research into the anatomy and functioning of the human brain has indicated that there are consistent differences between the brains of autistic and non-autistic individuals. According to research (Courchesne 1995), the cerebellum of children with autism is smaller and has more densely packed cells and other abnormal characteristics. Huebner (1992) found abnormalities to other parts of the brain including the hippocampus, brainstem and the frontal lobes although no conclusions have as yet been reached that have definitively supported the suggestion that these brain differences cause autistic symptoms. It is likely that there are several sites and types of neurological difference that cause autism. Scientists are also looking for abnormalities in the brain structures that make up the limbic system. Inside the limbic system, the amygdala is known to help regulate aspects of social and emotional behaviour.

Differences in neurotransmitters, the chemical messengers of the nervous system, are also being explored. High levels of the neurotransmitter serotonin have been found in a number of people with autism. Since neurotransmitters are responsible for passing nerve impulses in the brain and nervous system, it is possible that they are involved in the distortion of sensations that accompanies autism.

What causes normal brain development to go awry? Researchers are investigating genetic causes — the role that heredity and genes play in passing the disorder from one generation to the next.

It has also been suggested that autism may be triggered by something in the environment. In some cases a child is affected from birth, or shortly after birth. For this reason, researchers are exploring whether certain conditions, such as the mother's health during pregnancy, problems during delivery, or other environmental factors interfere with normal brain development.

Some families have noted differences in their child within the first year, and in other children clear symptoms have not been noticed until the middle of the second year. Some children seem to develop normally but then regress after their first year. There may be a history of severe trauma, related primarily to ill health, occasionally to an accident which the parents feel to be the triggering factor; while in other cases the cause is unknown. Possible environmental risk factors mentioned in research and by parents include exposures, before and after birth, to drugs, infections and heavy metals; metabolic disorders; genetic/chromosomal factors; exposure to viral infections; extreme reactions to vaccinations; or development of subclinical seizures. In most cases, however, there is no identifiable cause.

Autism may be caused by both genetic and environmental factors — something in the environment may trigger the disorder in children who are genetically susceptible. There is no shortage of theories about possible triggers — theories from mercury poisoning to vitamin A deficiency have been put forward to explain possible causes of autism in young children.

A new book by psychologist Simon Baron-Cohen (2003), defines autism as an imbalance between two kinds of intelligence — an intelligence based on 'empathising' with people, and an intelligence based on 'systematising' objects. According to Baron-Cohen, all individuals have both forms of intelligence but females, in general, are better at empathising and males are better at systematising. He regards autism as an exaggerated version of the male profile — an extreme need for rule-based systems, combined with an inability to intuit people's feelings and intentions. The book, titled *The Essential Difference*, raises some interesting questions for further discussion and offers a new framework for thinking about autism in both boys and girls. If Baron-Cohen is right, the current approach that sees autism as a medical condition requiring a cure may need to be reviewed. Autism may also be a mental style that people can learn to accommodate and even recognise as a possible gift. Though many of the characteristics commonly associated with autism may support Baron-Cohen's hypothesis, the model may be too simplistic. People with autism are not just extreme systematisers. They systematise in a distinct and unusual way that is not entirely logical. There is usually a preference for parts over wholes, a tendency to process information piece by piece rather than a gestalt approach of filtering information through general categories. Baron-Cohen agrees that the model may not capture all of the nuances of autism, but it does offer a possible explanation for the repetitive behaviours and restricted interests of people across the autism spectrum. According to current theories, most of the repetitive behaviours of individuals with autism are purposeless whereas Baron-Cohen suggests that these behaviours may be providing opportunities for individuals to look for predictable rules or patterns in the information being collected.

Most researchers believe that autism has a number of different causes. These different causes could all affect the same brain systems, or they could interfere with the development of communication and social functions in individuals. The communication and social functions are at the root of the problems and differences associated with autism, and form the basis for the current diagnostic procedures of looking at the triad of impairments.

There is also considerable interest in a number of possible physiological abnormalities affecting the gastro-intestinal tract, metabolism and the immune system. According to Jackson (2002, p 15):

> It is ... widely accepted that people on the autism spectrum have difficulties in the area of language, communication, social interaction and imagination and often engage in obsessive or repetitive behaviours and rituals. Many people on the spectrum also suffer from debilitating stomach and bowel problems.

Casein- and gluten-free diets have become popular, with documented reports of improvements both in the current literature and anecdotally from parents who have tried recommended diets. To date, however, there are no properly controlled studies reported in scientific or medical journals to support the outcomes from individual cases. Further investigation under properly controlled conditions is required.

While there is no consensus about what definitely causes autism, we do know that autism is *not* caused by parents or by the home environment as was suggested by some researchers from earlier decades.

There has also been enormous controversy over the past few years about the measles, mumps and rubella (MMR) vaccine being suggested as a possible cause of autism. See Chapter 2 for further discussion on the MMR vaccine.

Can autism be identified at an early age?

Early identification of young children with autism is important because it enables families to access specialised intervention at an early age and provides parents with information to help them understand their child's individual strengths and needs.

Research findings on the importance of intensive, early intervention for special needs children (McEachin, et al 1993; Koegal & Koegal 1995; Rogers 1996) have led to an increased focus on the early diagnosis of autism in children. A number of retrospective studies have provided insight into the benefits of the early identification of autism in young children and have concluded that early diagnosis of the condition is not only possible but can be relatively accurate. One of the difficulties faced by doctors and psychologists in diagnosing autism is that while autism is a neuro-biological condition, as Kanner originally hypothesised in 1943, it is also a condition that is not readily diagnosed medically; that is, there is no available medical test or procedure to identify the disorder. Early identification and diagnosis is based on the presence of a number of behaviours as well as the absence of a number of skills and developmental milestones.

Early signs of autism include:

- no pointing by age one;
- no babbling by age one, no single words by 16 months, no two-word phrases by 24 months;
- a loss of language skills at any time;
- no pretend play;
- little interest in socialising with peers;
- generally short attention span unless for special interest;
- no response when called by name, indifference to people;
- little or no eye contact;
- repetitive body movements, such as hand flapping, spinning or rocking;
- intense tantrums;
- fixations on a single object such as watching wheels spin;
- unusually strong resistance to changes in routines; and
- over- or under-sensitivity to certain sounds, sights, textures, tastes or smells.

Over the past ten to fifteen years a number of assessment tools have been developed to help identify autistic features in young children, thereby decreasing the reliance on clinical judgments. Experienced practitioners are now able to diagnose autism more accurately in young children of 2 or 3 years of age. However, early diagnosis is still difficult for children with very high or very low general ability, and in these cases a diagnosis may not be given until much later.

Prizant & Wetherby (1987) developed a framework to improve early assessment and diagnostic efforts. This framework included a profile of communication and symbolic behaviour to facilitate the early identification of autistic characteristics in young children. Ornitz, Guthrie & Farley (1977) studied the motor and perceptual development, speech and language of young children diagnosed with autism in their first two years of life through the use of a retrospective inventory. Dahlgren and Gillberg (1989) completed a questionnaire, the checklist for autism in toddlers (CHAT), with mothers of children diagnosed with autism and mothers of developmentally delayed children, to obtain information about early development and characteristics of children diagnosed with autism. Of the 130 items on the questionnaire, mothers identified 18 skills that, on average, distinguished children with autism from non-autistic developmentally delayed young children. These skills included difficulties with imitation of movements, strange reaction to certain sounds, limited play and lack of play with other children, 'empty' gaze, inability to attract adult's attention, preference for being alone and variability of behaviour. Gillberg et al (1990) used the questionnaire in an attempt to isolate symptoms specific to autism. They also found that young children with autism displayed abnormalities of play, aloneness and peculiarities of gaze and hearing. (See Appendix 2.)

Parents frequently ask questions about what causes autism and when it is first present in their children. Researchers have used parental home movies to help answer the question of when autism is first evident in young children. Studies have taken advantage of the fact that many parents take video footage of their child's first birthday parties. Video footage of young children who were later diagnosed with autism has been compared with footage of children without autism. Researchers used retrospective studies of home videos of children under 2 years of age to determine at what age autism could be first identified and what characteristics were first noticeable. They were able, with a very high degree of accuracy, to separate autistic from non-autistic children at 12 months of age (Adrien et al 1993; Osterling & Dawson 1994; Mars et al 1998). During the first year, deficits in communication, socialisation, motor development and attention were observed with these behaviours becoming more obvious during the second year. Adrien et al (1993) concluded that poor social response, lack of smiling, absence of appropriate facial expression, poor muscle tone, distractibility and limited attention were indications of the presence of autism in the first year and these become more pronounced in the second year.

Other researchers extended the original home movie studies to include videotapes of children as young as 2–3 months of age. Using sophisticated movement analysis, videos of children eventually diagnosed with autism or not diagnosed with autism were coded and evaluated for their capacity to predict autism. Children who were eventually diagnosed with autism were predicted from movies taken in early infancy (Teitelbaum 1998). This study supported the hypothesis that very subtle symptoms of autism are present in early infancy and argues strongly against vaccines as a cause of autism since vaccinations are typically given at a later age.

Recent American research has concluded that the size of a child's head at birth and subsequent growth spurts may assist in the early detection and treatment of autism. One of the key questions to evolve from the recent research is whether rapid brain growth is the cause or merely a symptom of autism.

Further information about the recent findings is available in Chapter 2 where there is a more detailed discussion of current trends in medical research.

How is autism diagnosed?

Autism is a neurological condition that may be diagnosed by a paediatrician, psychiatrist, neurologist or clinical psychologist. A diagnosis of autism continues to be based on an interpretation of an individual's observed and reported behaviours, which is not the most definitive scientific approach. The diagnosis is based on the presence of a pattern of behaviours and also a lack of skills in certain areas of functioning rather than any medical tests. This pattern of behaviours is consistent with the triad of impairments (see Figure 1.5).

There is no single behaviour, either by its presence or absence, that will indicate autism. For example, in the past it was commonly assumed that if a child was affectionate or provided good eye contact the child could not be autistic. This is not accurate, as it is the combination of a number of behaviours, their intensity, and the fact that they persist beyond the normal age that often leads to a diagnosis of autism. Although autism occurs in individuals within the broad range of intellectual capacity, many of the individuals diagnosed may also have additional learning difficulties. This adds to the problems in diagnosis, as it can sometimes be quite difficult to separate out the effects of autism and the effects of severe and multiple disabilities.

What information should you know about autism?

Autism occurs throughout the world in families of all ethnic, racial and social backgrounds. When Leo Kanner (1943) first described children with autism, he observed that many of the

Illustrations of autistic behaviour

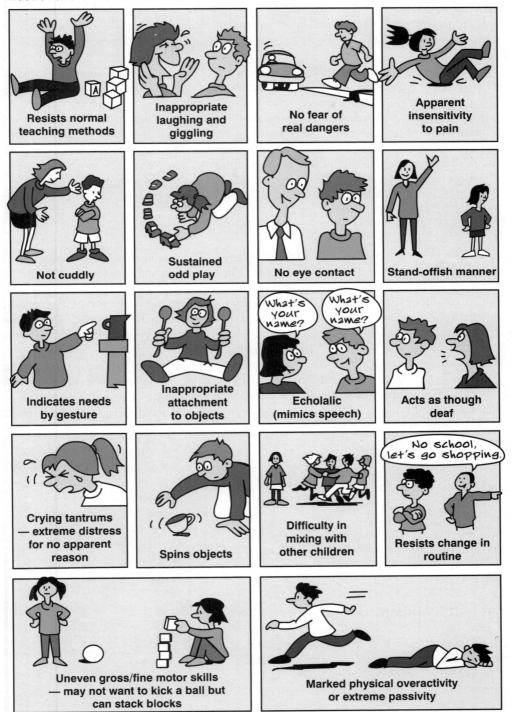

Figure 1.5 *Adapted from original by Professor J. Randle-Short, University of Queensland, Brisbane Children's Hospital*

children who attended his clinic came from well-educated families from the middle and upper social classes. As diagnostic services for autism have become more widely available, it has become apparent that autism occurs equally across all social classes and all cultures. A number of studies have found that the biological causes of autism are largely independent of cultural and racial factors.

The majority of the population affected by autism is male — approximately four males to every female. For Asperger's syndrome, the ratio is approximately nine males to one female.

The number of children diagnosed with autism appears to be increasing, partly due to improved diagnostic methods and partly because of the broadening of the autism spectrum. Early definitions of 'classic' autism were based on the set of characteristics described by Leo Kanner in 1943 but over the last ten to fifteen years the diagnostic criteria have changed to include children and adults with additional developmental problems and behaviours.

The most commonly used classification systems to diagnose autism are:

- Diagnostic and Statistical Manual of Mental Diseases of the American Psychiatric Association, Version IV (DSM IV); and
- International Classification of Diseases, Version 10 (ICD 10).

Some children with autism may develop epilepsy. The incidence of the development of epilepsy during puberty/adolescence is higher than in the normal population, possibly due to the fact that certain parts of the brains of people with autism are different.

Autism can occur with or without other disabilities. Children and adults with autism may also have other conditions that impact on how well they are able to function in society. Other conditions or disabilities associated with autism may include Down's syndrome, tuberous sclerosis, neurofibromatosis, cerebral palsy, Tourette's syndrome, Rett's syndrome, prematurity and seizure disorders. Some children with autism may also have a visual and/or hearing impairment.

People with autism may have intellectual abilities ranging from gifted to severely intellectually disabled. There are differing opinions about what percentage of people with autism also have some form of intellectual impairment. According to most accepted figures, approximately 70% of children and adults with autism have some form of intellectual disability ranging from mild through moderate to severe. However, when people with Asperger's syndrome are added to the equation, the numbers look quite different. Approximately 20% of people with an autism spectrum disorder (includes Asperger's syndrome, autistic disorder and other PDDs) would be classified as having some degree of intellectual impairment. These figures are illustrated in Figure 1.6.

What is the autism continuum?

The core features of autism range in severity. Each of the core features (communication, social interation, sensory impairment and restricted and repetitive interests and behaviours) may be presented along a continuum from severe to mild. People with autism will not necessarily present with the same degree of severity for each of the core features. For example, a person may present

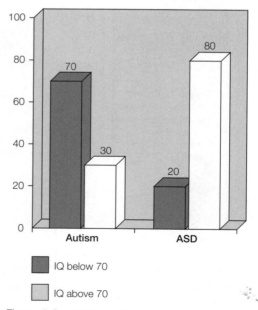

Figure 1.6 *Intellectual impairment and autism*

with a severe social impairment, moderate impairments in both expressive and comprehension skills and a mild degree of impairment in terms of his/her repetitive behaviours and restricted interests. Individuals with autism also grow and develop over time, and their place on the continuum in each of the skill areas will also vary over time. Figure 1.7, p 16, indicates the possible degrees of impairment in each of the key areas of development that relate to autism. Figure 1.8 provides an example of where a particular child falls on the autism continuum in each of the key areas of development based on a number of behavioural indicators.

The example of Jake shows just how difficult it is to determine where children fit on the continuum in terms of their skills and behaviours. Another person reading the example shown above, may have placed Jake differently on the continuum in each of the four areas and they would not be right, or wrong. The placement of children on the continuum is based on information about the child, observation of the child and an understanding of autism and normal development. This placement may vary if the child's behaviour changes in different situations, for different people or just generally over time.

Even today, nearly fifty years after Kanner first diagnosed children with autism, and with an accumulation of information and knowledge based on research of the condition, there is still a tendency to adhere to his rigid criteria without acknowledging the notion of an autistic continuum. This is partly due to the fact that the boundaries of the continuum have never been clearly defined, leading to some confusion when diagnosing children and adults with autism especially at both the profound and the milder ends of the continuum.

What treatments are available?

Parents who suspect that their child may have autism should contact their family doctor or paediatrician for a diagnosis. Referral to a psychologist for a developmental assessment will provide information about the degree of severity and appropriate educational interventions.

Autism affects a person's communication, social, sensory and play skills. However, with specialised intervention that takes into account particular learning styles as well as their strengths in visual processing, most children and adults make substantial progress. They can be taught skills that will enable them to function with varying degrees of support in the community. Research has established the importance of structured educational programs that teach functional communication, social and play skills and also provide children and adults with strategies to help them manage their behaviour and sensory deficits.

The most effective programs for children and adults with autism have a strong emphasis on the development of functional skills using visual supports to assist understanding as well as an emphasis on generalising these skills to different settings and different people. Parents play a major role in the intervention process, especially with young children with autism. Most intervention services aim to work closely with families in the development and implementation of individual programs in the home and the regular community.

As many children and adults with autism also have some form of sensory impairment in addition to the triad of impairments, it is important for intervention programs to assess children's sensory strengths and needs and implement specific programs that address these needs when working with children and adults with autism.

Families are encouraged to implement programs as consistently as possible while taking into account each child's individual strengths and needs as well as family circumstances. Parent training should also be an integral part of any treatment process.

See EK Gerlach, *The Autism Treatment Guide* (3rd ed) published in 2003 for detailed information about treatment options that may be available.

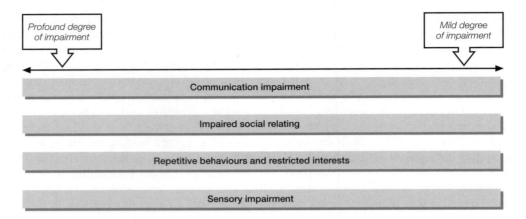

Figure 1.7 *Interpretation of the continuum of core deficits in autism. Developed by Louise Ulliana, Autism Spectrum Australia (Aspect), 2001*

Jake is a 4-year-old child with no functional language. He communicates his needs by taking his mother by the hand to what he wants. He does not respond to his name or to basic verbal commands without some form of physical prompt. However he is quite happy to accept social contact and will play alongside his mother with simple action response toys or sensory activities such as water, sand or bubbles. Jake does not tend to initiate any social interaction but will accept a hug and sit with his parents when they initiate the contact. Jake is obsessed with Thomas the Tank Engine and will sit and watch a Thomas video over and over again. He becomes extremely distressed when the video is turned off. Jake carries a small toy Thomas train around with him and does not like to put it down or give it to anyone else. Jake will sit and look at a book but only if it is about trains, especially Thomas the Tank Engine. Jake has a limited diet, will wear only certain clothing (he will not wear any shirts with labels or tags) and does not like the sound of the vacuum cleaner.

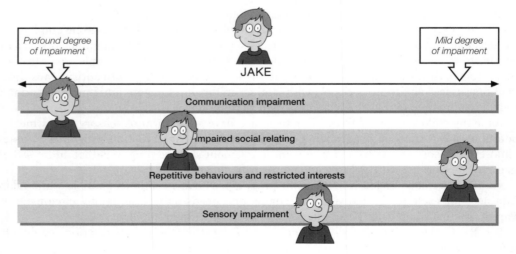

Figure 1.8 *Illustration of where Jake may be placed on the autism continuum in each of the core deficit areas*

Summary

Autism is a neurological disorder characterised by impairments in communication, social relating, and by the presence of repetitive and stereotypic behaviours and unusual responses to sensory stimuli. Children and adults with autism may show mild to severe disorders in both receptive and expressive communication, and in relating to people, objects and events. Children may have unusual play behaviours with toys and other objects, may have difficulty coping with changes in routine and may display repetitive body movements or abnormal behaviour patterns.

There are a number of possible causes linked to autism. Although the cause of autism is not known, the general consensus is that there is not one cause, but multiple causes, with a strong genetic underpinning and onset before 3 years of age. The controversy of the MMR vaccine as a possible cause of autism is topical.

Autism is classified according to either the World Health Organisation's International Classification of Diseases (ICD-10, WHO 1992) or the American Psychiatric Association's Diagnostic and Statistical Manual (DSM-IV, APA 1994). Both classification approaches incorporate the notion of a triad of impairments to describe autistic individuals.

Professionals face a number of issues in attempting to diagnose children with autism. Autism is a disorder that affects both males and females, with multiple genes and different genetic influences across families. Consequently, children and adults with autism vary widely in their abilities, intelligence and behaviour. Some children have no functional language while other children appear to have good communication skills but with a limited range of conversational topics, difficulty with abstract concepts and evidence of echolalic speech. Repetitive play skills, a limited range of interests, and impaired social skills are usually present in young children as well as unusual sensory responses (including a fascination with spinning objects, limited diet that only includes certain food textures, and sensitivity to the feel of certain materials such as playdough).

Intervention programs should focus on improving communication, social, cognitive, behavioural and self-help skills. Both home and classroom environments should be structured so that programs are consistent and predictable. Children and adults with autism learn more effectively and are less confused when information is presented visually as well as verbally. It is also important for individuals with autism to spend time interacting with non-autistic peers who are role models for appropriate communication, social interaction and behaviour. All programs should contain a generalisation component that will enable skills taught in one setting to be carried over to other situations and other people.

2

Current Trends

Autism has no single cause ... Today, researchers believe that several genes, possibly in combination with environmental factors, may contribute to autism.

There is currently no cure for autism. However, continued research has provided a clearer understanding of the disorder and has led to better treatments and therapies.

Autism Society of America Brochure 'Next Steps: A Guide for Families New to Autism', p 2

Professional interest in autism has increased dramatically over the past few years due to an apparent worldwide increase in the incidence of the disorder. This professional interest has provided parents and service providers with more information about the autism spectrum and has offered alternative treatment and educational possibilities. The diversity of the disorder has generated a considerable breadth of current concern and interest in autism research.

Current research trends include medical research into possible causes and treatments, educational practices that address the unique cognitive thinking and learning patterns associated with autism and alternative treatments that include vitamin therapy and dietary issues. In this chapter, we will address some of the most popular trends in medical research including the role of genetics in causing autism, improved diagnostic procedures that have presumably led to an increase in the numbers of people being diagnosed with autism, a possible breakthrough in the early identification of the disorder and the recent controversy over vaccinations and autism. The chapter will also address some of the most popular trends in educational practice including the use of visual supports, sensory issues, structured teaching practices, applied behaviour analysis, intensive early intervention, staff training and the importance of working closely with families. We will look at some of the skills commonly seen in autistic savants and also briefly outline some of the alternative treatments to autism that are now available.

What are the current trends in medical research?

As outlined in the previous chapter, autism spectrum disorders affect many more people than has generally been recognised, with as many as 60 per 10,000 children under 8 years of age classified with an autism spectrum disorder. For more classically defined autism, the numbers are between 10 and 30 per 10,000. The prevalence of autism in the adult population is not known but currently accepted research indicates figures as high as 93 per 10,000 when both children and adults are included in the population studies (Gillberg & Wing 1999). Diagnoses of autism and pervasive developmental disorders (PDDs) or autism spectrum disorders (ASDs) have increased since the disorder was first recognised. Moreover, the rate of increase has accelerated over the past decade from 3 in 10,000 to 1 in 500, 1 in 150, or even more in some studies. Methodological differences between studies, changes in diagnostic practice as well as public and professional awareness have been suggested as possible reasons behind the apparent increase in autism. 'Whether these factors are sufficient to account for increased numbers of identified individuals, or whether there has been a rise in actual numbers affected, is as yet unclear, although it is evident that significant numbers of people have ASD's as currently defined' (Medical Research Council Review of Autism Research December 2001, p 3).

While there has been debate on an apparent increase in autism, there has also been considerable interest in the role of genetics in autism. In the search to answer the riddle of autism, scientists are looking at the human genetic structure as one possible factor — genetics may not be the 'cause' of autism, but it may well be a contributing factor, along with many others.

Genetics and autism, is there a link?

The past decade has seen scientists make significant breakthroughs in understanding the genetics of autism. Researchers are focusing on specific chromosomal regions that may contain autism related genes. This involves the study of chromosomal abnormalities in individuals with autism and screening chromosomes for evidence of genes associated with autism.

Currently there are several major studies looking into the genetics of autism. These studies are linked to the International Molecular Genetics Study of Autism Consortium (IMGSAC), an international research project initiated in 1996 to identify the specific genes that may influence autism. One of the studies, from Oxford University, suggests that the search for the genetic link to autism can be narrowed to the regions of two specific chromosomes. If confirmed, these genes may make some people more susceptible to autism (IMGSAC, Centre for Human Genetics, Oxford University):

> The discovery of these regions … confirms the genetic component of autism, and will enable us to narrow our search down to specific genes and the factors they control. This should cast light on what is going wrong, and hopefully give us clues on how autism could be treated.

The picture that is emerging from genetic studies is, however, very complex and autism seems to be linked to many different locations on the genome. It is likely that several genes may be operating together to make certain people more susceptible to autism. Some scientists believe that what is inherited is an irregular segment of genetic code or a small cluster of unstable genes. In most people, the faulty code may cause only minor problems. But under certain conditions, the unstable genes may interact and seriously interfere with the brain development of the unborn child.

While there may be a genetic component to autism, it remains unclear what genes are involved — estimates run from as few as three to as many as twenty genes acting together. Among the most popularly indicated genes are those that regulate the action of three powerful neurotransmitters: glutamate (involved in both learning and memory), serotonin and gammaaminobutiric acid (GABA) (both of which have been implicated in obsessive-compulsive behaviour, anxiety and depression). Many other genes are also under consideration for the possible impact they have on a person's susceptibility to autism, including the genes that control brain development and immune system function. In a small number of cases, various single gene disorders and chromosomal abnormalities such as untreated phenylketonuria, tuberous sclerosis and fragile X syndrome, have been reported in individuals with autism spectrum disorders indicating that the phenotype may be derived from a number of different genetic components. 'It is entirely plausible that the autism phenotype may be derived from a number of different genetic components' (MRC Review of Autism Research, Dec 2001, p 3).

Researchers have found that the traits of autism, far more than autism itself, tend to run in families. Although few severely autistic individuals form relationships and have children, scientists have found that in many instances, some aspect of the disorder affects a close relative. For example, a sister may have difficulties academically at school, a cousin may have some very rigid behaviours and limited interests or an adult uncle may still live at home with parents, be very shy and anti-social with few, or no, friends.

There is increasing evidence of a genetic link to autism in some families, with several studies of twins suggesting that autism or at least a higher likelihood of some brain dysfunction can be inherited. One of the most effective ways of determining whether a particular syndrome or disorder is genetic is to examine the incidence in identical (monozygotic) and fraternal (dizygotic) twins. In research at the MRC Child Psychiatry Unit at the Institute of Psychiatry in London, it was found that in studies of identical twins using a strict definition of autism, if one identical twin had autism, there was a 60% chance that the second twin would also, and a greater than 75% chance that the twin without autism would still exhibit some autistic traits. On the other hand, if a fraternal twin is affected by autism the other twin is unlikely to have autism or any related disorder. Using a broader definition of autism (autism spectrum disorder), research has shown that when one twin has autism, approximately 92% of monozygotic (identical) and 10% of dizygotic (fraternal) twins will also have autism (Bailey et al 1995; Folstein et al 1977). These findings support the hypothesis that there is a strong genetic basis to autism. It also appears that parents who have one child with autism are at slightly increased risk of having another child with the disorder.

However, with researchers from around the world finding possible links to such things as genetics, vaccines, mercury poisoning and other potential causes, it is becoming more and more likely that autism is the result of a combination of factors that come into play in approximately 1–500 children. It is for this reason that no area of research can be ignored.

What about possible early identification?

Recent American research has concluded that the size of a child's head at birth and subsequent growth spurts may assist in the early detection and treatment of autism.

Children with autism appear to have accelerated brain growth within the first year of life, well before any behavioural indicators of autism appear. In a recent study from the University of California, San Diego (Courchesne et al 2003), more than half of the children diagnosed with autism had an enlarged brain by the time they reached 14 months of age. This may provide a powerful early indicator of autism in very young children. Researchers say that if the findings are verified in further studies, then head growth could be used along with other behavioural and biological clues to possibly make earlier evaluations of autism in children.

'If we understood what was making this change we would understand what makes autism a unique disorder,' said the study's lead author, Eric Courchesne, director of the Center for Autism Research at Children's Hospital Research Centre in San Diego and a professor at the University of California, San Diego. The researchers say abnormal growth in head size, and therefore the brain, during the first year of life may mean that an infant's brain is making jumbled connections that lead to the impaired functioning of autism. Rapid head growth can be brought on by other medical problems, although it also can occur in otherwise normally developing babies. Paediatricians typically track head growth.

The California researchers found that children later diagnosed with autism spectrum disorder, which includes mild to severe forms of autism, had bigger heads than 84% of other healthy infants. Their heads grew more quickly in the first year of life, and brain growth later slowed.

Those children later diagnosed with the most severe autism showed the greatest increase in early rapid head growth compared to those children with milder forms of the disorder. The increase was significant, considering that children with mild to severe forms of autism tended to have smaller heads at birth than about 75% of other newborns, according to the study.

Courchesne's 2003 study looked at the medical records of a number of children with autism and found that 'head size increased from the 25th percentile — based on the Centres of Disease Control and Prevention averages of healthy infants — to the 84th percentile in six to fourteen months. This excessive increase occurred well before the typical onset of clinical behavioural symptoms' (p 341). While the numbers in the study were small, Courchesne concluded that the rapid growth in head size 'may become a useful early warning biological sign for autism. That, in turn, allows the development of additional tests to verify the possible diagnosis of autism. It opens up the opportunity for a whole new realm of treatments at a much earlier stage'.

Dr Janet Lainhart, an associate professor of psychiatry at the University of Utah wrote in an editorial about the Courchesne study for JAMA (*The Journal of the American Medical Association*) that it is premature to conclude that increased rate of head growth is a universal feature of autism. She said the results needed to be confirmed in studies with a larger number of people with autism but the findings support the combined results of other research that point to increased rates of head and brain growth in early childhood in autism.

A key question to evolve from the University of California study is whether rapid brain growth, which may be too fast for vital neurological connections to form, is the cause or merely a symptom of autism.

What about MMR vaccinations and autism?

Measles, mumps, rubella (MMR) vaccine is a live vaccine that protects against these three diseases through the use of modified types of measles, mumps and rubella viruses. They protect against natural infection without causing the disease themselves. It is widely reco-mmended that all children be immunised at 12–15 months of age and again at 4 years of age.

In 1993, Dr Andrew Wakefield, a gastroenterologist at the London Royal Free Hospital, raised the possibility that the MMR vaccination caused autism in young children. He investigated autistic children whose parents blamed their problems on the MMR vaccination. He claimed to have found traces of the measles virus in the gut of young children and recommended that the components of the vaccine be given separately in order to reduce possible intestinal disturbances.

In 1998, the results of a second study were published in the prestigious British medical journal, *The Lancet*. In this paper, titled 'Ileal lymphoid-nodular hyperplasia, non-specific colitis, and pervasive developmental disorder in children', Wakefield claimed that the MMR vaccination may cause inflammation of the bowel, leading to decreased absorption of essential vitamins and nutrients and possible autism. Although the study was unable to prove any defi-nite association between the MMR vaccination and onset of autism, it sparked debate and raised a number of issues for medical professionals and parents. In a recently published paper, Wakefield wrote 'for MMR, autism, and inflammatory bowel disease, a significant index of suspicion exists without adequate evidence of safety' (*New Scientist* Feb 2001). He suggests that the bowel inflammation may make the gut leaky, allowing 'rogue peptides' from food to poison the brain. However, as Wakefield himself wrote in his original paper: 'We did not prove an association.'

Many parents of children with autism believe that childhood vaccines can cause autism. Some have heard stories of babies developing normally until they had the measles, mumps and rubella (MMR) vaccination and then regressing, losing skills and becoming withdrawn. Some talk from personal experience, adamant that their children changed dramatically within days of having their MMR shot, losing language skills and becoming difficult to manage.

Despite the lack of proof of any connection between the triple vaccine and autism, for some parents who see the first signs of autism soon after their children are vaccinated, it seems impossible not to blame MMR. The connection may be coincidental, however. Autism is usually detected in young children around 18 months of age. The MMR vaccine is first given when children are 12–15 months old. It therefore is inevitable that some children will be vaccinated just before the first signs of autism are detected.

Wakefield's studies have been widely criticised internationally for their weak methodology and a number of much larger and scientifically valid studies have been published since 1998, some of which have looked specifically at Wakefield's claims. These studies have included a study of primary school children in Australia (D'Souza et al 2000), a long-term study of children in Finland (Patja et al 2000) and a study in England that traced 498 children with autism to test if their condition could be linked to MMR (Taylor et al 1999). None of these studies found any link between inflammatory bowel disease, autism and MMR.

If MMR does trigger autism, it is most surprising that none of the studies found any evidence of a connection. At the very least, the research suggests that if there is a risk, it is minuscule. There is a much greater risk for children who will be left susceptible to measles mumps and rubella if they are not immunised. All three diseases can have serious complications including encephalitis. Encephalitis has long-term adverse effects on both physical and intellectual development.

Wakefield suggested that the components of the MMR vaccine be given separately. However, there is no evidence that giving the vaccine components separately is of any benefit and, in fact, providing the individual components sequentially leaves children exposed to possible outbreaks of serious diseases over a longer period of time.

There are a number of issues facing parents:

- Measles is a most unpleasant illness with a significant rate of severe complications including encephalitis, subacute sclerosing parencephalitis (SSPE), and long-term brain damage. The measles vaccine is very effective in preventing the disease.
- A measles outbreak can occur if immunisation levels fall below those required for herd immunity. It is no good therefore relying on everyone else to immunise their children and hoping that a child who is not immunised will be safe. Current statistics are overwhelmingly in favour of giving children the MMR vaccine to reduce risk of serious diseases.
- The measles vaccine does have some minor side-effects and there is always an extremely rare risk of encephalitis (less than 1:1million).
- The studies suggesting a link between MMR vaccine and autism have major methodological flaws. Several high quality studies have failed to demonstrate any link between MMR and autism.

Doctors are not pro-immunisation at all costs and closely monitor latest research findings for adverse effects from any vaccines.

In 2002, Wakefield published a second paper examining the relationship between the measles virus and autism. Once again the lack of appropriate research methodology has led to many questions about both the reliability of the research and the validity of the results.

In contrast, a number of studies have also been completed that refute a causal association between MMR and autism. In 1999, Taylor et al examined the relationship between the receipt of MMR and the development of autism in a controlled study. They examined the records of 498 children with autism and related disorders. The study examined the incidence and age at diagnosis of autism in vaccinated and unvaccinated children. The findings indicated that the percentage of children vaccinated was the same in children with autism as in children who were unvaccinated and the onset of 'regressive' symptoms of autism did not occur within 2, 4, or 6 months of receiving the MMR vaccine.

In 2001, Dales et al examined the relationship between the increase in the number of cases of autism in California and receipt of the MMR vaccine. The percentage of children immunised with MMR vaccine between 1980 and 1994 was compared with the incidence of autism during the same period. Although a dramatic increase in the incidence of autism in young children was reported, the percentage of children that received MMR vaccine remained the same.

In a similar study in England (Kaye et al 2001), the incidence of autism between 1988 and 1993 was examined and compared with the MMR immunisation rates. As in the Dales study, the incidence of autism increased but the MMR immunisation rates remained the same.

A number of expert review panels, including the Institute of Medicine USA, the World Health Organisation and the Medical Research Council, have considered the specific question of the potential link between MMR vaccination and autism. The reviews were unanimous in their conclusions that a causal link between the MMR vaccine and autism was not proven and that current epidemiological evidence did not support this proposed link. The Institute of Medicine report, however, noted that: 'this conclusion does not exclude the possibility that MMR vaccine could contribute to ASD in a small number of children, because the epidemiological evidence lacks the precision to assess rare occurrences of a response to MMR vaccine leading to ASD' (IMGSAC 2001, p 28).

The only scientific evidence against childhood vaccines comes from Wakefield. The evidence he presented was not entirely persuasive, if only because the children he studied were originally referred to him for intestinal problems. He did not look at children with autism with no history of intestinal problems.

What about the children whose symptoms appeared shortly after being vaccinated? A possible explanation is that the association is purely coincidental. The MMR vaccination is given around 15 months, about the same time that behaviour and language patterns are developing in young children to the degree that parents can notice when something is amiss. Most of the evidence suggests that autism is primarily caused by genetic factors. It may be that the disorder is present in infants but some of the communication, social and play impairments are still too subtle to be picked up until the infant is at least 12–18 months old.

The World Health Organisation continues to endorse the use of the vaccine, as does the British Medical Research Council and the Australian National Centre for Immunisation Research Surveillance of Vaccine Preventable Diseases (NCIRS).

Furthermore, the editor of eminent British medical journal, *The Lancet*, Mr Richard Horton, stated in February 2004, that the MMR/autism link was 'entirely flawed' and the research should never have been published. Dr Michael Fitzpatrick, a London GP with an autistic son, wrote in the *London Times*, 'Dr Wakefield is a scientist who has turned hypothesis into dogma, resolutely refusing to abandon his theory despite his failure to provide convincing evidence to support it' (March 2004, p 4).

If MMR has not caused an increase in autism, what has? The chances are that, in spite of headlines declaring a huge increase in the disorder, it has not increased significantly, if at all.

What has changed is the tendency of psychiatrists and paediatricians to diagnose autism, or autism spectrum disorders, more frequently. Children who would once have been diagnosed as developmentally delayed are now much more likely to be diagnosed with autism.

Researchers at Boston University School of Medicine looked at the evidence and concluded that this was what had happened. Their interpretation was that the major increased incidence of diagnosed autism was primarily a reflection of changes in diagnostic practices, such as more frequent identification, availability of services, and other similar factors.

Psychiatrists such as Lorna Wing brought about one of the main changes to diagnostic procedures. She first provided a clear definition of autistic spectrum disorder, and provided a label for individuals. Many of these individuals would previously have been condemned to life in an asylum.

In addition to recognising the importance of medical research in clarifying issues around the disorder and taking knowledge and understanding of autism forward, changes in educational practices over the years have led to greatly improved treatment options and successful outcomes for individuals with autism. As stated in Chapter 1, educational practices follow the lead of research and scientific theories, so that teaching practices of children and adults have evolved over the years in line with the scientific and medical findings.

What are the current trends in educational practice?

The distinctive characteristics of autism that cause the most difficulties and are the focus of most current trends in educational practice, revolve around the triad of impairments linked to autism — impairments in communication, impairments in social relating and impairments in the patterns of behaviour, interests and activities that are restricted, repetitive or stereotypic, as well as unusual responses to sensory experiences. The impairments linked to autism are covered in depth in Chapter 3.

Apart from these core deficits, there are a bewildering number of associated characteristics commonly seen in individuals with autism that have an impact on educational practices. These include impaired auditory processing skills, attention problems, impaired speech production and impaired cognitive functioning including weak central coherence and difficulties with theory of mind.

Many of the behaviours and characteristics that define autism are also found in individuals with other disabilities. What makes autism and the needs of people with autism unique is the pattern of these behaviours and the areas of functioning that are affected.

Educational practices that are most successful in addressing the needs of individuals with autism may vary in philosophy, procedures and intensity but all focus on accommodating the unique thinking and learning style of individuals, encourage exploration of both objects and people, encourage social initiation, and emphasise functional communication and social interaction in real-life situations (Janzen 1996; Attwood 2000; Quill 2000).

There is no evidence to support one educational model or practice over another but a number of factors have been found to influence successful outcomes and are key requirements for effective intervention procedures, especially for young children. These include intensive intervention as early as possible, structured teaching procedures that incorporate the unique learning styles of individuals and provide intensive one-to-one support, use of visual supports to augment language; planned change procedures that acknowledge the need for predictability and routine, an emphasis on teaching functional skills, a collaborative approach between parents and teachers, programs that support transitions and an emphasis on training professionals who are working with adults and children with autism in the most effective educational practices.

Children with autism usually demonstrate an uneven pattern of development with verbal and non-verbal communication skills and social skills being limited but visual spatial skills a relative strength. Teaching activities are most successful when they are matched to each child's current developmental level, individual learning style, strengths and interests.

First-hand accounts written by individuals with autism offer some insight into how the characteristics of the disorder affect their lives. Most accounts offer examples of how communication, social and sensory difficulties interact to cause problematic behaviours and social difficulties. Challenges in one area can cause or exacerbate difficulties in another. For example, a non-verbal student who screams and becomes aggressive in music class obviously has behavioural issues and communication issues but the screaming may be a reaction to sensory over-stimulation that occurs in that particular lesson. Viewing these challenging behaviours in light of the difficulties associated with auditory processing, regulation of attention and sensory system, speech production and cognitive function can help develop a better understanding of the individual's special needs.

Not all individuals with autism are affected by the entire spectrum of difficulties. Some of the higher functioning students with average to above average cognitive abilities and functional language skills may have sensory and auditory processing difficulties that will still compromise communication, social life, perception and behaviour. When trying to understand and support an individual with autism, it is important to know the person to ensure that his/her individual needs are addressed in whatever educational approach is introduced. The current most popular educational programs available for individuals with autism are discussed below. Remember that there is no program that can cure autism but all of the following programs have had success in teaching functional skills, managing problem behaviours and integrating individuals into their community activities to varying degrees.

What about applied behaviour analysis (ABA)?

Behavioural techniques have been used in the education of children with autism and severe learning difficulties for many years. During the early 1970s, Dr Ivor Lovaas and his colleagues used behavioural techniques with a group of 59 children with autism. The techniques were taught to parents in an intensive home treatment program. The approach is based on the premise that all behaviour is learned and is governed by what happens before (antecedents) and what happens after (consequences) the behaviour.

A person's behaviour is assessed through observations that focus on what the person does, when the person does it and at what rate, and what happens before and what happens after behaviour. Strengths and weaknesses are specified in this way. Skills to be taught are broken down into small steps and each step is then taught sequentially. The process of teaching each step involves:

- A — give a clear instruction, provide assistance in following the instruction (such as a prompt by demonstration or physical guidance) and use materials that are at the person's level of understanding.
- B — obtain a correct response.
- C — give positive reinforcement (a consequence that will lead the person to repeat the behaviour in the future).

Each step can be shaped through the use of rewards or positive reinforcement.

Many trials are given repeatedly in structured teaching situations and in the course of everyday activities. Instructions emphasise teaching a person how to learn, to listen, to watch and to imitate. As a person progresses, guidance is systematically reduced or faded to encourage independence and the person is taught to combine their skills in more complex ways and to practise them in different situations.

In an ABA program, problem behaviours are not reinforced and individuals are not allowed to escape from learning. They are constantly redirected to engage in appropriate behaviour. Each person's responses during every teaching session are recorded and the data used to determine the effectiveness of the activities and whether the individual program needs to be modified. Therapists' behaviour is also continually observed initially and then less frequently to ensure that the procedures are being correctly applied.

In order to optimise the benefits of an ABA program, intervention should take place for up to 40 hours per week for approximately two years and should be carried out by a team of trained people including supervisors, therapists, parents and peers.

According to Lovaas the following format will maximise the positive impact of the program:
- establish rapport with the child;
- extend receptive language, using highly structured speech;
- develop non-verbal imitation skills; and
- develop verbal imitation.

In summary, an ABA program is taught through a number of discrete trials in which correct responses are reinforced. New skills are shaped through prompting.

For more information: applied behaviour analysis (ABA) programs are available in most large cities or information about nearest available programs can be obtained from:

The Center for Autism and Related Disabilities (CARD)
Louis de la Parte Florida Mental Health Institute
University of South Florida
13301 Bruce B. Downs Blvd
Tampa Florida 33612-3899
Ph: (813) 974 2532
card-usf@fmhi.usf.edu

What about the Picture Exchange Communication System (PECS)?

The picture exchange communication system (PECS) is an augmentative communication system frequently used with children with autism (Bondy & Frost 1994; Siegel 2000; Yamall 2000). It was designed as a pictorial system to develop functional communication skills in young children based on basic behavioural principles and techniques such as shaping, differential reinforcement, discrete trial and incidental teaching models as well as other behavioural strategies. The aim of PECS is to teach children how to initiate communication through social exchange (Bondy 2001).

PECS initially assesses the child's preference for a small number of food items and some toys. The child is then taught, in a series of small structured steps, to exchange a symbol of an item for the item itself. A series of pictures, that are relevant to the child, are kept in a notebook (PECS board). The child is taught to use the PECS board to create a sentence by selecting picture cards, such as 'I want' card plus 'video' card, and handing the cards to a communicative partner as a request for the desired item. Initially two adults work with each child, one adult acting as the communication partner and the other prompting the child to pick up the symbol and give it to the communication partner. The child is then given the real object. This acts as a powerful reinforcement and encourages the child to repeat the action. PECS emphasises teaching a child to initiate requests, respond to questions and make social comments.

There are no prerequisite abilities, such as eye contact or verbal imitation skills, to begin a PECS program. According to Bondy & Frost (1998), the training expands to teach increasingly more complex communication and social skills. Of all children started on PECS, over 80% of the children acquired speech after 12 months training, and continue to use it independently or with augmentation.

The six phases of PECS are carefully structured to enable children to learn the concept of picture exchange, to actively find someone to give a symbol to as a request, to discriminate between several symbols, to use a portable communication book, and to construct simple sentences, both requests and comments. The PECS program aims to give children independence and to learn that communication is a two-way exchange that can achieve desired needs. PECS has been shown to facilitate the development of spoken language and to establish the basics of communication in advance of the emergence of speech (Bondy & Frost 1994; Schwartz, Garfinkle, & Bauer 1998). Other positive effects have been suggested from the use of PECS.

Anecdotal reports have indicated that the use of PECS may result in a decrease in problem behaviour and improved social behaviour (Bondy & Frost 1994; Peterson, Bondy, Vincent & Finnegan 1995) though none of the reported studies included an experimental research design to eliminate possible confounding variables such as maturation effects.

Because of the potential advantages and pragmatic features, PECS has been widely accepted in the autism community even without the empirically controlled investigations needed to support it (Charlop-Christy 2000; Yamall 2000). A recent study by Charlop-Christy, Carpenter, Le, LeBlanc & Kellet (2002), however, demonstrated the efficacy of the PECS protocol with three children with autism, the emergence of speech, and the collateral gains in social–communicative behaviours and concomitant decreases in problem behaviour. The findings support the use of PECS although the sample size was small and the study needs replicating with a larger group.

The PECS can be expanded to include the use of visual strategies to introduce the idea of making choices. Once children have learned that the exchange of symbols can be used to request, then the symbols can also be introduced to show children what choices are available and to encourage them to communicate their preferred choices. Choice boards can then be introduced for play and leisure activities as well as for basic needs.

Visual strategies are also used for timetables or schedules showing the sequence of daily or weekly routines. The use of visual sequences and timetables encourages children to become more independent and assists in the teaching of certain skills such as toileting, dressing, feeding, and in establishing routines. Visual timetables can be adapted to use in a home, preschool, school, the workplace or independent living setting. Timetables, sequence boards and choice boards assist the person with autism to become more independent and can help to make the environment better organised and predictable.

For more information, the *PECS Training Manual* by Bondy & Frost is available through large bookstores such as Amazon Books or contact a local speech pathologist with experience working with children with autism.

What is structured teaching or the Treatment and Education of Autistic and Communication Handicapped Children (TEACCH Program)?

Structured teaching is an approach to presenting information that emphasises the areas of strength of individuals in order to compensate for their areas of difficulty. It involves a systematic process of organising and structuring the environment to provide clear visual boundaries for those people who see the world from a different perspective. Information is presented in a visual, organised and clear manner that is individualised and developmentally based. The process capitalises on the visual abilities of people with autism to compensate for the difficulties they have in reading their environment.

'Structured teaching helps children "learn how to learn" by highlighting the important aspects of a learning situation and, thus, focusing their attention' (The Treatment and Education of Autistic and Related Communication handicapped Children TEACCH Program Manual).

Developed in the early 1970s by Eric Schopler, the TEACCH approach includes a focus on the person with autism and the development of a program around the individual's skills, interests, and needs. The major priorities include centring on the individual, understanding autism, adopting appropriate adaptations, and a broadly based intervention strategy building on existing skills and interests. In the TEACCH program, the person is the priority, rather than any philosophical notions such as inclusion, discrete trial training or facilitated communication. The program emphasises individualised assessment to understand the individual better and also 'the culture of autism', suggesting that people with autism are part of a distinctive group with common characteristics that are different, but not necessarily inferior, to others. Emphasising assessment and the culture of autism requires an understanding of people with autism as they are and building programs around each person's functional abilities. This does not suggest lower or higher expectations; it simply requires starting where people are and helping them to develop as far as they can go. This is different from espousing a model of 'normal' behaviour for everyone and requiring people with autism to fit into that mould, whether or not they are comfortable to do that.

Structured teaching is an important priority because, according to TEACCH research and experience, structure fits the 'culture of autism' more effectively than any other techniques that have been observed. 'Organizing the physical environment, developing schedules and work systems, making expectations clear and explicit, and using visual materials have been effective ways of developing skills and allowing people with autism to use these skills independently of direct adult prompting and cueing' (TEACCH). These priorities are especially important for individuals who have difficulties working independently in a variety of situations. Some individuals will benefit from regular educational programs, while others will need special classrooms for part or all of the day where the physical environment, curriculum, and personnel can be organised and manipulated to reflect individual needs.

Structured teaching provides information so the person knows exactly what to do, when to do it, where to do it and how to do it. According to Quill (2000), structured teaching approaches provide familiar, predictable and structured environments that reduce anxiety, promote independence and increase flexibility and tolerance for change. Learning to use a variety of visual systems independently is a crucial skill that may be applied to different activities and settings.

For more information:

The Treatment and Education of Autistic and Related Communication handicapped Children (TEACCH)

University of North Carolina at Chapel Hill

Chapel Hill

NC 27599-7180

Phone: (919) 966-2174

What about auditory training?

Auditory integration therapy (AIT) was originally introduced to treat hypersensitive hearing, deafness and other hearing problems. Two French physicians, Guy Berard and Alfred Tomatis, developed AIT.

Based on the results of an audiogram, people listen to electronically filtered music through headphones for a total of ten hours over a period of ten days. The theory behind the therapy is that it will help to correct hearing distortions, desensitise certain sound frequencies and improve dyslexia, attention deficit, hyperactivity, depression and autism.

Auditory training can be considered a form of sensory integration in which stimulation may sensitise or desensitise one or more senses. Theoretically speaking, if one or more senses are impaired in an individual, he or she may develop a distorted perception of the environment. There has been much research in the past fifteen years to indicate that many autistic individuals have sensory dysfunction in one or more areas. Although a number of studies (Bettison 1996; Rimland & Edelson 1995; Porges 2003) have looked at the effects of auditory training on children with autism, the treatment remains controversial and the benefits inconclusive. According to Rimland & Edelson, there appeared to be short-term improvements in eye contact, spontaneous speech, socialisation, and attention span as well as reduced sensitivity to certain sounds, although there is no concrete evidence to support any longer-term benefits.

For more information: The Society for Auditory Intervention Techniques (SAIT) is non-profit organisation that distributes information about auditory integration techniques and

other auditory based intervention to parents and professionals:
SAIT
PO Box 4538
Salem OR 97302
USA

What about sensory integration therapy?

Many children and adults with autism have a dysfunctional sensory system. One or more senses are either over- or under-reactive to stimulation. Such sensory problems may be the underlying reason for such behaviours as rocking, spinning, and flapping. Although the receptors for the senses are located in the peripheral nervous system (which includes everything but the brain and spinal cord), it is believed that the problem stems from neurological dysfunction in the central nervous system — the brain. Sensory integration techniques, such as pressure-touch, can facilitate attention and awareness, and reduce overall arousal.

Sensory integration refers to the integration and interpretation of sensory stimulation from the environment by the brain. It is an innate neurobiological process. In contrast, sensory integrative dysfunction is a disorder in which sensory input is not integrated or organised appropriately in the brain. Sensory dysfunction may produce varying degrees of problems in development, information processing, and behaviour. Dr A Jean Ayres developed a general theory of sensory integration and treatment based on studies in the neurosciences and those pertaining to physical development and neuromuscular function.

Sensory integration focuses primarily on three basic senses — tactile, vestibular, and proprioceptive. Their interconnections start forming before birth and continue to develop as the person matures and interacts with his or her environment. The three senses are not only interconnected but are also connected with other systems in the brain. Although these three sensory systems are less familiar than vision and audition, they are critical to our basic survival. The inter-relationship among these three senses is complex. Basically, they allow people to experience, interpret, and respond to different stimuli in the environment (Hatch-Rasmussen 1995).

For more information: Evaluation and treatment of basic sensory integrative processes is performed by occupational therapists and/or physical therapists. For more information about sensory integration therapy it is recommended that parents contact an occupational therapist either privately or through a community-based disability service.

What about speech–language therapy?

It is recognised that autistic children have difficulties with language, but it is clear that traditional approaches emphasising mastery of the formal properties of language are largely inappropriate — training children to speak is not going to bring about a transformation of their behaviour. The autistic child needs to learn not so much how to speak as how to use language socially to communicate.

That includes knowing how to hold a conversation, thinking about what the other person in a conversation understands and believes, and tuning in to the meta-linguistic signals of the other person, such as facial expression, tone of voice and body language. It is important to remember that communication is as much non-verbal as it is verbal, and autistic people have great difficulty understanding non-verbal language.

A speech pathologist specialising in the diagnosis and treatment of language problems and speech disorders may help a person learn how to communicate and socialise more effectively using strategies such as social stories to teach social relating skills and visual supports to augment speech. Visual supports also provide individuals with an effective means of communicating functionally.

What alternative treatment options are available?

Over the past few years, there has been an increasing awareness of autism. This has led to many research projects that are beginning to present interesting results and may eventually lead to a cure and, ultimately, the prevention of autism. Current research projects are looking at such diverse issues as more effective drug treatments for many of the common symptoms such as anxiety, hyperactivity, seizures, and obsessive behaviours; dietary treatments to assist with stomach and intestinal problems; auditory integration training and sensory integration therapy to assist with some of the sensory problems; and structured early intervention programs to provide intensive teaching of specific skills when children are first diagnosed.

Over the years, a number of treatments have been developed to assist some but not necessarily all children with autism. The most conclusive results to date have shown that the most effective treatment that helps every child to some degree is a structured early intervention and educational program that focuses on teaching individual skills in functional settings (Dawson & Osterling 1997). Other treatments may benefit some children or may improve certain aspects of their disability.

Janice Janzen, in her book *Autism. Facts and Strategies for Parents* (1999), provides a list of the most commonly mentioned treatments in autism literature. These include:

- structured education and early intervention;
- medication/drugs to treat specific symptoms;
- anti-yeast therapy;
- vitamin/dietary approaches;
- sensory integration therapy;
- occupational therapy;
- music therapy; and
- visual training.

It is up to parents to decide what popular treatments to try and to evaluate the success of chosen treatments for their child. For more information about individual treatments refer to Gerlach (2003).

What about vitamin therapy?

Vitamin B6 (pyridoxine) and magnesium have been an effective intervention for many autistic children and adults for over thirty years. According to Dr Stephen Edelson, of the Autism Research Institute, B6 and magnesium have received more scientific support than any other biological intervention for autism with a number of research studies showing that B6 and magnesium are beneficial to about half of autistic individuals. There has been documented evidence of improved behaviour as well as improvements in brain wave activity and metabolic processes. Anecdotal evidence from parents has supported these findings with parents reporting improvements in attention, learning, speech/language, and eye contact.

Magnesium should be given along with B6 to be most effective. Problems associated with magnesium deficiency include enuresis (bedwetting), irritability/agitation and sound sensitivity. Occasionally, an autistic person exhibits one or more of these behaviours when given B6 along with magnesium. In these cases, the person may need more than the recommended amount of magnesium. Magnesium is relatively safe although too high a dose will cause diarrhoea.

A comprehensive multivitamin/multimineral supplement is also strongly recommended since vitamins and minerals assist in metabolising B6 and magnesium.

There is some discussion on the side effects of high doses of B6. The only documentation of an adverse reaction to very high doses (higher than the recommended doses for autism) refers to peripheral neuropathy, but this is extremely rare. Peripheral neuropathy refers to tingling or numbness in the fingers and/or toes. Reducing the amount of B6 will usually eliminate the tingling or numbness within a day or two.

Low dosage of B6 and magnesium are relatively safe and inexpensive. It is recommended that, if parents try vitamin therapy with their child, they do not inform people beforehand but see if teachers, therapists and family members notice any changes in the child's behaviour as a result of the intervention procedure.

It is recommended that parents discuss with their family doctor the possibility of introducing a course of vitamin therapy to their child or adult's diet. The doctor will then provide information on recommended dosages and monitor any changes to the individual's health and behaviour.

What about special diets and medications?

There are a number of single case studies, observations and theories on the suggested role of vaccines, drugs, toxins, infections and diet as risk factors for autism. However, at this time the field is still relatively young and fragmented. Further study is crucial in this area to verify the individual findings and provide more rigour to the research process. There is very little recognised scientific research to support the suggestion that medications such as secretin or special diets are successful in treating autism. Most medical practitioners will recommend testing children for lactose and gluten intolerance and only then suggesting drastically altering diets if there is evidence of intolerance.

Current public debate about autism research has tended to focus on two issues, namely the suggested links between the combined measles, mumps and rubella vaccination and autism and the connection between bowel disorders and autism.

Gastro-intestinal problems

There is considerable interest in the possibility of significant gastro-intestinal problems in individuals with autism. According to some practitioners, altered intestinal permeability may result in problems in the central nervous system leading to developmental regression. It is not clear, however, whether such compromised gastro-intestinal function causes autism or whether it reflects one facet of the disorder in a small group of autistic people. There is no epidemiological evidence to support the incidence or prevalence of gastro-intestinal problems in individuals with autism. Further research in this area is needed before any definitive conclusions can be reached.

Inflammatory bowel disease

Inflammatory bowel disease (IBD) is a group of chronic inflammatory disorders of the small and large bowel, the most common being ulcerative colitis and Crohn's disease. The cause of IBD is not understood definitely but it is understood that there is most likely an immune mechanism as well as a genetic predisposition to the disease. The condition is relatively rare, and usually occurs in people between the ages of 15 and 30 years of age, although it also occurs in children. Common symptoms include diarrhoea, fever, stomach pain and weight loss.

Secretin

Secretin is a polypeptide hormone involved in the regulation of gastric function. It is normally prepared from the duodenal mucosa of pigs. It is used medically to test pancreatic function. A small amount is injected and the amount of bicarbonate which appears in the bloodstream is measured a short time afterwards. The bicarbonate secretin is required in order to neutralise the acid from the stomach and allow the enzymes in the duodenum to function.

As well as secreting bicarbonates, the pancreas secretes many other enzymes including lipases and especially peptidases. These peptidases will break down the peptides that, according to proponents of the opioid excess theories of autism, may be the major cause of the problems associated with autism. One way to decrease the problems caused by these potentially harmful peptides is to remove them from the diet. This is the basis for the gluten- and casein-free diets. Since secretin will stimulate the pancreas to produce these enzymes it could ameliorate the symptoms by this mechanism. It could also be acting in the brain itself or in the intestinal wall.

Secretin appears to have helped some people with autism with intestinal/metabolic problems that prevent them from digesting and processing certain food groups. According to anecdotal evidence, improvements have been seen not only in digestion but also in the communication, eye contact and attending skills of some individuals.

Gluten- and casein-free diet

The GF/CF diet has enabled many, many people to 'connect' with the world in which we live in a much clearer way. For Luke and others with Asperger's Syndrome, that connection has led to a much deeper understanding of himself and the social world.

(Jackson 2002, p 16)

There are a number of single case studies of clinical improvement in children with autism placed on gluten- and/or casein-free diets (Whitely, Rogers, Savery & Shattock 1999).

In allergy-induced autism, the symptoms usually become apparent during the first three years of life. Some children have autism that appears to have been triggered by intolerance to many foods and/or chemicals, the main offenders being wheat (gluten), cows milk (casein), corn, sugar and citrus fruits, although different substances may affect different children. The children also have many almost unnoticeable physical problems, namely excessive thirst, excessive sweating, especially at night, low blood sugar, diarrhoea, bloating, rhinitis, inability to control temperature, red face and/or ears and dark circles under the eyes.

The basis for the diet is quite simple and involves removing products containing gluten, casein, monosodium glutamate and aspartame.

Gluten is a protein that is found in wheat, rye, barley and oats. In order to eliminate this protein, alternatives must be sought for breads, baked goods, cereals, biscuits and pizza. Many flours and foods are produced from grains that do not contain gluten. Corn, rice and potatoes are three of the more commonly available alternatives, but health food stores also offer a variety of other choices.

Casein is the protein that is found in milk and milk products — all animal milk, not just cows milk. In order to eliminate this protein, alternatives to milk, cheese, ice cream and yoghurt should be sought. Additionally, casein is a common additive in the food industry, so care needs to be taken to read the labels and check listed ingredients of most foods.

For most people, the breakdown of dietary protein into smaller and smaller proteins and finally into individual amino acids is a process that is smoothly completed as food travels through the digestive system. However, for a person with autism, it has been found that a defect in the intestinal wall (leaky gut syndrome) permits incompletely digested components of the original proteins to pass from the intestine into the bloodstream.

In the case of two of the diet's most common proteins, gluten and casein, some of the components that are released into the bloodstream have opioid (morphine-like) properties. Gliadorphin-7 and other similar polypeptides are formed in the breakdown of gluten. Casomorpin-7 and other similar polypeptides are formed in the breakdown of casein. Recently, deltorphin and dermorphin have been targeted for their potential activity as well. All of these polypeptides contain regions very similar in structure to morphine. These proteins are transported to the brain where they bind to receptors causing an effect that is manifested in the symptoms of autism.

No effective test for this metabolic disorder is available at present. Some of the urinary analyses conducted on children with autism have found elevated levels of peptides but no test is available that provides conclusive evidence. A study by Whiteley et al (1999) failed to find any significant decrease in urinary peptide levels for those children who were on a gluten- and casein-free diet.

Some of the common indicators of intolerance to wheat and dairy products include eczema, bloating, constipation or diarrhoea, ear infections or a desire to binge on foods containing wheat and dairy such as bread or yoghurt. It is recommended that for those parents wishing to try the diet, it is introduced gradually and that they continue with the diet for at least three months before they assess their child for improvements.

By removing sources of gluten and casein from the diet of autistic children, it may be possible to alleviate and even eliminate some of the symptoms of autism. Before parents take any decision to drastically alter their child's current diet, they should consult with their family medical practitioner, obtain information about new diets, and then make an informed choice based on the needs of their child.

Although these treatments are yet to be fully tested, there is some anecdotal evidence to support them. The ideas are compatible with nearly all the accepted biological data on autism and are worthy of consideration. The dietary method must still be considered as experimental and no positive results can be promised or are claimed. The use of diet may well be far less harmful than other medical interventions or therapeutic regimes but care is still necessary during its implementation.

Why is diet such an important issue for individuals with autism?

Diet is such an important issue because most children and adults with autism have a very limited and usually inappropriate diet. Because of their restricted interests or obsession with certain fast foods, food is also often used as a way of motivating these individuals to learn new skills.

In recent years, there has been an increased interest in the effect of certain diets and food groups on the behaviours and skills of children and adults with autism. While research has reached no definite conclusions as yet on the effects of certain foods, because parents and professionals aim to provide a healthy and balanced diet for children and adults with autism they usually try to include all of the recommended food groups whenever possible.

One of the difficulties in achieving this aim is that most individuals with autism have very limited and restricted interests that include what they eat and drink. They are also visual learners who respond to easily recognised and widely advertised labels and logos. Children and adults with autism are often advertisers' dream customers because they respond to the visual hype rather than the quality of a product. They therefore tend to prefer easily recognised and available fast foods that are usually bland in taste and are visually stimulating. This presents a nightmare for parents and professionals. Parents are sometimes forced to use inappropriate foods as rewards to motivate their children to learn new skills and to maintain their interest during structured teaching sessions. At the same time, parents are usually very aware of current general concerns around diet and childhood obesity.

While certain foods may initially be used to motivate individuals with autism to learn new skills, the longer term aim is to expand their interests and awareness of other food options and to gradually move away from inappropriate diets to a more balanced and varied diet that includes a range of foods. However, initially when teaching a new skill it is essential to start with images that are easily recognised as well as images that will be motivating for the individual in question. Unfortunately, some individuals are motivated by offerings of certain fast foods and it is necessary to start with these foods as rewards. The aim is to gradually move towards offering more acceptable rewards that may include a range of activities, objects and healthy food.

Summary

Encouragingly for parents and professionals, autism has become an area of interest for international research. Research into causes and interventions has expanded and improved technology has enabled families to access the latest information about the disorder and to regularly confer with each other.

Information is now available about possible causes, some of the common problems associated with autism (such as sensory differences, cognitive differences, attention deficits, and verbal processing problems) as well as many treatment options. There is increasing interest in autism, especially the perceived increase in the incidence of the disorder, the possible genetic links to autism and also in a number of alternative treatment options.

Educational practice has varied over the years with improvements in understanding the individual thinking and learning styles of people with autism. Knowledge about possible causes of autism and the strengths and deficits associated with an autism spectrum disorder have led to a better understanding of the unique needs associated with the disorder.

While the most popular treatments involve some form of educational intervention, there has been an increase in the number of alternative treatments available to individuals and families.

CHAPTER

3

Impairments Linked to Autism

Autism is a neurobiological disorder of development that causes discrepancies or differences in the way the brain processes information.

Janzen 1999, p 7

Discrepancies in how the brain processes information present in many different ways among the autistic population but there are also many similarities, especially in those areas of development that are primarily affected by autism. As Janzen (1999) states, autism affects the individual's ability to communicate effectively and to relate and interact appropriately with others and with the environment. Autism also affects people's ability to process and react to sensory stimuli and to think and learn in similar ways to their neuro-typical peers.

Unfortunately, there is no simple way to describe autism. Autism presents differently in each individual and to 'know' one person with autism certainly does not mean that one would therefore 'know' autism. Nevertheless, the pattern of behaviours is consistent with the idea of a triad of impairments developed by Wing & Gould in 1979.

What is impaired communication?

People with autism have a pronounced communication deficit. This deficit does not relate to one particular aspect of communication but affects both expressive and receptive language skills and the expression of both verbal and non-verbal behaviours.

The communication deficits range along a continuum from limited comprehension and no functional language to literal understanding of language and reasonable conversation skills.

People with autism:

■ may have no speech or very limited speech and lack typical communicative gestures;

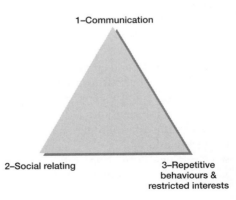

Figure 3.1 *The triad of impairments*

35

- may use speech but revert to inappropriate, non-verbal behaviours when confused or anxious;
- may speak in complete sentences but be unable to initiate or maintain a conversation;
- may guide an adult by the hand to a desired object rather than ask for something, or may do things independently, or do without, rather than request assistance;
- may use repetitive sounds or repeat certain words, phrases, chunks of dialogue, or questions over and over;
- may have unusual vocal quality (tone, pitch, speed of speaking);
- may reverse pronouns (using 'you' instead of 'I', for example);
- may not consistently follow verbal directions;
- may perseverate on certain topics or have difficulty maintaining a topic that is interesting to a peer or other conversational partner;
- may not respond to own name;
- may interpret what others say in a very literal, concrete way (for example, 'it's raining cats and dogs' is understood literally);
- may have difficulty 'reading' non-verbal messages in facial expressions and gestures;
- may show little attention and response to verbal instructions;
- may present with echolalia, repeating words spoken by other people (often with little meaning);
- may 'recite' long passages from books or videos but be unable to respond to questions that would indicate an understanding of the recited material;
- may have difficulty with comprehension;
- may misunderstand or respond inappropriately to figurative, metaphorical language and 'turns of phrase' used by others; and
- may become frustrated, non-compliant and aggressive or 'tune-out'.

Communication often involves speech but it does not depend solely on it. Quill (2000, p 14) describes it thus:

> Communication is a reciprocal, dynamic process. It is the instrumental force propelling social knowledge, relationships and a sense of self. An effective communicator has an inherent motivation to interact, something to express, and a means of communication. Unlike language, which is symbolic and rules based, communication is social and constantly changing.

Communication includes the act of getting a message across, sharing ideas, thoughts and feelings, thinking and analysing information/stimuli. Many different skills are required in order for a person to communicate successfully. Individuals with autism may have difficulties attending to situations, processing information and formulating appropriate responses using whatever language they have. According to Quill (2000), 'communicative interactions require moment-to-moment integration of multiple contextual, language, social, and emotional elements as well as an ability to adjust to the behaviours of others'.

A person with autism may have difficulty:
- establishing or shifting attention;
- following rapidly changing stimuli;
- taking in information;
- processing information;
- storing information;
- retrieving information; and
- sending information (Hodgdon 1995).

Children and adults with autism have problems understanding and using all forms of communication including:

- speech;
- sign language;
- body language including facial expression;
- tone of voice;
- gestures; and
- vocalisators (vocal sounds other than words).

Some of the difficulties may be so subtle and well disguised in a more able person with autism that no obvious communication deficit is noticeable to the casual observer. A young adult, for example, may participate in a conversation with a family friend, but tend to talk about things of interest to him and try to dominate the conversation. He may quickly lose interest if the topic changes.

> Nick works as a bus driver for a large company. He is very interested in transport and collects magazines about cars and trains. He also likes to memorise bus and train timetables and likes to talk about the latest bus and train models. Even at weekends, Nick loves to visit the train and bus museum and take train and bus rides around the city. He tends to dominate social conversations talking about his interests and not really listening when other people try to talk about other topics.

Some people with autism never develop speech. As well as being 'non-verbal', they may also have difficulty in developing or understanding other forms of communication such as signing, gestures or pointing. Other individuals may not use speech but communicate their needs non-verbally.

A young child may not communicate verbally that he is thirsty but may scream loudly, may drag a parent by the hand to the fridge or may independently go and get his cup and bring it to an adult.

> When Ingmar wants to go outside and play on her trampoline, she does not ask, sign or point to the door. She goes up to her mother, hits her and tries to push her towards the back door. If this does not work, Ingmar usually starts to scream and bang her head on the floor. Eventually her mother realises what Ingmar wants. Ingmar is now learning to point to a picture of a trampoline when she wants to go outside.

While some individuals with autism communicate non-verbally, many individuals will develop speech and language, to varying degrees. They need to be taught to use speech as well as gestures, facial expression and body language to communicate functionally. They have to be taught how to:

- request things such as food, objects or attention;
- protest at unwanted or uncomfortable situations and express concerns and fears;
- greet familiar and unfamiliar people appropriately;
- ask and answer questions reliably;
- comment on objects and events;
- interact socially with familiar and unfamiliar adults and peers;
- label objects and actions; and
- express choices.

In routine situations, the expressive and receptive skills of the person with autism may appear far better than they really are. This leads people to overestimate an individual's abilities and underestimate the severity of their communication impairment. Sometimes it is difficult to determine whether an individual comprehends language or is responding to visual cues. For example, if a child runs to the door on the command 'let's go to the park', he may actually be responding to the visual cue of mum picking up the car keys or picking up her handbag.

Many young children with autism successfully communicate their basic needs non-verbally. They can take a person to the cupboard when they want food, will push a parent to the door when they want to go outside and will even learn to turn the TV/video on for themselves. They begin to encounter problems however when other people start to put demands on them or have expectations of them that they do not understand. They may be expected to conform to certain rules, routines or directions without anyone teaching them what these rules, routines and directions are. This leads to confusion, anxiety and even frustration as the children try to understand what is expected of them. Communication impairment in autism may be described as a problem of both receptive and expressive language. Even with very young children, it is important to introduce the concept of visual supports to provide clear and simple messages to children about what is expected of them.

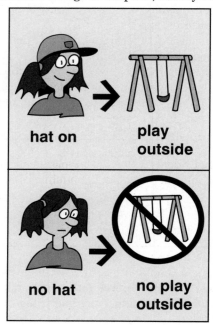

Figure 3.2 *Visual representation of message*

For example, Figure 3.2 shows a visual strategy providing a clear message to children that if they want to play outside they must wear a hat. This is a common rule for both preschools and schools.

What are the speech production problems associated with autism?

To fully understand the communication impairment of children and adults with autism requires a basic understanding of the normal speech process. Language involves the ability to form words (syntax) and understand the rules associated with putting words together in a particular order (semantics). Learning to use language effectively involves more then merely learning word meanings and grammatical rules. People must also learn how to use language appropriately (pragmatics). Children and adults who understand the pragmatics of language are sensitive to the social rules that govern communication and are able to shape their speech and language behaviour accordingly.

In addition to difficulties with the form (syntax or grammar) and the content (semantics) of language, children and adults with autism have severe problems with the pragmatics of language. Problems associated with the pragmatics of language include poor looking and attending skills, an inability to take turns or interpret gestures and body language, a limited ability to initiate conversational topics, and a limited ability to respond appropriately to the attempts of others to communicate socially. Children and adults who do not use language appropriately often suffer frustration, rejection and isolation.

The communication impairment in children and adults with autism is pervasive and affects both verbal and non-verbal skills. When speech and language skills do develop, they are obviously different from the speech and language of their peers. Immediate or delayed echolalia is often present and pronoun reversal is also common. Many individuals are unable to label objects or use and understand abstract concepts until quite late, if at all. Most individuals are literal in their understanding of language. This can be most confusing and at times even embarrassing. For example, when a young man with autism was told by his mother to stop humming 'because the noise was driving her mad' the young man was really confused because 'noises don't drive'.

Allan had no idea how to control the volume of his voice. He always spoke very loudly no matter where he was. This proved embarrassing for the people with him and he was asked by his teacher to lower his voice. Instead of talking more quietly, Allan bent down until he was close to the ground and kept talking at the same volume. He thought that he had 'lowered' his voice.

Individuals with autism typically engage in idiosyncratic speech or jargon as they attempt to communicate with familiar adults and peers. These particular speech patterns or utterances are usually non-communicative except to those people who are familiar with the individual. Abnormal speech intonation and affect are also symptoms of communication impairment in individuals with autism. Speech may be characterised by rises at the end of sentences or a monotonous, flat tonal quality. Pitch, rhythm, intonation, pace and articulation may be irregular and there may be little use of non-verbal communication such as facial expression or gesture.

What is impaired socialisation?

The American Psychiatric Association (1994, p 70), defines the social impairment of autism as including 'a marked impairment in the use of multiple nonverbal behaviours such as eye gaze, facial expression, and gestures to regulate social interaction'; 'a lack of spontaneous seeking to share enjoyment, interests or achievements with other people (e.g., by a lack of showing, bringing, or pointing out objects of interest)'; and a 'lack of social and emotional reciprocity'.

These non-verbal social–communicative behaviours, along with imitation deficits (usually shown by an inability to imitate simple actions, sounds and words), are among the most important indicators of autism in children. During the first twelve months of life, infants typically begin to use and respond to eye gaze, gestures and facial expressions of familiar adults in initial attempts to socialise. They develop these skills to initiate social interactions, engage in simple turn-taking activities, make basic requests and share interests with others.

The non-verbal social–communicative skills in children with autism 'are characterised by significant difficulty with nonverbal joint attention skills, some difficulty with social turn-taking skills, and less difficulty with nonverbal behavioural regulation skills. These fundamental differences define impaired social reciprocity' (Quill 2000, p 8).

Social impairments are one of the core deficits associated with a diagnosis of autism. In addition to the core social–communicative deficits, the diagnostic criteria outlined by the American Psychiatric Association in the DSM-IV (1994) includes a 'lack of varied, spontaneous make-believe play or social imitative play appropriate to developmental level' and a 'failure to develop peer relationships appropriate to developmental level'. For children with autism, the acquisition of social skills is qualitatively different from other children. They fail to develop normal reciprocal or interactive social relationships with others.

Young children with autism may treat people as tools or objects — they may take a person by the hand to procure a wanted object, to open a cupboard, fix a broken toy or pour a drink. Some children with autism may be able to respond appropriately to people in familiar situations or to very familiar people, but become confused and anxious at other times. They may appear rude because of their inability to understand and use the more subtle aspects of social interaction. Many parents of young children describe their children's interactions as needs-based — the children attempt to interact only when they need something, rather than because they want social contact with a familiar adult.

Both children and adults with autism have difficulty interacting socially with others and their behaviour does not encourage interaction from others. Most individuals appear to be socially isolated. Their behaviour reflects this through poor eye contact and an apparent lack of desire to share activities with others. However, the opposite is often true, especially for younger children, who may attempt to socialise or who watch others with great interest but have no idea how to initiate interaction or join in play with their peers. Individuals with autism frequently want to socialise. They just do not know how to initiate appropriate forms of interaction. They also fail to understand other peoples' points of view (social empathy) or that other people have their own beliefs, desires and intentions that guide their behaviour. This lack of empathy — often seen as selfishness — is not inappropriate behaviour, but rather a lack of the skills needed to respond in any other way.

Over the past ten years, 'theory of mind' has become a popular explanation for many of the social deficits in autism. This theory links the fundamental cause of social isolation with a failure in 'meta-cognition' or the concept of 'thinking about thinking'. People with autism appear to lack an awareness of other people's minds as being distinct from their own. They are unable to understand the feelings, beliefs and desires of other people and tend to interpret most information only in terms of how it relates to themselves.

People with autism:

- may not differentiate between familiar and unfamiliar people;
- may lack joint attention;
- may appear rude at times by approaching strangers inappropriately or by ignoring another person's attempts to communicate/interact, etc.;
- may behave as though other people do not exist;
- may appear disinterested in other people unless they need those people to get them what they want;
- may have a flat affect, showing little facial expression except for extremes of anger, frustration or joy;
- may avoid looking at others;
- may have difficulty taking turns in activities and sharing objects and toys with their peers;
- may not engage in parallel play, interactive play or symbolic play;
- may be observed on the periphery of social activities, watching but not joining in;
- may fail to develop appropriate peer relationships;
- may engage in unusual and inappropriate requests for attention from peers such as pushing a student or hitting a peer;
- may show more interest in objects that people;
- may be unintentionally aggressive in an attempt to be social;
- may cope badly with being teased;
- may show little empathy to the feelings of others;
- may appear very self absorbed and 'in a world of their own';
- may have limited play skills: playing with few toys and displaying no imagination in play or interest in playing socially with others;
- may prefer physical play such as tickle games, and rough-and-tumble activities;
- may have difficulty shifting attention between people, objects or activities in the environment;

- may exhibit inappropriate affect for a particular situation such as laughing when someone is hurt; and
- may lack self-esteem.

People with autism are often described as 'living in a world of their own', showing little interest in, or awareness of, others. They may avoid eye contact or look through people as if they are not there. Some people with autism avoid physical contact and will stiffen or walk away if someone approaches. They may also become distressed if touched. Others may be completely oblivious to other people and fail to respond if touched. However, many people with autism are affectionate and enjoy physical contact with others though usually only if they initiate it or on their terms.

It is extremely difficult for individuals with autism to understand and express emotion. Their facial affect is often blank or 'flat' and they fail to read or understand the facial expressions of others. Their social skills are limited, and social interactions are mechanical or stilted in nature.

What do repetitive behaviours and restricted interests mean?

The third characteristic of the triad of impairments outlined by Wing is the most difficult to describe and to understand. Although autism is typically identified by a number of ritualistic and idiosyncratic patterns of behaviour, it remains the least understood and most obscure characteristic. The ritualistic patterns of behaviour in autism are defined by the American Psychiatric Association in the DSM-IV (1994) as:

> ... preoccupation with one or more stereotyped and restricted patterns of interest that is abnormal in intensity and focus, apparently inflexible adherence to specific, non-functional routines or rituals, stereotyped and repetitive motor mannerisms, and persistent preoccupation with parts of objects.

This characteristic of autism manifests itself differently in children and adults and may also be referred to as an impairment of imagination and social understanding.

In young children it is usually seen in the way children play, or don't play, so that it presents as an absence or abnormality of imaginative, pretend play. Young children with autism do not develop play skills in the same way as other children. Their interest in play is restricted to repetitive, stereotypic actions that do not involve any social interaction with others. For example, children tend to have a limited interest in toys, will only play with certain toys and objects and play tends to be repetitive, anti-social and not age appropriate.

In adults, the problem may be shown as an inflexibility of attitude, a perseverative interest in certain topics, an inability to imagine consequences of actions and an inability to understand the thoughts and feelings of other people. Adults may be very rigid about how things should be done, may collect information or talk constantly about one topic such as dinosaurs, train timetables or the solar system and have no understanding that other people are not interested in the same topics and are bored with the conversation.

Repetitive behaviours vary from simple actions such as spinning wheels, lining up objects, tapping, rocking and flapping hands to more complex behaviours such as insistence on following routines, obsessions with certain objects and activities (collecting bus tickets, computers, naming dinosaurs,) and obsession with facts (cricket scores, models of cars and car numberplates and position of planets in the solar system).

Over a number of years, in a series of books and journal articles, Wing (1980, 1988, 1996) described the range of impairments of imagination and social understanding in children and adults with autism. She outlined a problem understanding other people's point of view, an inability to generalise concepts, difficulty imagining the future and difficulty planning ahead. With limited ability to anticipate future events, people also tend to lack the ability to organise themselves. This leads to dependence on routine and on events happening in a predictable, consistent order without change. Most individuals with autism will defend routine and sameness rigorously because their sense of security is dependent on it.

Most individuals relate abnormally to objects and events in their environment. They may be obsessive about their immediate environment, requiring things to remain unchanged, from the position of objects to the order of routines. Even slight disruptions to a routine, or changing the position of a particular object can result in severe behavioural or emotional reactions.

> Jane became extremely distressed when she arrived home 10 minutes late from her supported work program to find that her T.V. show had already started and she had missed the opening credits. Watching the credits was part of her usual evening routine and she had to struggle to cope with the change to her usual routine for the remainder of the evening.

People with autism find it difficult to interpret and process new information, preferring things to remain constant and unchanged. A high level of stress may result from any minor change in a routine, activity or surroundings. Individual reactions to stress may vary from withdrawal into their own world and the introduction of rituals and obsessions, to aggression against themselves or others. Such inflexibility can lead to a very rigid lifestyle for the individual and for those around them.

Some people with autism develop bizarre attachments to objects. They may be distracted, to the exclusion of all other objects within their environment, by particular items, such as a special toy, a piece of string, or a favourite item of clothing that has to be kept near at hand at all times.

Some children become intrigued or obsessed with one part of an object such as spinning the .

> Carlos always carried a piece of string that he would twiddle and flap in front of his face. He learned to put the string in his pocket during work time or place it on the desk in front of him. He was allowed free time during the day to play with his string. Carlos could cope as long as he could see or touch his string.

wheels of a toy car, opening and closing the doors of a cupboard, smelling the pages of a book or looking at the words on the back of the cereal packet. They fail to understand the real or major functions of objects. They engage in repetitive motor movements such as spinning objects, hand-flapping, rocking or pacing. Some people become absorbed in watching the movement of certain objects for hours, such as spinning fans, lights flashing or leaves moving in the wind. Reaction to sensory stimuli may vary from over-sensitivity to a total lack of response.

People with autism:

- may show fear of strangers or new activities by avoiding or resisting contact;
- may develop a strong attachment to certain objects, routines or rituals and may stay involved with them for long periods and become upset if interrupted;
- may show an inflexible adherence to non-functional routines and rituals;
- may display unusual body and hand posture and stereotyped and repetitive motor mannerisms such as flapping, rocking, spinning or toe walking;
- may become upset about changes to normal routines or repeatedly ask questions about when events will occur;
- may be very concerned about completing work perfectly and may be unwilling to attempt work that cannot be completed without error;

- may become distressed if familiar routes are not followed when out in the community;
- may be extremely neat and continually return objects to their correct place in the house;
- may show an intense level of interest in one area (dinosaurs, Thomas the Tank Engine, electrical appliances, train timetables);
- may listen to the same story or watch the same video over and over again;
- may 'act out' a character or sequence from TV in a repetitive way;
- may not understand that an object can be used for more than one purpose (for example, pretending that a banana is a telephone or a block is a car);
- may be motivated to remain in control of situations and be successful at manipulating people into allowing this control to be maintained;
- may have disturbed sleep patterns;
- may have difficulty toilet training; and
- may respond to toys and objects in an unusual and repetitive way (spinning wheels, lining up objects, opening and closing doors).

These problems usually result in specific behaviours that include repetitive and unusual manipulation of objects and toys, frustration and disruptive behaviours when routines and rituals are disrupted, insistence on sameness, challenging behaviours when the environment is changed and preoccupation with parts of objects.

What is impaired sensory information processing?

In addition to the triad of impairments, many children and adults with autism also have a sensory impairment that affects the way they respond to sound, sight, touch, taste, scent and pain. Sensory disturbances in autism are not recognised as part of the formal diagnostic classification in the current diagnostic manual of the American Psychiatric Association (DSM-IV) although sensory impairment was mentioned in the earlier version (DSM-III). This is despite the fact that feedback from practitioners and parents confirm that abnormal responses to sensory stimuli are common in autism. There is little constructive research to date in the area of sensory impairment and autism, although it is an area of great interest and relevance, especially for individuals with autism and the parents and practitioners who are regularly living and working with them.

Kanner, in 1943 (p 250), first talked about autism as a 'biological impairment like physical or intellectual handicaps'. He also mentioned the perceptual difficulties and overreaction to loud noises and moving objects he noticed among the children he was observing. In the 1960s and 1970s a number of researchers looked at the perceptual and sensory processing problems associated with autism. Schopler (1965) observed abnormal responses to visual, vestibular and auditory stimuli among a group of children and Ornitz (1970) labelled autism as a disorder of sensorimotor integration and later also identified problems with the modulation of sensory input and motor output (Ornitz 1973). Sensory input occurs before motor output. The central nervous system receives the input that it then organises and processes before responding appropriately to a particular situation. For example, we put something on our tongue to taste it and the sensory information is processed — we either swallow the substance or we spit it out.

More recent research (Bauman & Kemper 1994) has found developmental abnormalities in the cerebellum and limbic regions of the brains of people with autism that supports the idea that individuals with autism have problems with the sensory integrative process including the modulation of sensory input. There are also a number of personal accounts of unusual sensitivities to certain stimuli by individuals with autism, including Grandin (1986, 1995) and Williams (1992, 1994) that describe the difficulties these young adults had, and continue to have, with sensory information processing.

People with autism may show unusual responses to sensory experiences (including sound and touch but also taste, vision, smell and pain). They may over-react or under-react to sensory stimuli — perceiving ordinary sensations as extremely intense or weak. Children and adults with autism are often unable to make sense out of the information that comes to them through their eyes, ears, nose, vestibular, proprioceptive (muscles and joints), touch and taste organs. This has consequences for their intellectual, motor and emotional development and affects their functioning in communication and social interaction.

A person with sensory sensitivities:

- may show unusual or inappropriate responses to sounds, textures, visual and auditory stimuli;
- may be unusually sensitive to their surroundings and be unable to screen out irrelevant stimuli (dog barking outside, ticking of a clock);
- may vary from day to day in their capabilities and abilities to attend and respond;
- may ignore some sounds but over-react or be very sensitive to other sounds;
- may play with, seek out, ignore or react negatively to objects or toys that make certain sounds;
- may place fingers in ears, become distressed, hum or sing to block out certain sounds;
- may actively avoid eye contact, or offer fleeting contact lacking in social intent (some individuals with autism have reported that it is painful to look directly at other people);
- may use peripheral vision (look from the corners of their eyes) rather than central vision — therefore giving the impression of not looking or making eye contact;
- may focus intently on the small visual details or patterns of walls, furniture, objects, toys, prints, pictures or body parts while not seeing the whole picture;
- may show intense interest in light or shiny reflective surfaces (for example, may filter light through fingers or stare at light or reflections in glasses, watch water going down the plug hole);
- may be fascinated by certain visual patterns such as drain covers or car hubcaps;
- may explore by smelling or mouthing objects, people and surfaces;
- may have eating problems that could be related to the smell, texture or flavour of food — often having strong preferences and refusing unfamiliar foods;
- may chew or eat things that are not food (pica);
- may have delayed or limited response to obvious pain;
- may seek out vibrations or engage in repetitive movements such as rocking, bouncing, flapping arms and hands, or spinning without becoming dizzy;
- may exhibit extreme aversion to certain textures by screaming or avoidance;
- may have unusual fears or phobias;
- may crave activities that provide sensory feedback such as swinging or jumping;
- may be resistant to being hugged or cuddled;
- may exhibit withdrawal or challenging behaviour in chaotic environments with visual or auditory challenges such as large shopping centres, crowded places;
- may hold or move hands or body in unusual (often-rigid) postures;
- may have difficulty with position of body in space, and motor planning;
- may walk on tiptoes; and
- may indicate marked preference to be alone.

The central nervous system receives information from all of the senses. These senses work together to enable people to function, learn and perform a myriad of everyday tasks and activities. 'Our senses give us the information we need to function in the world' (Kranowitz 1998).

Stimuli from both inside and outside the body send information to the senses that enable people to function in the everyday world (Kranowitz 1998). Smell, touch, hearing, sight and taste are the five senses that respond to stimuli from outside the body. They are known as the far senses because they take in information from the environment.

Three other important sensory systems are the tactile, vestibular and proprioceptive systems and these are recognised as the near senses. The near senses are more refined and relate to how the body perceives itself. The tactile sensory system processes information about touch; the vestibular sense processes balance, movement and gravity information; and the proprioceptive sense processes information about the body's position in space.

A person's response to particular sensory experiences may fluctuate from one day to the next. Some days they may seek out certain sensory experiences, on other days they may avoid that same experience.

People with autism show many unusual responses to sensory experiences and they may over-react (hypersensitivity) or under-react (hyposensitivity) to sensory stimuli. Although research in this area is still relatively new, it is known that the problems lay, not in the sense organs themselves, but in the way that the brain processes the sensory information it receives from the sense organs. These processing difficulties impact on the individual's social, emotional, communicative, cognitive and motor development.

It is not clear how extensive the abnormalities in sensory development are, although it appears that children and adults may range from mildly affected in one particular sense to severely affected in many sensory areas.

Sensory problems include either hyper- or hypo- sensitivity, overload, synesthesia and fluctuation.

Hypersensitivity

Hypersensitivity indicates a heightened response to a particular sensory experience, as the sensations are registered too intensely. The nervous system is highly stimulated by even a weak sensation.

> James continually smells things including food, objects he picks up, and even other people but has no overt reaction to any other sensory stimuli. He appears hypersensitive to smell.

Hyposensitivity

Hyposensitivity indicates a dampened response to a particular sensory experience, as the sensations are registered less intensely than normal. The nervous system is poorly stimulated by even a strong sensation. See Figure 3.3.

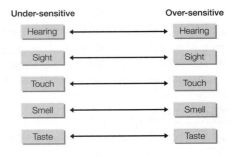

Figure 3.3 *People with autism may be hypersensitive or hyposensitive to stimuli in any of the outlined sensory areas*

Overload

Overload suggests an inability to filter out what is unimportant or to selectively attend to certain things. Some people have difficulty attending to more than one channel of sensation concurrently so that they are unable to listen and look at the same time. This is one possible explanation for why many people with autism display poor eye contact.

> Jessica is visually sensitive and loves to sit and watch the clothes dryer spin around. She becomes distressed by certain sounds such as the vacuum cleaner or even the toilet flushing, especially when she is trying to watch her favourite video or the ceiling fan rotate. She is unable to filter out certain sounds in her environment and concentrate on what she is seeing. Jessica has sensory overload because she is unable to block out stimuli that is not relevant.

Synesthesia

Synesthesia refers to a crossover of the senses; for example, seeing an emotion through certain colours or experiencing loud sounds as flashes of colour. Wendy Lawson, an adult with Asperger's syndrome states that most people she sees have a colour 'aura' that is related to how she feels about them.

Fluctuation

For most people with autism, their sensory issues will fluctuate over time. For some people with autism there may be fluctuations from day to day in how they perceive things and how they can process information from their senses. Some days an individual may seek out certain sensory experiences while on other days those same experiences may be avoided.

> Stephen may react differently to a particular sound or taste from one day to the next. He sometimes becomes extremely distressed when taken to a large and noisy shopping centre but on other occasions may cope very well in the same situation. Sometimes he will eat chicken or fish but other days he refuses to eat any meat or vegetables at all. Stephen's response to sensory stimuli fluctuates from day to day.

There is also evidence to support the hypothesis that an individual may be affected by sensory stimuli in different ways at different times.

Many of the accounts published by individuals with autism relate to problems in processing sensory information or to problems of sensory overload. Many parents talk about their children coping with sensory input throughout the day at school but then turning into absolute monsters when they get home and any demands are placed upon them. Many children with autism try to behave appropriately and conform at school but then need down-time when they get home to enable them to cope with their sensory overload.

Temple Grandin, an adult with Asperger's syndrome who has written extensively about her experiences growing up with an autism spectrum disorder in her book *Emergence Labelled Autistic*, talks about her life (1986, p 32):

> I ached to be loved — hugged. At the same time I withdrew from over-touch as from my over-weight, overly affectionate, 'marshmallow' aunt. Her affection was like being swallowed by a whale. Even being touched by the teacher made me flinch and draw back.

What other problems are often associated with autism?

In addition to the four impairments outlined above, a significant number of individuals with autism have other problems including cognitive deficits, auditory processing problems, attention problems and abnormal mood swings. These deficits exacerbate language, social and behavioural impairments.

What are cognitive deficits?

The majority of individuals diagnosed with autism have an intellectual impairment of varying degree. All areas of cognitive development in an individual, however, are not impaired to the same degree. Some people have a peak skill or exceptional ability in one or more areas of cognitive functioning.

Over the past few years, there has been increasing evidence to support the concept of a particular thinking and learning style among people with autism. This style is quite different to the way that most people think and learn and provides possible explanations for many of their difficulties and their behaviours. People with autism display 'a pattern of strengths and weaknesses' in the acquisition of social and communication skills (Mundy & Sigman 1989). Understanding this pattern of strengths and weaknesses is fundamental to future research and intervention approaches.

In 1991, Rogers & Pennington proposed a developmental model for autism and highlighted several domains that appeared to differentiate people with autism from other groups. These clinical domains were: imitation; emotional perception and responses; joint attention and communication; theory of mind; and executive function. Understanding autism, and how people with autism differ from their peers, however, is not that simple. Many people with autism eventually develop joint attention behaviours, speech, some level of sharing of experiences and affect. Many higher functioning people with autism, or Asperger's syndrome, also develop reasonable theory of mind skills but may not pick up higher order aspects of theory of mind such as irony. There is wide individual variability in the development of social interaction skills in autism, and many individuals develop social knowledge, interest and reciprocal social relations. Many individuals with autism want to relate socially to others, they just do not know how to go about it.

It appears that early indicators of autism in young children include both joint attention disturbance (Mundy 1995; Mundy & Markus 1997) and poor imitation of motor movements (Rogers & Pennington 1991). In higher functioning or older individuals with autism, the signs change to include difficulties in the pragmatics of language (Happe 1993; Surian, Baron-Cohen, & Van der Lely 1996), theory of mind (Baron-Cohen 1995) and attention difficulties.

A number of cognitive skills are disordered in people with autism that differentiate them from their peers. These skills affect their ability to understand abstract concepts; understand the overall message by processing information rather than focusing on specific detail (weak central coherence), plan ahead and sort through options before choosing an appropriate response (executive function deficits), and understand the thoughts and feelings of others (theory of mind deficits).

Most individuals with autism have difficulty understanding abstract concepts. Both children and adults tend to think in concrete terms and fail to understand abstract or metaphorical concepts. They take figures of speech literally and do not pick up on the nuances of language or non-verbal cues such as gestures, facial expression and tone of voice.

For example, a child with autism who is told by his teacher to 'pull his socks up in class' may actually stand in the classroom and pull up his socks rather than understand the metaphor that he needs to improve his work.

Central coherence refers to our drive to find meaning in the big picture. People with autism are often more concerned about isolated details and fail to grasp the overall message or purpose of an activity or event. The term 'central coherence' was introduced by Frith (1989) to explain the ability of individuals to extract the most relevant information from a story or conversation in order to form a 'whole' picture rather than the individual elements of the story. Frith has suggested that this ability to see the whole picture is disturbed in autism. According to Francesca Happe, a London-based psychologist, autism is characterised by a cognitive style biased toward detail rather than more general information. She calls this 'weak central coherence'. Happe (1994) found that people with autism are remarkably good at detail, especially visual details, but usually miss the bigger picture. They frequently notice when someone has moved a piece of furniture, put the television remote control in the wrong place or dropped a small piece of thread on the floor. They may have sensory problems and focus on the hum of the ceiling fan, hear the sound of a radio playing softly a few rooms away and are unable to block these out to concentrate on more immediate issues.

The ability of individuals with autism to focus on detail, rather than the bigger picture, has advantages in some tasks. Shah & Frith (1993) demonstrated that children with autism are unusually proficient at certain activities that require them to focus on specific details. Children with autism tend to do well in the block design sub-test of the Wechsler Intelligence Scale for Children (WISC) or in tasks where embedded shapes have to be detected inside a larger design.

Because of their weak central coherence, individuals with autism tend to have an idiosyncratic focus of attention, often focusing on particular details of an object or picture rather than the overall meaning.

> Jenny has difficulty looking at a picture book with her mother and her teacher because she is obsessed with numbers and becomes totally focused on looking at, and counting out loud, the individual page numbers. She shows little interest in any story or picture book unless it is a counting book.

Executive function refers to 'the ability to plan and organise tasks, monitor one's own performance, inhibit inappropriate responses, utilize feedback, and suppress distracting stimuli' (McAfee 2002). Most individuals with autism exhibit executive function deficits in their ability to plan, control their actions, process information and filter through options before making a response.

According to Ozonoff (1995), executive functioning is mediated by the frontal lobes of the brain. He quotes Luria's (1966) definition of executive function as 'the ability to maintain an appropriate problem-solving set for the attainment of a future goal'. Deficits in executive functioning can lead to many difficulties at home, at school, and in the work environment. Hughes et al (1994) listed a number of deficits associated with executive functioning that are commonly seen in individuals with autism. These included deficits in:

■ planning;
■ impulse control;
■ organised search; and
■ flexibility of thought and action.

Whiteley, Rogers & Shattock (1998) explored a number of characteristics of autism where the principles of executive function deficits apply. Many people with autism have described the problems they encounter when attempting to switch from one sensory mode to another. Donna Williams (1996), a woman with Asperger's syndrome, discussed the difficulties she has when she is focusing on processing visual information, to then have to take in and make sense of any incoming auditory stimuli. Courchesne et al (1994) provided convincing evidence that people with autism do have great difficulty in switching their attention from one perceptual mode to another. If a person with autism is in visual mode, it takes a long time for them to switch to auditory mode. The control of the switching system may be described as an executive function.

The behaviour of people with autism is often rigid, inflexible and perseverative. They are often impulsive and while they may have a large store of knowledge, it is usually around one or two topics, and they are unable to apply this knowledge in a meaningful way. They often seem narrowly focused on detail, and cannot see the whole picture. Grandin (1995, p 37) offered an example of executive function deficit in autism: 'I am unable to hold one piece of information in my mind while I do the next step in the sequence.'

Children with autism find it especially difficult to make choices. Making choices is about filtering through options and, when the ability to filter through information is affected, such a process becomes extremely difficult.

> When presented with a large tin of assorted biscuits and told to choose one, Sarah will tend to take the same one every time even though she does not appear to like it. She will only take one small bite and then hand it to the nearest adult. She does not seem able to look at all of the biscuits and consider her options and then choose a different variety from her original selection.

Many psychologists have drawn attention to the problems people with autism have in planning future activities. Planning involves a consideration of a variety of possible activities. The ability to filter through a range of possibilities, visualise, consider and reject possibilities, and then make choices is expecting a lot from individuals where the basic processes are impaired.

The possible impact of executive function deficits on individuals with autism suggests the need for particular teaching strategies. For example, it may be necessary to break tasks down into clearly defined steps, use sequencing to teach specific skills and identify the main idea in any new information.

What are auditory processing problems?

Individuals with autism typically have problems processing auditory information. An auditory processing problem occurs when a person hears speech sounds but is unable to perceive the meaning of the sounds. Sometimes a lack of speech comprehension may be interpreted as an unwillingness to comply. However, in actual fact, the individual may not be able to retrieve the meaning of a sound at the appropriate time. Language skills are usually impaired on some level, as autism is fundamentally a communication disorder.

For children and adults with mild autism, the language disorder may present as difficulty with higher-level language skills, such as understanding idioms, humour or limited social interaction skills. These individuals usually have reasonable grammar (with the exception of problems with irregular past tense verbs, irregular plural nouns, or reflexive pronouns, for example) and so are able to participate in mainstream classes. Their differences, however, are apparent upon close examination and may include few or no friends, limited interests and difficulties with new situations.

For many people with mild autism, reading skills often appear normal. They develop functional reading skills because of their excellent visual memories. Many high-functioning individuals with autism can read fluently because they have memorised all of the words in the story. Many of these individuals, however, do not develop adequate phonological awareness to sound out new or unfamiliar words. An auditory processing problem is the reason for the difficulties associated with phonological processing. The development of phonics knowledge requires normal auditory processing skills, because the person has to hear the sound to develop sound/symbol association skills (for example, 'b' says 'buh' as in 'baby'). Even children who are not autistic but who have an auditory processing disorder will usually have reduced phonological awareness. Individuals with autism are often good at masking these difficulties because they have such a vast sight word vocabulary. A second problem with reading is that many children and adults may read fluently but have little (or no) comprehension of what they have read. Poor comprehension is also related to the auditory processing problems associated with autism. Reading comprehension develops because the reader is able to listen to himself/herself read, and then process the information that was read.

Auditory processing problems are linked to several autistic characteristics. Autism is often described as a social–communication problem. Processing auditory information is a critical component of social communication. Problems associated with auditory processing difficulties include anxiety or confusion in social situations, inattentiveness, and poor speech comprehension.

Many people with autism have difficulty understanding and following directions. These difficulties are related to the need for explicit instruction. They do not learn indirectly as do their peers. They have to be taught new skills, rather than receiving information incidentally by observing, imitating and modelling what others do. Parents, teachers, and health professionals need to teach children and adults with autism essential skills and then teach them to generalise these skills to new events and situations.

What about problems with attention?

Children and adults with autism are unable to regulate and maintain attention to a variety of activities or events. They experience difficulties:

- orienting;
- selecting;
- shifting;
- sustaining; and
- integrating.

Orienting attention

Orienting attention refers to the ability to determine the source of information being received. For example, when a person takes in information through one or more of their senses they may have difficulty working out the original source of the information (such as where the sound they hear is coming from). Sometimes a person may not know what type of information they are attending to — it could be sound, smell or light.

Selecting attention

Selecting attention refers to the ability to work out what details to attend to. Some people with autism tend to be over-selective and attend only to small details rather than the bigger picture while other individuals tend to take in all of the information, both relevant and irrelevant, without editing, and still others fail to take in any information at all.

Shifting attention

Shifting attention refers to the ability to change the focus of attention from one activity/object to another. Situations that require constant shifts of attention present major problems for people with autism. Courchesne et al (1994) noted that impairment in shifting attention became more pronounced when there was more than one modality involved. For example, a child may be listening to the teacher talking but then have to shift attention when she writes on the blackboard. This requires having to shift attention from an auditory to a visual stimulus.

Sustaining attention

Sustaining attention refers to the ability to remain focused. Many people with autism have difficulty attending to something long enough to take in the necessary information. Motivation plays a part in a person's ability to sustain attention over a period of time. If the topic being discussed happens to be within the narrow range of interests of the person with autism, the focus of attention may be maintained for an extended period of time, even several hours.

Integrating attention

Integrating attention refers to the ability to process information from a number of different sources. Many people with autism are unable to integrate several types of information at the same time. For example, a person with Asperger's syndrome may prefer to stand next to another person during conversation, rather than face-to-face, because of difficulties integrating information from two different sources (sight and sound) at the same time.

Individuals with autism will miss much of what is happening around them because they fail to pay attention to the important and relevant details. Strategies need to be implemented to assist them to establish and maintain their focus.

What are abnormal mood swings?

Abnormalities of mood are seen in the erratic emotional responses of individuals with autism. They may show little variation in their emotions, or they may have incredible mood swings from happiness, to anger, to fear, or sadness. These emotional states may be unrelated to what is happening in their environment. A person may laugh when hurt or cry when watching a favourite cartoon. Many individuals may fail to show fear in dangerous situations and yet have an excessive, irrational fear of certain objects.

What are autistic savants?

Along with the widely recognised impairments/deficits of autism, some individuals with the disorder also display unusual but quite remarkable abilities that place them well above their neuro-typical peers in certain areas of development. These splinter skills are very rare and individuals who have them are known as autistic savants.

'Autistic savant' is a term used to describe individuals with autism who have extraordinary (or splinter) skills not usually seen in the general population. Autistic savants possess astonishing skills that provide a marked contrast to their other skills. An autistic savant, for example, may be intellectually disabled and be unable to function generally in the community without high levels of support, but also possess an incredible genius in some aspects of their development. The estimated prevalence of savant abilities in autism is 10% whereas the prevalence of savant skills in the neuro-typical population is less than 1%.

Some people with autism display remarkable abilities with a few demonstrating skills way out of the ordinary. At a young age, when other children are scribbling with crayons, some children with autism are able to draw detailed, realistic pictures in three-dimensional perspective. Some children with autism have visual memory abilities that enable them to put together complex jigsaw puzzles, without even looking at the picture. Some children begin to read very early, perhaps before they learn to speak. Some individuals with a keenly developed sense of hearing play musical instruments they have never been taught, repeat a song they may have heard only once or name any musical note they hear. Some people with autism memorise complete movies, pages of a telephone book or have highly developed calendar skills. Still others may exhibit unusual mathematical abilities that allow them to calculate square roots, prime numbers, multiplication and division of large numbers or even what day of the week it was on a particular date in time. Other savants may possess advanced memory skills, artistic abilities or talents, while still others may be able to play chess or possess perfect pitch.

These abilities, known as 'islets of brilliance' or 'savant skills' are rare.

There are many different savant skills that have been documented over the years in individuals with autism. Recent studies have shown that a probable explanation for savant abilities is damage to the left central nervous system and higher memory structures. This damage forces the right brain and lower memory structures to compensate. In particular, all forms of savant skills are associated with phenomenal memory, which leads to the recognition of patterns in everything from musical rhythms to calendar counting.

What is the impact of an autism spectrum disorder?

People with autism are affected to differing degrees in each of the above areas — and of course the impact is multiple. Each deficit in autism has links with every other impairment in the disorder. It is therefore difficult to pinpoint which deficit is the cause of a particular behaviour.

As a result of these interconnecting factors, autism can have a profound and complicated impact on even the most simple and everyday activities. Each minor change, different activity, set of instructions or social exchange can overwhelm an individual with new information. Children and adults find it difficult to make sense of their surroundings, take in information from their environment, process that information and understand what is required in response. Most children with autism experience problems with many of the basic, everyday activities such as sleeping, eating, dressing, toileting, shopping, having a haircut, visiting others, schooling and having dental or medical checkups.

When working intensively with children and adults with autism, it is essential to have at least a basic understanding of how they think and learn. Individual skills may be either above average or very delayed, and these skills are often learned out of the normal sequence.

> Peter is a 6-year-old boy who loves to 'read' books. He can read all of the words but does not understand the meaning of what he reads. He also likes to draw detailed pictures of trains and planes. However, he still has difficulty feeding himself with a knife and fork. Sometimes he can complete quite complex tasks but other times he is unable to complete the simplest activity.

People with autism have a different way of taking in information, processing that information and formulating responses. The learning style of people with autism does not conform to the way that most other people learn — they have a unique way of functioning that can be most confusing. They often behave in unexpected and inappropriate ways and do not respond to conventional means of intervention. For intervention to be successful, it is necessary to understand why people with autism think, learn and behave the way that they do.

Dr Lorna Wing (1980, p xi), a renowned London psychiatrist and pioneer in the field of autism, wrote: 'An autistic child can be helped only if a serious attempt is made to see the world from his point of view, so that the adaptive functioning of much of his peculiar behaviour can be understood in the context of his handicaps.'

Once we understand the basics of autism and how people with autism think and learn, it is possible to identify the cause of many learning problems and to provide more appropriate and effective teaching strategies in response.

Summary

A diagnosis of autism is based on disordered development in a number of key areas. These areas, known as the triad of impairments, include disordered communication, social relating and repetitive behaviours and restricted interests. In order for a diagnosis of autism to be obtained, deficits in each of these areas must be present. The deficits, however, may range from mild to severe in each of the areas and present differently in each individual.

In addition to the triad of impairments, many children and adults with autism also present with a sensory impairment. The sensory impairment may affect any of the far senses (smell, touch, hearing, sight and taste) and/or the near senses (tactile sense, vestibular processes and proprioceptive sense). People may have a fluctuating response to sensory stimuli and a particular smell, sound, taste, feel or light may elicit a heightened response (hyper or over-sensitive response) or a dampened response (hypo or under-sensitive response).

In addition, most people also have cognitive deficits that interfere with their ability to cope and function independently. Cognitive deficits include limited ability to understand abstract concepts, weak central coherence, executive function deficits and theory of mind deficits.

Because of the many difficulties associated with autism, people who have the disorder experience problems with even the most simple everyday tasks and activities.

The most effective programs for people with autism are those that recognise and acknowledge the individual learning styles, interests and abilities these children and adults have and use their particular strengths to teach functional skills.

CHAPTER

4

Impairments in Communication

Communication is a range of purposeful behaviour that is used with intent within the structure of social exchanges, to transmit information, observations, or internal states, or to bring about changes in the immediate environment.

Stokes 1977

Communication is primarily the sending and receiving of a message and sharing ideas, thoughts and feelings with others. It is a two-way process that requires both expressive and receptive communication skills. Communication requires a person not only to speak and express their ideas and needs to others, but also to understand what other people are saying — to comprehend speech and other forms of communication such as gesture, body language and environmental cues.

According to Quill (2000, p 14), 'communication is a reciprocal, dynamic process. It is the instrumental force propelling social knowledge, relationships, and a sense of self. An effective communicator has an inherent motivation to interact, something to express, and a means of communication.' This is illustrated in Figure 4.1.

Hodgdon (1995, p 7) put it this way: 'Effective communication does not just happen. It takes considerable effort from both the sender and the receiver of information to ensure that communication attempts accomplish their intent.'

The process of sending the message is referred to as 'expressive' communication. The process of interpreting or understanding the message is 'receptive' communication. Whenever there is a problem with either the expression or reception of a message, a communication breakdown is said to occur.

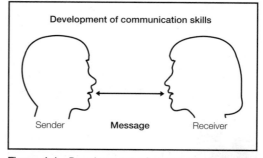

Figure 4.1 *Development of communication skills*

Appropriate communication is not just what is said, but how language is used and responded to in everyday functioning. Language is based on a series of rules and is symbolic. Communication is a social process that is constantly changing and evolving. Communication can be verbal or non-verbal, as long as some intent, evidenced by anticipation of outcome, is inferred. Not all vocalisation or speech would qualify as intentional communicative behaviour. Some young children with autism may make repetitive squealing sounds that are self-stimulating for them rather than actual attempts to communicate. Communication occurs in many different ways and may involve the use of behaviour, actions, sounds and/or words. For speech to be considered communication, it should take place within a social context.

When social–communicative interactions are observed among individuals with autism, however, they appear disordered. Deficits observed among children with autism include limited imitation; failure to engage in joint sharing of attention; limited use of non-verbal behaviours such as pointing, gestures and facial expression; impaired ability to maintain reciprocal interaction; and lack of pretend play. According to the American Psychiatric Association in the DSM-IV (1994), the diagnostic criteria for autism include 'marked impairments in the ability to initiate or sustain a conversation with others' and 'stereotyped and repetitive use of language and idiosyncratic language'.

Because social relations are difficult for children and adults with autism, it is not surprising that their effective communication is significantly impaired. Social interaction and communication are closely related and interdependent and should be considered together when developing and implementing specific programs. Quill (2000, p 14) says 'Children with autism struggle to understand the intents, internal states, and meaning behind others' social, communicative, and affective behaviours; therefore, their ability to participate in social communicative interactions is profoundly impaired.'

There is widespread support for intensive intervention during early childhood. This is a period when so much of a child's learning takes place. The most intensive period of speech and language development occurs during the first few years of life, when the brain is developing and maturing. These skills develop best in a stimulating environment, full of different sounds, sights and constant exposure to the speech and language of many other people. The basis for speech development lies in the infant's desire to communicate and interact with the world. Children with significant communication disorders may be discouraged from communicating because of the great effort required. Sometimes parents, peers and teachers even anticipate their needs. There is little or no motivation for children to develop their communication and social skills if their needs are being constantly anticipated and met by parents and teachers. This is especially true for young children whose needs are usually simple and easily anticipated by familiar adults. These children do not learn that communication and social interaction will usually achieve things for them, thus encouraging them to try to interact with others.

What are the early signs of communication?

Early signs of communication occur in the first few days of life when an infant discovers that crying brings food, comfort or companionship. Infants learn to recognise the sound of their mother's voice and quieten to the sound of their mother singing or talking softly. By 3 months of age, babies begin to recognise different speech sounds and by 6 months most children recognise the basic sounds of their native language. As the speech mechanism and voice develop, infants begin to make controlled sounds. This usually begins with repetitive 'cooing' and develops into babbling and then repetitive syllables such as 'ba, ba, ba' or 'da, da, da'. Eventually, babbling turns into jargon with the tone and cadence of speech but without meaning. By about 12 months of age, children are saying a few words even though they do not understand the meaning. Words are generally repeated because they create a positive reaction from the people around them.

After 12 months of age, speech develops quickly. Children increase their vocabulary and, by age 2, begin to string words together to make simple sentences such as 'go play', 'more juice' or 'music on'. Children realise that words symbolise or represent different objects and actions.

By age 3, children engage in representational or pretend play, their vocabulary increases and they begin to master the rules of language. These rules include the rules of phonology (speech sounds), morphology (word formation), semantics (word and sentence meaning), prosody (intonation and rhythm of speech) and pragmatics (effective use of language).

The early communicative skills of children with autism are characterised by significant impairments in verbal and motor imitation, non-verbal joint attention skills and social turn-taking skills.

What are the main categories of communication disorders?

The autism spectrum is broad and accommodates children and adults with a wide range of related problems. It is a difficult disorder to diagnose, especially when so many of the associated behaviours are not clearly defined and paediatricians are reluctant to label individuals. The communication deficits in autism are pronounced but vary along a continuum in terms of severity. Not only is autism difficult to diagnose but it is also a disorder in which the causes of the problems are not always obvious or clear-cut.

Communication skills disorders are grouped into two major types. The first type is typical language-based learning disorders that are due to problems in spoken/written language and include expressive, receptive, processing and articulation language disorders. Most routine speech and language evaluations examine these areas.

The second type is autism spectrum disorders and includes non-verbal communication problems — in particular, problems with socialisation, empathy, theory of mind, pragmatics of language and representational play. They may occur with and without additional verbal speech problems.

Further, autism spectrum disorders may be broken down into two groupings. First is the pervasive developmental disorders (PDD) as defined in DSM-IV. Examples of how communication is affected in PDD include:

- Autistic disorder — Severely disordered verbal and non-verbal language; unusual behaviours.
- Asperger's syndrome — Relatively good verbal language; with milder non-verbal language problems; restricted range of interests and relatedness.
- PDD-NOS — Non-verbal language problems not meeting strict criteria for other PDDs.

The second grouping includes other labels that are commonly used by professionals to describe and diagnose children and adults with autistic features. These labels are not listed in the DSM-IV diagnostic manual. The most commonly used labels include:

- semantic pragmatic disorder;
- non-verbal learning disabilities;
- high functioning autism;
- hyperlexia; and
- aspects of ADHD.

Semantic pragmatic disorder

The semantics of language refers to an individual's ability to understand the meaning of words, phrases and sentences and to use these words and phrases appropriately in speech. The pragmatics of language refers to an individual's ability to know what to say in different social contexts.

Semantic pragmatic disorder is, therefore, a language difficulty that affects the way a person acquires and uses language. People with semantic pragmatic disorder present with the following difficulties:

■ understanding the language of others and using language to express themselves, for example, using clear, well-formed sentences;
■ dealing with new situations or new people;
■ developing vocabulary;
■ interpreting the thoughts and feelings of others;
■ interacting appropriately with others; for example, taking turns in conversation, using appropriate body language, maintaining eye contact or keeping to a topic of conversation; and
■ comprehending written material; for example, reading abilities may be exceptional for the person's age however they will present with difficulties understanding what they are reading.

Children with semantic pragmatic disorder may also tend to memorise language that they hear around them. Their speech usually sounds repetitive or inappropriate in conversation. They may also have obsessive interests or topics of conversation and may become distressed by unfamiliar situations or people. Semantic pragmatic disorder is considered to be on the autism spectrum by some professionals, while others consider it purely as a stand-alone language disorder.

Non-verbal learning disabilities

Individuals experience difficulties integrating information in the following areas:
■ non-verbal communication;
■ spatial perception development; and
■ motor coordination development.

High functioning autism

High functioning autism is considered by some practitioners to be synonymous with Asperger's syndrome while others recognise it as a milder form of autism, without developmental delays.

Hyperlexia

Hyperlexia has been described as a preoccupation with letters and words at an early age, and exceptional word-recognition skills with delayed comprehension of meaning (Healy 1982).

Aspects of ADHD

Impulse and control difficulties in ADHD may lead to difficulties with empathy.

What causes communication problems in autism?

Although the cause of speech and language problems in autism is unknown, it is believed that the difficulties arise from a variety of conditions that may occur either before or after birth. These conditions interfere with the individual's ability to interpret and interact with the world.

Children and adults with autism experience difficulties with the form, content, and use of language. They also have difficulty understanding and using all forms of communication including speech, sign language, body language, tone of voice, gestures and vocalisations.

Kanner (1943, p 242), who originally described the fundamental deficit in autism as 'children's inability to relate themselves in the ordinary way to people and situations', proposed that their communication difficulties were based primarily in the area of social communication. Certainly, the communication difficulties associated with autism are closely linked to impairments in social relating. Aarons & Gittens (1992) claim that children tend to acquire language because of an innate desire to communicate, initially seen in their interactions with parents. They claim that if the motivation to communicate is impaired, as it is in children with autism, then this would be a contributing factor to their delays in acquiring language.

Some researchers tie the communication problems of people with autism to an impaired ability to think about thoughts or imagine another individual's state of mind (Baron-Cohen 1995; Wing 1996). In addition to this, there is an impaired ability to symbolise, both in communication and in play. In other words, people with autism tend to be very literal and concrete, both in their thoughts and actions, and have difficulty communicating feelings and emotions or using their imagination in pretend play.

The difficulties associated with autism do not relate to one particular aspect of communication but affect both expressive and receptive language skills. The majority of people diagnosed with autism have both receptive and expressive deficits in non-verbal communication such as eye contact, imitation, understanding and use of facial expressions and gestures such as pointing. They also have difficulty using verbal communication to relate to others and may have problems with word and sentence meaning, intonation and rhythm. The problems vary, depending on the intellectual and social development of the individual.

Some people with autism are unable to communicate verbally while others may have extensive vocabularies and talk at length about topics of interest. Because their communication development is uneven, most children and adults with autism communicate in ways that are not typical of normal development. Many children's language is echolalic (repetition of something previously heard) to begin with. Other children say things that have no functional content (such as repeatedly saying 'bananas in pyjamas' or 'Oh! What a feeling, Toyota'). Some individuals may use sophisticated language forms but be unable to comprehend relatively simple concepts. For example, someone may be able to discuss in great technical detail how a computer works but be unable to answer a simple question such as what he would like for dinner or whether he would like to invite a friend to the movies.

> Su-lien likes to sit at the station and read train timetables. She can tell you when each train is expected to arrive and depart from Central Station. She lives at home with her mother, however, and is unable to walk down to the corner shop to buy her the bread and milk because she would need to cross the road and watch out for oncoming traffic. She does not know how to request the items she wants to buy and has no idea how to pay for them.

One of the social–communicative deficits of autism is evident in children's inability and lack of motivation to share a focus with another person. They may not understand what is being said to them, or they feel threatened by the presence of other people, and therefore may respond inappropriately or not at all. They have difficulty engaging in joint attention — they find it difficult to do something with another person, to share information about something of interest, or to share their feelings. Tager-Flusberg (1996, p 169) notes that difficulties with joint attention and the lack of understanding of the social intentions of others, have a profound impact on communication skills as the 'essential motivation to communicate lies in the desire to share intentions, thoughts and emotions with others'.

What are the most important functions of communication?

When working with children and adults with autism, it is important to keep in mind the primary functions or purposes of communication. These primary functions are:

- to *regulate behaviour* (communication is used to request, protest or satisfy immediate physical needs);
- to *promote social interaction* (communication is used to initiate, respond to, maintain or terminate social interactions); and

- to *promote joint attention* (communication is used to direct another's attention to an object, event or topic, to comment or to give information to others).

In most children, these three functions are developed by approximately 12 months of age. Children with autism, however, use language to communicate for a narrow or restricted purpose or function. They tend to communicate to request things or to indicate refusal.

Children and adults with autism may need to be shown the importance and relevance of social communication for it to become meaningful. Parents and teachers should use motivating activities or objects if they wish to encourage individuals to develop a desire and intention to communicate with others.

> Joseph loves water and will happily spend hours splashing around in puddles or playing in the dog's water bowl. In order to motivate Joseph to request, to share toys and to take turns, his mother set up structured play sessions while he was in the bath and then encouraged him to play at the water trough with his sister sharing and taking turns with the toys.

> Cameron is obsessed with movies and videos, especially action movies. He loves to talk about his favourite scenes and movie actors. Cameron finds it difficult to talk with his class-mates at school but when his teacher introduces movies as a topic of conversation, he is able to communicate with his peers and participate in the conversation quite comfortably.

There are a number of important elements individuals with autism need to learn in order to communicate more successfully. These elements include:

- an understanding of cause and effect;
- a desire to communicate;
- someone to communicate with;
- something to communicate about; and
- a means to communicate.

An understanding of cause and effect

It has been suggested that the desire to communicate is a type of cause and effect relationship. The implication is that a child must understand that another person can make something happen and that the child also has the power to affect another person's actions through some form, such as communication. Children with autism have difficulty understanding cause and effect relationships and so this skill is often one that has to be specifically taught to young children. With very young children, it is important to begin with real objects that may be presented during play situations. Children initially learn that they can affect what an object does by manipulating it (pop-up toys, push-button toys, and musical toys). Once this is established, they learn that they can also affect different situations and people by using communication (by requesting, questioning and refusing), in its many forms, to manipulate situations.

A desire to communicate

Several strategies may be used to provide the support and intent needed to develop a desire to communicate in an autistic child. For example, hiding objects, then labelling them as they are discovered, withholding turns or objects 'by accident', placing desired objects out of reach, making packaging difficult to open and introducing games or activities requiring active participation and particular responses.

Someone to communicate with

It is through play that most children begin to really develop the basics of social interaction and the skills they require to communicate with others. There are many early childhood texts that discuss theories of play development in young children and the importance of play in promoting development and teaching skills. Parten, as early as 1932, formulated a series of stages that children normally pass through as their play skills develop. Children and adults with autism, however, do not follow normal patterns of development. Most children with autism do not naturally gravitate to other children in order to engage in social play. They are more interested in certain objects than in other people. There is little interest in playing and interacting socially and in developing friendships or shared interests. It therefore becomes important to teach social play skills to children with autism in order to promote their awareness of, and interest in, other people. Play techniques such as modelling, prompting, imitating, use of visual supports and reinforcement are effective methods to teach essential early communication and social skills.

> Kylie's teacher at preschool showed her how to share toys with another child by modelling a turn-taking activity and also prompting both children to wait for their turn. The teacher used simple hand gestures such as 'stop' and 'give me' to encourage the children to wait. Kylie learned to wait for her turn and to share the toys because the teacher showed her what to do.

> Ricky's mum started to imitate his actions when he engaged in repetitive play actions such as spinning wheels or lining up blocks. Ricky thought it was funny and laughed. He wanted the fun to continue so he started to imitate his mum's actions and before long they were taking turns in play. Ricky's mum was able to expand the play so that soon they were building block towers and knocking them down. Ricky's mum was therefore able to engage him in social play activities by showing him that it was fun to play with someone else.

Something to communicate about

In young children with autism, most early attempts to communicate, both verbally and non-verbally, revolve around their basic needs or restricted interests. Communication is therefore limited and needs-based. It is essential to see communication as part of a broader program focusing on a range of skills, interests and behaviours. Communication enables the child with autism to be less withdrawn and isolated. An interest in social play and a range of play skills forms a basis for communication and social interaction. It is through play that young children develop the desire to communicate. They also have things to communicate about and the support to develop their communication skills confidently and independently.

A means to communicate

Individuals may communicate in a number of ways. Some individuals may choose to use different communication forms in different situations. For example, a child may use a gesture, such as pointing to the cupboard to indicate that he wants a biscuit. However, the same child may show a photograph of the car to indicate that he wants to go out or vocalise by screaming when frustrated.

What means of communication are available?

The following means of communication may be used by autistic children:

■ Motoric — includes direct physical manipulation of a person or object. For example, taking a parent's hand and dragging them over to the cupboard to indicate 'want biscuit'.

- Gestural — includes pointing, looking or showing a desired item. For example, bringing an empty cup to a parent to request a drink.
- Vocalisation — includes crying, sounds or word approximations to communicate. For example a child may cry to indicate hunger or a child or adult may stand close to another person and vocalise 'dk-dk-dk' to indicate drink.
- Sign language — includes using a conventional sign language system such as Makaton, Signed English or Auslan as an alternative method of communication. Sometimes individuals will develop their own gestures or 'signs' to communicate basic needs.
- Real objects — uses real objects to indicate what is wanted. For example, handing the cover of a favourite video to another person to indicate 'want video'.
- Photographs/remnants — uses colour or black-and-white photographs of favoured objects or the remnants of commercial packaging as a means of communication. For example pointing to the remnant of the milk carton to indicate 'want milk' or handing another person a photograph of the local park to indicate 'let's go park'.
- Line drawings — uses two-dimensional drawings that represent objects, actions or feelings, to request. For example, showing a picture of an angry face to indicate 'not happy'.
- Written words — uses written or printed words to communicate. May include use of technical, computerised communication aids.

What is expressive communication?

Expressive communication is the ability to use speech or other forms of communication to say something. In order for us to communicate effectively, we need skills in both verbal and non-verbal areas of language.

Verbal communication skills include:

- the ability to use and understand words, phrases and sentences, including abstract concepts and idioms (semantic language);
- the ability to understand spoken words and ideas and also to express ideas with spoken words;
- the ability to process and derive meaning from sounds and words, including the ability to distinguish between similar words and to pick out the main voice from the background noises — 'what we do with what we hear' (auditory processing of language); and
- the ability to speak each word clearly (articulation of language).

Non-verbal communication skills include:

- the desire to initiate shared social interaction and two-way communication (this is an aspect of theory of mind);
- the ability to communicate in a social setting, such as knowing what to say, where and when to say it and the give and take nature of conversation (this is an example of the pragmatics of language);
- the ability to know what is, and what is not, important;
- symbolic play skills; and
- the ability to read the non-verbal transmission of information via facial expression, body language, and tone and prosody of voice.

All people with autism are impaired in their ability to express themselves verbally and non-verbally. Individual levels of expressive communication may range from mild to severe along a continuum of impairment.

According to Professor Michael Rutter (1984, p 194):

... abnormalities of language loom large in any description of the phenomena that characterize the syndrome of autism. Yet there continues to be widespread misunderstanding of what these abnormalities comprise. Often there is a focus on the presence of language delay, but delay occurs in a host of different disorders. Autistic children are indeed usually slow to gain skills in the understanding and production of spoken language, but so are children with a variety of other handicaps. It is not the limitations of language capacity that are pathognomonic to autism but rather the particular patterns of deviance.

Professor Rutter concluded that the speech and language development of children with autism had particular characteristics that placed them apart from other communication disorders. These differences centre around oddities and abnormalities associated with social development. This supports the current view that the communication impairment in autism is a social–communicative problem. Because the intrinsic impairment in autism is in reciprocal social interaction, it is the *communicative* aspect of speech and language that is very much the primary area of investigation and remediation.

Table 4.1 outlines the verbal and non-verbal impairments in expressive communication that are a major factor in how well individuals with autism are able to communicate and interact socially. The severity of the communication impairment, impacts on the individual's ability to engage in reciprocal social interactions.

Table 4.1   *Outline of the different degrees of expressive communication impairment in people with autism. Adapted from the work of Louise Ulliana, Autism Spectrum Australia (Aspect)*

Degree of impairment	Verbal	Non-verbal
Profound	Those people at the severe end of the continuum are non-verbal and use mininal communication in any context apart from challenging behaviour such as screaming. Rarely initiate or use any type of communication in any situation (except challenging behaviour). Vocal sounds are not recognisable as words & tend to be self-stimulatory.	People at the severe end of the continuum may not use gestures to communicate with others, may actively avoid eye contact and have a very flat affect with little facial expression.
Moderate	Verbal skills are limited but people may initiate communiction occasionally. They use some learnt phrases and single words and tend to use non-verbal ways to communicate. Echolalia is common.	Will tend to use some gestures or take person to what is wanted or get things independently. Starting to point and may give eye contact fleetingly.
Mild	Talkative, have wide vocabulary and use grammatically correct sentences. Subtle impairments are evident like not being able to adjust volume of voice or style of language according to the situation (the way you speak to a policeman versus your family) Conversations are one-sided.	At the mild end of the continuum, a person may stare at others without looking away or may stand too close and invade personal body space.

How do people with autism learn language?

Individuals with autism have a particular learning style that forces them to take in and store information in whole chunks. They do not break down information into smaller manageable units that may be analysed and processed. For this reason, most individuals have better expressive communication than receptive communication skills because they rote-learn chunks of information without actually understanding the meaning. They take in the information in unanalysed chunks and then retrieve the complete chunks without editing the information for relevance or meaning. For example, a person may memorise the steps involved in making a cup of tea. If the sequence is changed to make a cup of hot chocolate or coffee, the person may not be able to comprehend the changes. They may be unable to complete the task unless they are taught to incorporate the changes into their learned sequence.

A child may learn the dialogue of a favourite video and repeat the words and actions without understanding the meaning of what is being said. The same child may repeat back what is said to him when asked 'do you want a drink?' rather than answer the question. This is an example of echoed speech or echolalia.

What is echolalia?

Children and adults with autism learn to repeat (or echo) whole phrases or sentences yet they are typically unable to understand the separate components of those sentences. Echolalia (the repetition or echoing of words said by others) is common in autism.

Echolalia should be seen as a language acquisition strategy. Research suggests that echolalia is used to assist communication — to make sense of what others say and to develop functional language skills. It is important to treat echolalia as a sign of emerging linguistic awareness, not as an undesirable behaviour. There is a difference between echolalia and obsessionaland perseverative language. According to Roberts (1988), children with autism use echolalia as:

- a coping strategy;
- a means of assisting comprehension;
- a means of initiating or maintaining social contact;
- a means of requesting, rejecting, protesting, and commenting;
- a strategy to provide processing time and rehearsal; and
- a language acquisition strategy resulting in the eventual development of a more flexible system of rules.

Approximately 75% of verbal children with autism go through a period of marked echolalia. Some children never move on from that and remain echolalic through adulthood. Echolalia assists a person to make sense of what that person hears and to express verbally. Echolalia is used to request, comment, affirm something or as a turn-taking strategy.

Echolalia may be immediate, delayed or mitigated. Immediate echolalia occurs when the individual repeats the question, 'do you want a drink?' instead of answering the question with a 'yes' or 'no'. In delayed echolalia the individual may say 'do you want a drink?' whenever he or she is really asking for a drink. An individual who sometimes echoes words, phrases or sentences is displaying mitigated echolalia. Delayed echolalia and rote memory are closely related. Echolalia may be due to the chunk or gestalt learning style of autism. As mentioned above, children with autism learn spoken language in unanalysed chunks using rote memory. They then echo these chunks when language is required, often without understanding the meaning of what they are repeating. Mitigated echolalia seems to be a transitional stage as children move from predominantly echolalic speech to predominantly spontaneous speech.

Echolalia may increase during unstructured, unpredictable or transitional periods or when tasks or situations are unfamiliar, difficult or challenging. Echolalia also increases during activities or situations that cause anxiety, fear, distress or excitement or when the language used by the communication partner is too complex.

Should people with autism be taught to sign?

Signing is an alternative form of communication that is often recommended for non-verbal children and adults, or for individuals with specific language impairments. It is frequently recommended to augment spoken language, or as an alternative to speech.

Some children and adults with autism may never develop functional language and may therefore need to rely on alternative communication methods. These methods can help them to understand what is happening around them and to communicate their needs and desires to others. Signing may be introduced with some children to augment speech and then faded (stopped) as the children begin to use speech to communicate their needs. Natural gesture and visual supports are usually a more successful and less demanding way of augmenting speech with children with autism. These systems form the basis of an alternative communication system if functional speech does not develop.

There are a number of arguments for and against introducing manual signing for people with autism. Signing does provide the individual with an alternative to verbal communication. This eliminates frustration and provides a means of expressing basic wants and needs. The disadvantage of this argument is that the use of signing, as an alternative to speech, is very limited as few people recognise and understand manual signs.

Signing is a visually based system of communication that caters to a strength of individuals with autism. It is widely documented and accepted that people with autism have relative strengths in processing visual information rather than auditory information. Signing is one method of presenting information visually. Signs, though visual, are transient and non-permanent. The transient nature of signs does not allow time for individuals to take in the information, process it and then formulate a response before the sign has disappeared. Most people with autism have processing difficulties and require additional time to understand information. Visual systems that are non-transient and permanent, allowing additional processing time, are more effective for people with autism.

Although manual signs are considered a visual communication mode, the gestures and hand movements used in signing are abstract, arbitrary symbols. Most individuals with autism have comprehension difficulties and prefer concrete, easily recognised images (such as real objects and photographs) to assist them in any communicative exchanges. Unlike manual signing, visual systems that rely on photographs, pictures and written words, provide symbols that are universally understood and easily recognised by anyone using them. This enables people with autism to communicate efficiently and effectively with different people and in different situations.

Signing is not appropriate for those individuals with autism who engage in repetitive, self-stimulatory motor movements (such as handflapping). These repetitive motor movements interfere with the signing process and make it difficult for signs to be correctly interpreted. A person may inadvertently be reinforced for repetitive motor movements that are misinterpreted as a poorly executed sign. Manual signing requires the user to have reasonable imitating skills (Carr & Dores 1981; Carr, Pridal & Dores 1984) and no fine motor coordination difficulties (Seal & Bonvillian 1997). Studies by Hughes (1996), Seal & Bonvillian (1997) have shown that problems associated with imitation and fine motor deficits, often seen in individuals with autism, make it difficult for them to use manual signing as an augmentation or alternative communication system.

A major problem associated with the use of manual signs as a means of communication, is the fact that signs are not widely used or understood in the general community. Manual signs, therefore, are not empowering or effective for people with autism.

Manual signs are not universally recognised, even by people who sign, because there is no one system of manual signs used by everyone. Many people with autism do not spontaneously sign, but only sign when prompted. They will memorise certain signs, but do not use signs to communicate without a physical or verbal prompt. Manual signing is not readily used or understood outside of the hearing impaired community, and is therefore not a viable or functional alternative to speech for children and adults with autism. In effect, individuals who have a non-transient, gestalt, concrete, learning style are trying to learn a transient, analytical, abstract system of communication.

While autism is recognised as a disorder of communication and social relating, parents tend to place a lot of emphasis on teaching children to talk. Many parents feel that once their child is able to speak, many of the associated problems of autism will disappear or will be easily managed. In actual fact, the comprehension deficits of autism, the inability of children and adults to process information or understand language, are as much, if not more, of a problem for most individuals with autism.

What is receptive communication?

Receptive communication or comprehension is the process of interpreting or understanding a message that is sent by someone else.

For most people with autism, their receptive skills are more impaired than their expressive skills. Many parents and teachers overestimate the comprehension skills of people with autism because they assume that their comprehension level is about the same as their expressive skills. Schuler, Prizant and Wetherby (1997) stated that it is easy to overestimate how much speech children with autism understand because of their use of situational cues and their ability to memorise daily routines.

Table 4.2 outlines the impairments in receptive communication that are a major factor in how well individuals with autism are able to understand what is happening and how well they read their environment. The severity of the comprehension impairment impacts on the person's ability to function independently both at home and in the general community.

Difficulties with comprehension in social situations can lead to a number of problems for children and adults with autism. Individuals will frequently display:

■ anxiety because they do not read the current situation and become stressed that they will 'do the wrong thing';

Table 4.2 *The different degrees of receptive communication in people with autism. Adapted from the work of Louise Ulliana, Autism Spectrum Australia (Aspect)*

Degree of impairment	Impairment
Profound	People with autism often fail to alert to the human voice.
	May not respond consistently to own name being called.
	Often the speaker needs to repeat the most basic one and two word phrases several times and use physical assistance and gestures to support.
	They may not acknowledge another person's voice or respond to simple requests without physical and gestural prompts.
Moderate	Individuals may respond to simple instructions and statements that are part of the routine. ('Time for breakfast', 'Put on your sun screen'. 'Let's mow'). May respond to 'Want' questions.
	Respond better when familiar people speak rather than unfamiliar people.
Mild	Have concrete and literal understanding of language. Difficulty understanding:
	■ words that have more than one meaning
	■ sayings like 'line up', 'shake a leg' & 'he's over the hill'
	■ abstract (non-concrete) concepts
	■ relevant parts of a message — tend to get stuck on details rather than the major point — underlying or implied meanings.
	Many people with mild receptive language difficulties appear to have good understanding of language and are able to understand as long as most concepts are concrete rather than abstract.

- an insistence on sameness and ritualistic behaviour because any changes mean that any previously learned strategies will no longer be effective;
- inattention since it becomes difficult to remain focused on something that is not understood;
- rude and obnoxious behaviour because they may not understand the rules of conversation or pick up any of the non-verbal cues from the current social situation;
- preference for certain objects than for people because objects are much more predictable; and
- a sense of isolation and withdrawal from the situation because of poor relating and conversational skills.

What strategies work to develop social–communication skills in autism?

Many children with autism have specialist intervention from a speech pathologist to evaluate their communication skills and develop and implement ongoing speech and language therapy. The emphasis in all programs should be to develop functional communication skills; that is, skills that are useful and necessary in everyday life.

For some individuals, the goal may be functional speech while for others it may be more realistic to achieve communication through gestures or the use of visual supports.

The following suggestions may help to move children and adults with autism along the continuum of language development:

- Use modelling, contingency management, visual strategies and feedback to teach communication skills when appropriate during the day. For example, in a supported work environment, it may be possible to pair a disabled adult with a non-disabled peer who can model appropriate social, communication and work behaviours; to have certain leisure activities that are contingent on the person appropriately requesting the activity either verbally or non-verbally; to provide visual supports in the form of choice boards, sequence cards and timetables in the work environment; and also to encourage staff members to respond positively to any client's attempts to communicate.
- Shape appropriate behaviour rather than use extensive prompting techniques. For example, break down some tasks and activities into smaller steps and use visual sequence cards to show individuals how to accomplish each step independently. Use this method to teach children and adults how to initiate and respond to interactions from their peers and also skills that they will need to be able to participate in general group activities.

> When Andrew first arrived at work he would have liked to join his work colleagues for a cup of coffee and chat before starting work. He felt uncomfortable because he had never been taught how to make his own coffee and had no idea how to approach his peers and initiate a conversation. He was quite comfortable in a one-to-one situation but did not know how to participate as a member of a group. Andrew's supervisor showed him how to make coffee using a visual sequence and his co-workers encouraged Andrew to join in by reinforcing his attempts to participate.

- Structure opportunities to learn, practise and master critical social and communicative skills throughout the day. For example, it may be possible to introduce structured sharing and turn-taking activities in the playground at school, to introduce small group projects in the classroom where children have to work together, and to introduce opportunities in the classroom for individuals to discuss favourite topics in small groups in a relaxed atmosphere.
- Select language sequences that correspond to the person's developmental level and encourage generalisation to other situations and settings. It is important to use language that the

individual can understand and imitate and that is age and developmentally appropriate. Language may be either verbal or non-verbal but must be functional to encourage its use in a variety of situations and settings. For example, a preschool child should be taught how to request help, how to greet others, how to share and take turns in play and how to imitate actions, sounds and words. These skills should be encouraged at home, at preschool and in the general community and the child provided with opportunities to practise these skills.

The following text discusses some points to consider when developing communication skills in children and adults.

■ The relevance of the other person (partner) in the communication process

Children and adults should learn appropriate ways to interact with another person, to accept approaches from another person and to enjoy the communicative process. Communication partners may also need to be trained to simplify their language, initiate communication and interaction, and respond to all attempts by the person with autism to communicate.

■ Teach the use of more appropriate ways to communicate

People with autism need to be understood if their attempts to express themselves are to be successful. Alternative, socially acceptable, ways of communicating messages may need to be taught. For verbal children, modelling of appropriate language is one method of teaching communication. For all children, whether verbal or non-verbal, training in alternative forms of communication such as using visual systems will assist communication development.

■ Create a desire to communicate

Try not to anticipate every need or respond too quickly to requests as this enables children and adults to avoid communicating.

■ Communication development through play

Play sessions may be used to teach communication skills in a fun, non-threatening situation that is highly motivating for young children.

■ Functional language

Emphasis should be placed upon developing language that will be useful to children and adults in everyday life. Initially this may include words, pictures or signs such as 'help', 'more', 'bye', 'go', 'up', as well as food and drink words. All of these should be taught in the situation in which they are most likely to occur. Visual supports in the form of objects, remnants of food packaging or photographs may be introduced to assist in making choices and indicating simple needs and wants.

■ How to assist understanding

Simplify language when communicating with children and adults with autism. Leave out words that are not necessary for the meaning, such as 'the', 'and', 'a' and descriptive words like adverbs and adjectives. In addition, to simplifying language, present only one idea at a time and also incorporate other cues such as gestures, modelling, pictures and signs. Use even more cues to assist during unfamiliar situations or when introducing abstract ideas.

■ Teach in functional situations

Teach communication skills in the situations in which they will be used. If teaching the word or picture for 'water', success is more likely if you wait for the appropriate time and place (such as bath-time, swimming in the pool, drinking water) and introduce the word then.

■ Set up situations to practise skills

This may include holding back a desired object until children and adults attempt to communicate, placing objects out of reach or behind locked doors, and pretending not to understand or anticipate what the person wants. In order to avoid frustration, you may need to initially prompt or shape the required response to ensure the person understands what is expected.

■ Use total communication

When implementing any system, it is important to aim for total communication, pairing speech with the pictures/signs used in the system, aiming for communicative competency above everything. It is also important to use natural gestures such as pointing and indicating, facial expression, body language, and the volume and intonation of the voice, as well as contextual/environmental cues/information, to assist understanding.

■ Manage obsessional and perseverative language

Try not to let perseverative and obsessional language dominate all interactions. Teach rules about when, and with whom, it is appropriate to talk about favourite topics. Use this interest to develop conversational rules (waiting, listening, stopping, taking turns etc). Remember that the opportunity to talk about favourite topics may be used as a reward. Sometimes talking about obsessive topics is a way of reducing anxiety or of engaging in a conversation without knowing normal conversational rules.

■ Use visual strategies

Not all people with autism will acquire the verbal skills to enable them to achieve even basic needs using words alone. Visual supports may make it easier for them to communicate their needs and wants. Visual systems support the development of more complex verbal skills and understanding of language.

What are visual supports?

Visual supports provide a means of communication for children and adults who have difficulty using and processing verbal information. They consist of real objects, remnants of packaging, photographs, computer graphics programs (line drawings) or written words. Figure 4.2 is an example of a visual support that incorporates line drawings and written words to enable a child with autism to let his parent or teacher know what activity he would like to choose.

The long-term goal for all children and adults with autism is to provide them with an effective and efficient communication system that will enable them to successfully participate in their life activities. Visual supports are designed to assist individuals accomplish their goals.

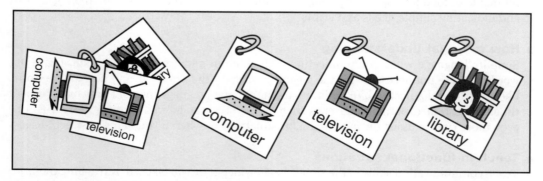

Figure 4.2 *Examples of visual symbols incorporating the written words*

Visual supports should be considered as a part of a communicative repertoire but should not necessarily be seen as an alternative to spoken language, especially not for children and young adults. Visual systems are used to augment language and to help with the understanding of rules and routines. The aim is to encourage the development and use of speech as the primary form of communication, but also to set the foundation for an alternative method that is reliable and user friendly for those individuals who may not develop functional language. Evidence suggests that the use of visual supports actually enhances the development of speech in people with autism.

There are numerous visually based methods to assist communication in people with autism. Visual supports may be used to accompany and augment spoken language to assist in the understanding of speech. They can also be used to help preverbal children to express their needs by requesting what they want. Visual strategies may be used to enhance communication, augment language, facilitate learning, support behaviour and promote independence for people with autism.

Special care should be taken to establish what forms of communication each person understands and responds to most effectively. Messages may be conveyed through tone of voice, gestures, body language, speech, pictures and words. Introducing a visual communication system that is appropriate and comfortable for a particular person helps to establish a relationship of mutual respect and enables the person with autism to feel valued.

Visual supports may be used to convey information because children and adults with autism typically perceive and interpret visual information more effectively than auditory information. Visual information is both concrete and non-transient (that is, visual information remains available over a period of time allowing time for the information to be processed). Most people with autism have superior visual spatial skills relative to their other skills and so tend to respond more effectively when visual supports are included (Hodgdon 1995).

Communication techniques

Experienced practitioners working directly with children and adults with autism have used a number of communication techniques successfully over the years to maximise the benefits from using visual strategies. These techniques include the following recommendations.

Be positive

Praise often and honestly and be specific when praising. 'Good looking' is better than 'Good boy'.

Show as well as tell

Remember that visual skills are often superior to auditory skills. It is therefore important to maximise visual information. Many people with autism 'think in pictures' rather than in words and have highly developed visual skills relative to their auditory processing abilities. By modelling what a person should do, it ensures that the person is receiving a very clear message that is easily understood.

Teach listening skills

When giving a direction, ensure that the person is attending and that they have understood the message. Most children and adults do not follow directions because they do not understand the meaning of what is said. Obtain their attention first — this may involve getting down to their eye level, with a child, and perhaps touching them. It is important to be consistent and expect them to respond when the message is simple and understood. Initially it may be necessary to support a request with some form of visual augmentation and assist people to carry out the directions once they have been understood.

Know what you want people to do

Be very clear about what people should do and why. Be sure that any request is reasonable and relevant and within the person's capabilities.

Provide adequate information to forewarn of changes

Tell people in advance what is going to happen next. This may be done verbally (if appropriate) or visually. Inform them of any changes, involve them in plans and explain what behaviour is expected. Use simple language, pictures and gestures, daily schedule boards, visual timetables, sequences routines and picture wallets to provide information.

Use language that is simple, clear and concise

Giving too much verbal information or too many directions may lead to frustration and confusion. Many children and adults with autism comprehend only a limited amount of verbal information. Use a calm clear voice. Loud, excited voices are difficult for people with autism to listen to. Do not engage in baby talk or use an unnaturally high-pitched voice with young children. Remember that language does not always need to be presented verbally. Many requests can also be made non-verbally. For example, pointing or gesturing or showing a photograph of what a person is supposed to do provides a very clear message.

Tell people what to do and avoid telling what not to do

Use statements that will provide information about what is acceptable behaviour. Negative statements only tell a person what is not acceptable and do not provide necessary information to help them understand what to do differently and more appropriately.

Be as neutral as possible when giving directions

The tone of the voice, facial expressions or the difference of a word can change the meaning of a question, direction or statement.

Avoid asking questions with a choice

Unless a person is actually being given a choice, directions should be given to be followed or to provide information. Do not ask a child if they want to do something unless prepared to accept 'no'. Avoid using questions unless absolutely necessary as they are particularly difficult for the person to interpret. For example, it is better for a child with autism to be told 'It is time to come inside when the bell rings' rather than 'Are you ready to come inside now?'

Teach children and adults to respond immediately

Teach immediate responses to learned words, phrases, environmental cues or questions — these help set expectations and permit people to function more appropriately in a variety of settings. However it is also important to remember that people with autism may require up to 15–20 seconds to process information and formulate a response.

Exaggerate facial expressions

Children with autism often fail to use facial expression as a means of communication and their expressions may not match their thoughts. Use exaggerated expressions to model correct facial expressions in different situations. For example, a child with autism may laugh and giggle when another child falls and hurts himself. In that situation, it is important to model an animated response such as frowning and looking concerned and say: 'You fell and hurt your knee.' At other times, a more natural (not exaggerated) facial expression may be more appropriate to ensure the person is focusing on the verbal directions rather than concentrating on interpreting different expressions.

Label feelings

Children and adults with autism have difficulty recognising the feelings of others and expressing their own feelings. Use photos, books and social stories for older children. Social stories describe social situations, assist children with autism to make sense of these situations and teach them how to behave or respond. Introduce visual supports and discuss emotions in the context in which they may occur with children and adults (see Figure 4.3). This should never be done in a negative way. Criticising or attaching negative labels to children and adults only reduces their self-esteem and self-confidence.

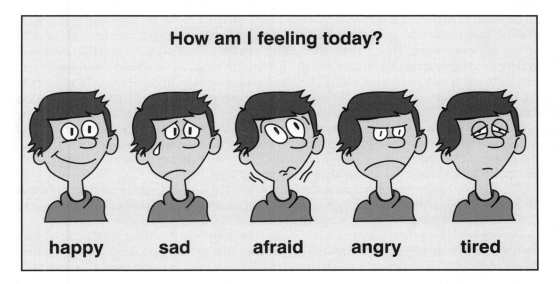

How am I feeling today?

happy   sad   afraid   angry   tired

Figure 4.3 *How am I feeling today?*

Avoid reprimands

Use rules that are consistent and neutral. Reprimands do not benefit anyone. Rules may be presented in a variety of different ways depending on the form of communication each person responds to. Support words with visual cues. Present important information visually by drawing pictures, pointing to real objects or photos and using gestures.

So what should I do to help my young child?

Dawson & Osterling (1997) reviewed early intervention programs for young children with autism ranging from intensive, one-to-one discrete trial approaches to programs in inclusive environments using naturalistic procedures. They concluded that the level of success achieved across all programs was fairly similar; all of the programs generally were effective for about half of the children.

There is no one treatment that has been found to successfully improve communication in all children and adults with autism. The most successful interventions are those that are introduced early, during the early childhood years, are individualised, target both communication and social interaction and involve both parents and professionals. The most important thing for parents of young children with autism to remember is that they must be involved in whatever intervention approach they choose. They should be prepared to work side-by-side with therapists and teachers to provide a consistent program that meets the needs of their child in all possible settings.

Summary

The communication problems associated with autism vary according to the intellectual and social development of the individual. Some children and adults are unable to use spoken language whereas others may have extensive vocabularies and are able to talk about topics of interest in great depth. Most individuals have difficulty effectively using language as well as problems with word and sentence meaning, intonation and rhythm.

Most individuals with autism do not give eye contact and have short attention spans. They are often unable to use gestures to communicate either through sign language or pointing to an object they want. The advantages and disadvantages of signing as an alternative form of communication, or even to augment speech, have been discussed.

Some individuals have poor intonation and pitch so that their speech is either high-pitched or very flat and robotic. They may be unresponsive to the speech of others and fail to respond to their own name giving an impression of a hearing problem. Some children and adults also have difficulties with the correct use of pronouns in speech, especially the use of 'I' when talking about self. For example a child may say: 'You want to go toilet' instead of 'I want to go toilet'.

Learning long lists of labels, dates or other factual information is not a functional form of communication. It may be highly motivating to people with autism as an obsessional interest. It is more relevant, however, for people to be able to approach another person to communicate needs, desires and feelings in daily life.

Autism is recognised as primarily a social disorder that Kanner (1943, p 242) described as 'children's inability to relate themselves in the ordinary way to people and situations' with communication difficulties based largely in the area of social communication.

The whole of the difficulties in communication that people with autism must contend with mean that they tend to be very literal and assume that words mean exactly what they say. They may become confused by what is meant by certain phrases such as 'John cried his eyes out.'

In attempting to understand the impairments in communication linked to autism, it is important to look at the functions of communication and to think about ways to encourage communication in children and adults with autism.

All individuals with autism have comprehension impairments, whether they have Asperger's syndrome or autism. Comprehension impairment includes difficulties empathising or understanding the thoughts and feelings of others, selectively attending to speech, interpreting context as well as words and with abstract concepts of language.

Priorities should be directed toward assisting children to communicate in ways, either verbally or non-verbally, that are useful in everyday life. This includes introducing visual supports into everyday routines to assist each person with autism to understand what is happening around them. Information about visual supports has been provided and the use of visual supports in augmenting speech was discussed.

CHAPTER

5

Impairments of Social Relating

Social skills represent the ability to accommodate or adapt to ongoing situations and social interactions. Unlike cognitive and language development, which are rule based, social development is constantly changing.

Quill 2000

Social development includes using eye contact, facial expression and body language to connect with others. It also requires an ability to wait, share and take turns in games and every-day social situations; to interpret and respond appropriately to other people's actions, thoughts and emotional states; to understand and acknowledge other people's viewpoint; to respect ownership and to co-operate with others in group situations. In order to maintain proper social etiquette, individuals also need to understand correct social distance; vocal quality; conversation skills that include starting, maintaining and finishing a conversation; an interest in, and awareness of other people's favoured topics of conversation; how to obtain someone's attention and request assistance and also reasonable grooming and hygiene.

The requirements for appropriate social functioning are enormous and place a lot of pressure on people with autism who are not naturally social. Many researchers consider impairments in social functioning to be the major deficit of people with autism, and certainly the social problems encountered by people with autism are both complex and pervasive. Most of the early research into autism focused on the social isolation of individuals. Kanner (1943) referred to extreme autistic withdrawal and in later work he described extreme isolation as a defining characteristic (Kanner & Eisenberg 1956). Rutter (1978) discussed the social problems associated with autism and described a failure to develop relationships as being partly due to an apparent lack of interest in people.

What are social skills?

During the first year of life, infants learn to use and respond to eye gaze, gestures and facial expression in social situations, especially to familiar adults. They develop early non-verbal social–communicative skills. These skills enable them to initiate social interactions and to engage in reciprocal turn-taking. They also begin to make basic requests and to share interests with others. Infants also respond to the attempts of others to engage them in social interactions. These early non-verbal social–communicative functions form the basis for reciprocal social interaction skills, joint attention skills and behaviours designed to regulate others.

Imitation also plays an important role in the development of cognitive and social skills. Imitation is critical for the emergence of symbolic play and is necessary for sustaining social interactions. Most infants first show interest and motor responses when adults imitate their behaviour and the motivation to continue the social contact sustains the imitation exchanges. During the first year of life, infants progress from repeating motor and vocal actions within their repertoire to imitating novel actions. By age 2, children begin to imitate a sequence of new actions and they learn to imitate actions that they have observed previously.

What is an impairment of social relating?

Autism typically affects a person's ability to communicate, form relationships with others and respond appropriately to their environment. Most individuals with autism have problems interacting and communicating socially, imitating others and playing imaginatively.

Autism is seen as an impairment of social relating. According to the American Psychiatric Association (1994 DSM-IV, p 70), social impairment in autism may be defined by 'a marked impairment in the use of multiple non-verbal behaviours such as eye gaze, facial expression, and gestures to regulate social interaction; a lack of spontaneous seeking to share enjoyment, interests and achievements with other people (including a lack of showing, bringing or pointing out objects of interest); and a lack of social and emotional reciprocity'. Baron-Cohen, Allen & Gillberg (1992) stated that the limited non-verbal social–communicative behaviours and poor imitation and atypical play behaviours of children are the prime indicators of autism. Impairment in these skills, however, varies significantly among children and adults with autism.

Impairment of social relating may be summarised as:

- lack of empathy with other people and awareness of the role others play in the social interaction process;
- lack of initiation in interactions and response to the attempts of other children and adults to interact;
- lack of listening and imitation skills;
- limited acceptance of other people's point of view;
- limited acceptance that the individual may be wrong;
- limited acceptance of change;
- limited ability to read the social cues expressed by other people — the looks, body language, hints, facial expressions and voice intonation; and
- limited desire to relate to other people.

The severity of these behaviours varies from one individual with autism to another along a 'social' continuum. The social continuum provides an indication of a person's social skills at any point in time, from severe to mild. It is important to note that an individual may vary along the continuum over time and an individual may appear at one place on a continuum in one skill and be placed quite differently in other skills.

What is the social continuum for autism?

Wing and Gould (1979), felt that many children did not exactly fit Kanner's description of extreme autistic withdrawal, but still had significant problems in communication, social relating and imagination. Wing and Gould recognised that the core characteristics of autism varied between individuals according to intellectual disability and degree of disability and also varied within individuals over time according to age.

Individuals at the severe end of the social continuum appear aloof and indifferent to others, including their peers, and are lacking many of the basic social skills such as sharing, waiting and turn-taking. At the milder end of the continuum, individuals may appear quite gregarious, seeking the company of others but approaching them in an odd, repetitive way and taking little notice of their needs or interests.

Social impairments affect the ability to relate to others in different ways. There is not one autistic stereotype. The three typical stereotypes that epitomise the range of social interaction seen in autism are identified as aloof, passive, and active but odd. Some people with autism may display all three types of behaviour, depending on the circumstances.

The individual who is classified as aloof or withdrawn tends to avoid social interaction but may form simple attachments to familiar adults. The passive person also tends to be solitary, attending a range of different activities but failing to join in unless pressured to do so. Many passive individuals will engage in repetitive behaviours such as flapping, rocking or tapping. The active but odd individual, who appears more outgoing, typically will engage others in a one-sided conversation or ask repetitive questions while paying little or no attention to the answers.

As suggested by Wing & Gould, not all individuals with autism and Asperger's syndrome are withdrawn, lacking emotion and empathy, or want to avoid social situations. Many children and adults feel quite intense emotions and would like to socialise but they do not understand how to express feelings or manage and understand different social situations. Wing & Gould outlined three groups of children as a result of a study in 1978. Wing & Attwood, in 1987, expanded the study and grouped children according to how they handled themselves in social situations:

■ Group 1 — children who are generally observed on the periphery of social situations, either watching other people socialise or appearing oblivious to interactions that are happening around them. They appear to be aloof and withdrawn.

■ Group 2 — children who are fairly passive. They also watch interactions but seldom initiate social approaches. They will willingly respond if others initiate and are easily led into activities. Although they want to have friends, they often misinterpret casual remarks and are easily hurt by rebuffs and being left out.

■ Group 3 — children who are actively involved in social situations, with no awareness of the effect of their behaviour on others. These children will relentlessly pursue their own interests without picking up the cues of boredom or reluctance from others. Their abilities are frequently overestimated because they have reasonably good social and communication skills. In 1996, Wing added an additional group:

■ Group 4 — children who are overly formal and stilted and who try very hard to behave by sticking rigidly to rules of social interaction. These children do not really understand the rules and have difficulty adapting to subtle differences in behaviour in different situations. They are excessively polite and formal. This group is more pronounced among adolescents and adults.

Figure 5.1 illustrates these groups.

What are the social deficits associated with autism?

The earliest descriptions of the social deficits associated with autism are by Kanner (1943) and by Kanner & Eisenberg (1956). Their findings contain references to at least twelve different aspects of social impairment among the group of children studied. These deficits include lack of 'apparent affection', withdrawal from people, lack of attention to people, non-communicative use of language, lack of communicative gestures, treating people as inanimate objects, lack of eye contact, lack of appropriate social behaviour, attention to non-social aspects of people, and lack of awareness of the feelings of others. Most of these findings have been corroborated and supported by later studies.

Wing & Gould's (1979) survey found that the social impairment associated with autism could be distinguished into three types: social aloofness, passive interaction, and active-but-odd

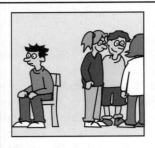

Withdrawn
Actively avoids being with others
(particularly peers) sometimes moving
them out of the way as if people are
objects. May use others as tools to get
something that is wanted.

Profound degree
of impairment

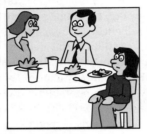

Passive
May accept social contact but does not
spontaneously approach others to
initiate contact. Has learnt basic social
etiquette like greeting skills. May attend
a wide range of activities without
complaint.

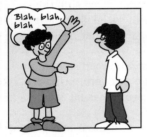

Outgoing
Seeks company of others, however
approaches others in odd, repetitive
way, not paying attention to the
response of others or their point of
view.

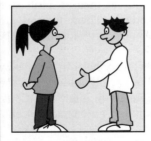

Formal
Very rule driven, rigid and literal in their
behaviour and communication. They
are uncomfortable in unfamiliar social
situations and tend to stick to familiar
timetables, very polite and socially

Mild degree
of impairment

Figure 5.1   *Degrees of impairment*

interaction. Their study highlighted that not all children with autism show withdrawn social behaviour and many do approach and attempt to interact with others, but in inappropriate ways. Hopkins & Lord (1981) concluded that children's social impairments change according to whom they are with and also over time as they develop. Their study also found that people with autism do take account of other people's behaviour.

According to Janzen (1996), a number of factors closely associated with social deficits in children with autism include:

■ an inability to understand the perspective of others and how one's own perspective impacts on others;

■ an inability to identify and make sense of social information generated through facial expression, gestures, language nuances, etc.;

- an inability to formulate an appropriate response in varied and ever-changing social situations; and
- an inability to show social judgement.

In addition to the factors above, the following factors also impact on the social skills of children and adults with autism:

- an inability to share objects and information with another person (joint sharing of attention);
- an inability to sort out relevant versus irrelevant details from the information they take in;
- an inability to think in abstract terms (literal thinking);
- an inability to see the whole picture rather than focusing on the smaller details (this difficulty generalising perceived details into concepts and meanings to form a larger 'scheme of things' is known as weak central coherence); and
- a limited ability to communicate with others either verbally or non-verbally.

The effects of these deficits have a huge impact on how individuals relate to other people and are usually seen in their inflexibility because social rules are learned in a rigid way, with little understanding that there may be a range of acceptable behaviour. If told what to do, the individual will tend do it the same way exactly with no variation. This inflexibility makes it difficult to adapt to changes and to interact socially.

In addition, there is little understanding of what is acceptable behaviour privately and publicly. Without an understanding of the perspective of others, children and adults with autism do not feel embarrassment or automatically learn social and cultural rules and taboos.

> Peter was taught to ask people their name as an introduction. 'Hello, my name is Peter, what is your name?' Peter now approaches anyone that he does not recognise and introduces himself, even total strangers that he passes in the street. He has not been taught how to discriminate between 'friends' and 'strangers' or when it is, or is not, appropriate to introduce himself to people.

Individuals with autism have limited organisation and management skills, especially in unstructured situations such as free time, breaks, weekends, parties and holiday time.

They have difficulty initiating interactions, entering ongoing interactions or engaging in social conversations. They seem unable to read the subtle body language or social cues in others. They do not tend to pick up indications of boredom or embarrassment or to understand a desire to change the subject or end a conversation.

Even the most capable individuals with autism have difficulty expressing and interpreting the range of emotion and social and cultural rules that are normally acquired automatically. According to Janzen (1996, p 45) 'Their natural innocence, honesty, guilelessness, and their lack of social judgement make them vulnerable to exploitation. They are often misunderstood and easily hurt when they are corrected or teased.'

Most people with autism are unable to focus on what is relevant information in a group activity in order to share common experiences. They also tend to misunderstand social overtures, humour and jokes.

People with autism appear to have a heightened focus on details rather than an ability to see the whole picture — a cognitive style termed 'weak central coherence'. Many young children with autism, for example, will focus on spinning the wheels of a toy car or opening and closing the doors of a toy bus rather than observing that the other children in the group are all working together to build a road or rail system out of blocks that they can share and have fun together. A young adult may focus on reading the labels and logos on the side of the bus shelter after school rather than join in with the students to organise their social activities for the weekend ahead.

Jordan loves numbers and is fascinated by math textbooks or computer magazines. He loves to sit and read his books at lunchtime at school. He is not aware of what his peers are doing and does not join in their general discussions. He will only participate as long as the discussion is about computers otherwise he loses interest and prefers to look at his magazines.

People with autism are unable to look beyond the details of a particular situation to look at things in context. For example, on a task that looks at different emotional states, children with autism will often mistake emotions such as fear or surprise because they focus on the small detail of an open mouth or wide open eyes and fail to look beyond that detail to the bigger picture or the general context.

Limited or lack of joint attention skills may also be considered as a social deficit associated widely with autism. Joint attention is the ability to use eye contact and gestures such as pointing to share information or experiences with others. Joint attention is not usually fully developed in a child until around 18 months of age. Prior to that, however, most typically developing children at about 9 months will begin to visually follow when a familiar person points to something and

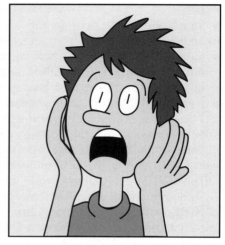

Figure 5.2 *Misunderstanding emotions*

verbalises 'Look at _____!' By 12 months of age, most children will attempt to obtain an object that is out of reach by pointing, verbalising and giving eye contact to gain a person's attention. Most children will look from the desired object to the adult in an attempt to communicate that he/she wants the object (protoimperative pointing). Soon after, most children begin to point to interesting objects, verbalise and look at an adult, not necessarily to obtain the object, but simply to direct the adult's attention to the object or event of interest (protodeclarative pointing). Children also begin to bring items to an adult just to share information.

Most children with autism are impaired in their ability to share attention and engage in pretend play. These abilities vary in intensity from person to person. The impairments affect their ability to sustain a shared interest in social interaction and to use specific joint attention skills, such as pointing and showing. The importance of joint attention is underscored by data suggesting these skills are important to later language skills (Kasari 2002).

Marco loves to play outside. He likes to sit in the garden and collect leaves and twigs which he then likes to 'post' through the small hole in the fence. When his Mum sits outside with him Marco is happy to respond when his Mum points out the flowers and a butterfly but he does not initiate any interaction himself.

Whalen & Schreibman (2003) effectively trained and targeted joint attention behaviours in children by integrating the training into existing interventions. The study provides evidence that children with autism can be trained to engage in joint attention activities and demonstrates that there is the potential to improve their social interactions and language acquisition.

Problems associated with theory of mind may be considered a social deficit commonly seen in children and adults with autism. It is believed to be an innate drive that develops from birth and is often considered to be a social tool that affects the way a person will understand and interact with others. The theory of mind account of autism, however, suggests that people with autism find it difficult to conceptualise and understand the thoughts and feelings of others.

Many of the tasks used to test theory of mind included both autistic and non-autistic children and children with a developmental delay. The theory of mind phenomenon was found to be unique to those children with autism. The information gained has helped practitioners to develop and understand the nature of the triad of impairments of autism. It has also led to an understanding that people with autism lack the ability to think about thoughts and to self-reflect. Unlike typical children and adults, who have the ability to 'mind read' situations, events and activities, individuals with autism are not able to think about other mental states and are 'mind blind'. It is this 'mind blindness' that may impair people with autism and Asperger's syndrome from relating to and understanding the behaviour of others. According to Baron-Cohen (1995), theory of mind does not appear to be related to intelligence, although people with Asperger's syndrome exhibit the problem to a lesser degree than people with autism.

By not understanding that other people think differently from themselves, people with autism may have difficulty relating socially and communicating with others because they may not be able to anticipate what other people may say or do in various situations. They may also have difficulty understanding that their peers or family even have thoughts and emotions, and this may make them appear to be self-centred, eccentric and uncaring.

Research has shown that not all aspects of socialisation are impaired in people with autism and, according to Happe (1999), 'autism may be best thought of not as an impairment of sociability, but as an impairment of social ability'.

It is necessary to teach individuals with autism to understand and acknowledge the thoughts and feelings of other people if they are to learn to socialise more effectively. Social stories, a concept developed by Carol Gray, are widely used to teach both children and adults with autism to understand themselves and others better. The short stories describe different scenarios and provide strategies to help an individual to understand a situation and also provide appropriate responses for the situation. By introducing social stories to children and adults with autism, they may be motivated to start asking questions about other people and at least recognise that different individuals think in unique ways. Social stories also provide individuals with concrete information about how they should act and react in particular situations.

What are social stories?

'Social stories are short stories that describe social situations in terms of relevant social cues and often define appropriate responses' (Gray 1993). Social stories were first developed to assist children with autism to make sense of social situations and to teach them how to behave or respond in particular situations.

Social stories are widely used today to help people with autism to understand reality; to communicate key information; to give pointers on how to behave in particular situations; and to provide positive feedback when an individual is doing well. Social stories describe social situations in terms of relevant social cues, and often define appropriate responses. They present information as clearly as possible while minimising teacher–student interactions involved in traditional teaching methods. They also provide information about what a person may know, think or feel in different situations.

They are written in response to the needs of children and may be identified as necessary through:

- recognition that certain situations may be difficult for a particular child;
- a child's response to questions about social situations that indicate that the child is misreading a particular situation; and
- social skills assessments and curricula.

Based on the identified needs, social stories may:

- describe any situation in terms of the relevant social cues and correct responses in a non-threatening format;
- personalise or emphasise social skills covered in any social skills training program;
- translate goals into understandable steps;
- explain the fictional qualities of stories and movies and help to identify realistically appropriate from inappropriate interactions depicted in those stories;
- teach routines, as well as helping children to accommodate changes in routines;
- teach academic material in a realistic way that assists children to relate learned material to real situations; and
- other possibilities, limited only by creativity.

Children, parents and professionals can write social stories. Social stories are effective for children functioning within a wide range of abilities. It is not necessary for children to be able to read before they can be introduced to social stories. They may be presented pictorially or be recorded on audiocassette for non-readers.

A parent or teacher may read social stories to a child; a parent or teacher and a child may read them together; or a child may read them independently. Stories should be read often, especially just prior to the targeted activity, in order to reinforce and remind the child of the preferred behaviour. Social stories may be presented in many different ways. A particular story may be presented as a booklet, a small card, a wall chart or a piece of paper that fits in the pocket when folded. An example of a social story is set out in Figure 5.3.

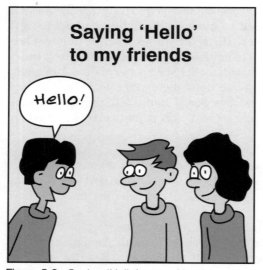

My name is Maria.
I have just started my new school.
I have some new friends.
My teacher told everyone in the class my name.
She was happy when I smiled and said 'hello' to everyone.
I feel happy when I say 'hello' to my friends.
My friends are happy when I smile and say 'hello'.
My friends smile back and talk to me.
I look at my friends, smile and say 'hello'.
I also say, 'How are you?'.
Every morning when I go to school I say 'hello' to my friends.
My teacher is very happy that I have met some new friends.
I am very happy that my classmates like me.

Figure 5.3 *Saying 'Hello' to my friends*

What strategies are useful in teaching social skills?

Because individuals with autism may be socially isolated and fail to learn social skills in the usual way, these skills usually have to be taught through constant repetition, exploration, support and practice.

The first step in teaching social skills is to ensure, beyond doubt, that the person with autism has accurate and specific social information — that they are aware of what is happening in a particular situation or setting, and that they are informed about what will be expected of them. This helps to alleviate any unexpected surprises, stress and anxiety. This information can be provided in a social story.

> Whenever Georgie's family go to visit their cousins, Georgie's mum, Jo, marks it on Georgie's weekly timetable beforehand to give her time to process the information and prepare herself for the visit. She then has time to ask questions about when they will be going, how long they will stay, who will be there and what will happen when they get there. Jo sits down with Georgie and they write a social story together to help answer all of Georgie's questions. Jo has time to give Georgie all of the information she needs to feel comfortable and relaxed.

The second step in teaching social skills is to develop the following:
- tolerance of the intrusion of others;
- an awareness of, and interest in, other people (how we depend on them and what we can obtain through them);
- ability to share both objects and experiences (joint sharing of attention);
- looking and attending skills;
- turn-taking skills;
- self-awareness and the awareness of others as separate individuals; and
- play and leisure skills.

Strategies that may be employed with children with autism to teach some of the social skills listed above (and that they will need to interact socially with their peers) should include the following:
- teaching and practice of social skills simultaneously in both structured and natural settings;
- using reinforcers that occur naturally as these are the most motivating and effective rewards over time;
- incorporating structure and routine into teaching techniques;
- not making unexpected changes to routines unless these can be fully explained, and the child prepared, ahead of time;
- introducing visual supports such as gestures, pictures or cue cards to augment any instructions and ensure that everyone is consistent in using the correct supports;
- pairing non-verbal cues such as visual supports, with verbal cues where possible; and
- practising and generalising targeted social skills so that they become part of children's normal routine then using the skills in different situations.

Teaching young children to socialise involves some different strategies from those outlined above and may include the following:
- Set the scene. Choose an area with no distractions and set out a number of fun activities, especially activities that incorporate skills in taking turns and imitating.
- Support the children rather than direct or isolate them. The constant presence of an adult may make children seem unapproachable to their peers. Rather than isolating a particular child, a teacher may model appropriate play and social skills by interacting with a child as part of a small group.
- Pair a child who is socially withdrawn with a more confident child who has good social skills.
- Introduce small group activities that focus on learning and reinforcing social skill development. Prepare activities that involve sharing, turn-taking and interactive play.
- Teach appropriate skills before setting up structured situations with other children to practise social skills. Preparation is most important.
- Introduce visual supports to assist children with autism to understand what is expected of them in a particular situation. These supports will also assist other children in their attempts to interact with children with autism.

- Visually augment the play materials to make it easier for children to follow the steps of the activity.
- Provide a 'Finish Box' to assist children to make the transition from one activity to another. Children can 'post' the completed activity (or the visual symbol of the activity) into the box before starting the next task.
- Encourage other children to play with a child with autism by always being positive about the child's attempts to interact.
- Prepare the group by discussing autism and provide simple explanations for the child's behaviour.

> Sally is still learning how to talk. She doesn't always understand what we're saying so we need to show her what we want her to do.
> Carlos is not sure how to use the outside play equipment so we need to allow him extra time to climb and be careful not to push him.

- Provide strategies for the other children if the child with autism is aggressive towards others.

> Billy is learning how to share. He doesn't understand the toys are for everyone. If he is using something, it's very important that you don't snatch it from him when it is his turn.

- Give the child with autism some responsibility in the group. In some cases, complete adult assistance may be necessary to finish a task but the other children will still see that the child with autism is included as a useful member of the group.
- Provide other children with some concrete information about what they can do to assist a child with autism to function as a member of the group.

Note: Adapted from *Learning Language and Loving It* by Elaine Weitzman (1994)

> Billy has limited play and social skills. He wants to join in and play with other children but does not know how to initiate interaction. In the classroom, Billy's teacher explains to the other children: 'Billy has difficulty understanding when you ask him to play with you. Show him what you want him to do and then wait for a few seconds to give him time to answer you.'

What is bullying?

As children move from the protection of home into the community at preschool, school and eventually the workplace, they are faced with a series of new challenges to deal with. Because of the unique characteristics associated with autism, one of the many problems children and adults face is persistent bullying. Bullying occurs in all environments and most people are subjected to some form of bullying. Children and adults with autism, however, seem to be prime targets for bullies because of their social isolation.

According to Gray (2000) in *The Morning News*, Vol 12, No 4, bullying may be defined as:

- repeated negative actions (possibly coupled with negative intent) toward a targeted individual or individuals over a period of time or as a single event;
- an imbalance of power, either physical, verbal, social and/or emotional, within an interaction; and

- the possibility of contrasting differences in the immediate or delayed effect of the individual or individuals involved.

There are a number of different roles that people play in the bullying action. Gray (2000) nominates three different social groups that are commonly associated with bullying:

1. The social majority are children and adults who demonstrate effective social skills and who are able to establish and maintain friendships among their peers.
2. The targets of bullying are usually individuals who lack positive self-esteem and find it hard to form relationships with others.
3. People who bully others need to be in control, lack empathy for others and defy authority. They will use direct confrontation or indirect gestures, rumours or exclusion.

Bullying is a common experience for many children and adolescents. Surveys indicate that as many as half of all children are bullied at some time during their school years, and at least 10% are bullied on a regular basis. According to Nansel et al (2001), at least one in six American children in sixth to tenth grade are moderate to frequent victims of bullying.

What are the main types of bullying?

According to Dan Olweus (2003, p 9), a researcher into bullying behaviours, 'a student is being bullied or victimised when he or she is exposed, repeatedly and over time, to negative acts on the part of one or more students. It is a negative action when someone intentionally inflicts, or attempts to inflict, injury or discomfit upon another'.

Bullying may take different forms and can be either verbal or physical. Verbal and written bullying are the most common forms of bullying that occur throughout life. They include name-calling, negative comments, intimidation, being laughed at and teased. Physical bullying refers to interactions where there is harm inflicted to a person's body or possessions. It includes pushing, scratching, biting, damage to personal property or physical gestures used as threats. Social bullying refers to a group effort to emotionally harm another person. It includes verbal or written innuendos or accusations, telling gossip or secrets to humiliate or shame someone, spreading rumours, ostracising or excluding a person.

Boys tend to engage in physical intimidation or threats, regardless of the gender of their victims. Bullying by girls is more often verbal, and is usually aimed at other girls. It is important for people to understand and recognise the difference between bullying and normal conflict. Table 5.1 illustrates this.

Research studies have shown that persistent bullying of children and adults can leave long-term scars including low self-esteem and depression. Children who are bullied experience real suffering that interferes with their social and emotional development, as well as their school

Table 5.1 *The difference between bullying and normal conflict.* From Olweus (2003) *Bullying at School: What We Know and What We Can Do,* Schwab Learning

Normal conflict	Bullying
Happens occasionally	Happens repeatedly
Accidental	Done on purpose
Not serious	Serious threat of physical, emotional or psychological harm
Equal emotional reaction	Strong emotional reaction from victim
Not seeking power or attention	Seeking power or control
Not trying to get something	Used to gain material things or power
Remorseful	No remorse and blames victim
Tries to solve problem	No attempt to solve the problem

performance. Some severely bullied victims have contemplated, and even committed, suicide to escape their tormentors.

Children, adolescents and adults who bully thrive on controlling or dominating others. They are also more likely to engage in other antisocial and delinquent behaviours such as vandalism, truancy and illicit drug use that may continue into adulthood.

Bullying causes children to become fearful and anxious, and also leads to feelings of isolation and loneliness, rejection by their peers, and an increase in chronic illnesses of unknown origin.

Individuals targeted by bullies tend to fit a particular profile. Bullies often choose people who are passive, easily intimidated, and have few friends. Victims may also be smaller or younger, and have a harder time defending themselves. People with autism are often the victims of bullies because they tend to have few friends to defend them and are unable to defend themselves.

Why is bullying a problem for people with autism?

The unique characteristics associated with autism place autistic children and adults at a high risk of bullying. While there is little research evidence to support the high incidence of bullying that occurs among children and adults with autism, anecdotal evidence suggests that the incidence of bullying and the odds of being a target of bullying are much higher among this population. Individuals with autism are socially isolated, have poor social skills and the syndrome places them at extremely high risk of frequent, chronic bullying.

One of the outstanding characteristics of autism is an inability to communicate well. People with autism fail to read the non-verbal signals other people give off so miss many of the social cues that provide information about how to behave in a particular situation. For example, a person with autism may not be able to differentiate between a smile and a frown and may respond inappropriately by laughing when someone is unhappy. Many people with autism are obsessed with certain rituals and are unable to cope when rituals are broken. These types of behaviours can lead to bullying and teasing.

Bullies often target children with disabilities, and children with hidden disabilities, who look average but are socially naïve, are targeted even more.

How do people with autism cope with bullying?

'Bullies who are not stopped are more likely to have criminal records in young adulthood than youth who don't bully. Bullying, therefore, is a serious problem for both the bully and the victim. Both bullies and victims need positive adult intervention to make the bullying stop. Remember that bullying is a learned behaviour that can — with adult intervention — be prevented or stopped!' (Snyder et al 2003)

There are a number of strategies that can be introduced to assist the person with autism to cope with bullying:

- Initially, determine whether a child or adolescent is aware of being bullied and what effect the bullying is having on their physical and emotional wellbeing.
- Identify how the person responds and reacts to being bullied. What coping strategies are they currently using? One of the first indications of bullying having an impact on a person is reflected in changes to their behaviour.
- Once it is established that a person is a victim of bullying, a number of strategies may be implemented to support them. This may include involving peers and friends to protect them and provide social support. For example, if bullying is happening at school, a buddy system may be introduced to provide protection and support for the child being bullied.
- Understanding the intentions of bullies may assist the person being bullied to avoid potentially explosive situations and also help determine how to react to the bullying to minimise its impact.

■ Social stories and comic strip conversations can be used to help a person with autism to understand what is happening when bullying occurs and also to explore ways of responding to bullying. Comic strip conversations are useful in solving problems around particular incidents of bullying. Developed by Carol Gray, a comic strip conversation is a conversation between two or more people that incorporates the use of simple drawings. They provide a visual representation of a conversation in order to enhance the person's understanding and comprehension. The illustrations can include symbols, drawings and written words. A specific structure is followed to organise a social exchange and build in predictability. Comic strip conversations are most helpful when there is a need to convey important information, when there is a misunderstanding, or to solve a problem, such as bullying. A comic strip conversation may also be used to teach a social skill. The illustrations usually consist of stick figures and bubbles where the figures' words and thoughts are written. When a person gains experience with using comic strip conversations, colours can be associated to express feelings such as green for happy, blue for sad, or black for anger. The conversation usually begins with small talk, just as any conversation usually does. The person with autism takes the lead in a comic strip conversation, and the parent, professional, or peer serves as a guide to the conversation. Comic strip conversations focus on what people in the situation may be thinking. Often the person with autism may have difficulty interpreting what someone else may be thinking, or they may interpret something that was said literally. This presents an opportunity to assist them in understanding the situation or another person's perspective. Finally, the conversation is summarised and, if necessary, concluded with the identification of a new solution.

Victims of bullying should be taught how to respond to bullying attempts. They need to remain calm and avoid becoming anxious and distressed. They should try to focus on something positive and try to ignore the bullying. Focusing on something positive or visualising a favourite picture or place can have a calming effect (see Figure 5.5).

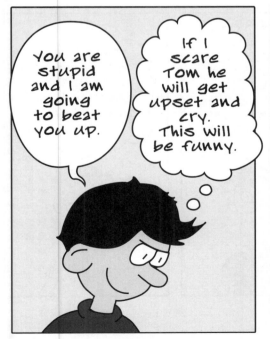
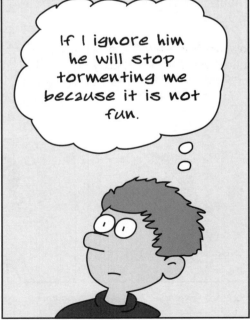

Figure 5.4 | *Example of a comic strip conversation*

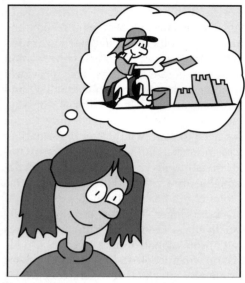

Figure 5.5 *Focusing on something positive*

- Victims of bullying may engage in self-talk to remind themselves to remain calm and positive. Children and adults can role-play scenarios to help them know what to say in a stressful situation and how to say it.
- It should be stressed to victims of bullying that they have to tell someone in authority, a friend, a teacher or a parent. They need to ask for help so that programs can be implemented to stop the bullying from continuing.

People with autism cannot hide their disability, nor should they have to. A person with a physical disability is offered protection and other people are aware of their needs, limitations and rights. Individuals with autism, however, are often misjudged and have unrealistic expectations placed upon them. Sometimes individuals may appear to be disruptive, lazy and wilful when, in fact, they are struggling to understand what is happening around them and trying to fit in and conform to our expectations. These people are easy targets for bullies.

Bullying is just one of the problems facing individuals with autism as they struggle to cope socially in a world that does not tend to recognise their unique talents. They are expected to conform to a social environment that is quite foreign to them. The struggle that individuals with autism have trying to fit in and manage in society can be likened to being dropped into the middle of an isolated foreign country and not speaking the language.

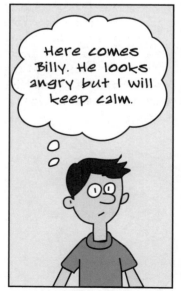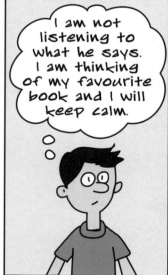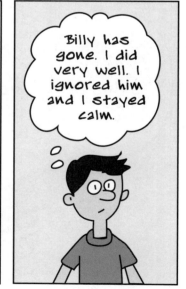

Figure 5.6 *Example of a visual strategy*

Summary

Social impairment is recognised as one of the major difficulties associated with autism. People with autism fail to develop normal reciprocal or interactive social relationships with others. They often avoid looking at others or 'look through' them as if they are invisible. Their interest in other people is usually on a needs basis and is limited to using people as tools to help them obtain something they want. Some individuals with autism may avoid physical contact and become distressed if someone gets too close or touches them. Others, however, may be completely unresponsive to physical contact and appear quite apathetic.

Some people with autism are very affectionate but it is usually 'on their terms' and only when they initiate it. Most have difficulty understanding and expressing emotion. Their facial expression appears blank or neutral and they also find it difficult to read or understand the facial expressions of others. Their social skills are poorly developed, and social interactions, when they happen, appear odd because they look rote learned and mechanical in nature.

Typical social development differs from the impaired social development of people with autism. People with autism have problems interacting and communicating socially, imitating others and playing imaginatively. Autism is seen as an impairment of social relating.

Wing & Gould recognised that the core characteristics of autism varied between individuals according to intellectual disability, degree of disability and according to age. The three typical stereotypes that epitomise the range of social interaction in autism are identified as aloof, passive, and active but odd.

We explored some of the social deficits associated with autism and offered strategies for teaching social skills to children and adults with autism. One of the most popular and successful strategies for teaching social skills is the use of social stories.

Many individuals with autism have been exposed to different forms of bullying throughout their lives. Bullying is a common problem for most people but individuals with autism are extremely vulnerable and are often targeted by bullies. The biggest single problem at school reported by people with Asperger's syndrome is bullying and teasing.

When a person with autism is bullied, it is important to ensure that the person understands the bullying situation and has strategies in place to help them to cope. If the person is not able to cope alone, a social support system should be established to provide assistance and visual strategies, such as social stories and comic strip conversations, should be introduced. It is important to take into account the person's readiness and ability to understand the instructions and techniques when planning specific coping strategies. That way, the strategies adopted will be most effective. Social stories and comic strip conversations can be introduced to help individuals with autism understand and manage bullying behaviours.

CHAPTER

6

Restricted, Rigid and Repetitive Patterns of Behaviours or Interests

This type of behaviour ranks high on the list of problems that cause parents the most worry and despair. If not handled properly, a child's insistence on routine can come to dominate the life of the whole family.

Wing 1996, p 99

Since Leo Kanner first described the syndrome of infantile autism in 1943, the observation that children with autism have an obsessive need for sameness has prevailed. All subsequent descriptions of autism have concurred with his original observation that children with autism have stereotyped, restrictive motor movements and repetitive, rigid behaviours.

The core deficits associated with the restricted, rigid and repetitive patterns of behaviour or interests are shown as a preoccupation with particular objects or topics, an adherence to non-functional routines, an abnormal attachment to objects or the use of objects, and stereotyped and repetitive behaviours.

The spectrum of repetitive behaviours includes:

- motor stereotypies such as head banging, handflapping and spinning;
- compulsions or rituals accompanied by severe anxiety at any change, tactile and olfactory explorations and lining up toys; and
- repetitive ideations relating to a restrictive, intrusive and narrowly focused range of interests.

Where do these patterns of behaviour fit in a diagnosis of autism?

According to Wing and Gould (1979) and Wing (1988, 1996) autism is diagnosed by a series of criteria, and they placed great emphasis on the social nature of the three areas of difficulty:

1. impairment of social communication;
2. impairment of social interaction; and
3. impairment of social imagination and understanding.

The third element of Wing's triad, referred to as impairment of imagination and understanding, was described as:

- a delay or absence of 'pretend or imaginative' play;
- a reliance on routines and familiar experiences;

- a dislike of new experiences and resistance to change;
- inflexibility of thought;
- a single-minded pursuit of special interests; and
- difficulty understanding other's point of view.

Wing (1996, p 44), stated that 'children with autistic disorders do not develop pretend play and imaginative activities in the same way as other children ... They act out a sequence of events that they have invented. This looks convincing at first but prolonged observation shows that the child goes through the same sequence over and over again, without any changes.' Some children also act out scenes from favourite videos that initially appear to be imaginative, but the actions are limited and repetitive rather than inventive.

What does impairment of imagination mean?

Play lies at the very heart of learning and socialisation (Piaget 1962; Vygotsky 1964) and also provides a means of encouraging exploration of objects, social discovery, self-discovery and imagination. According to Beyer & Gammeltoft (2000), the development of play skills enables children to explore their environment by becoming more aware of their own bodies and familiar with a range of toys and other objects. Play also provides opportunities to learn new skills from familiar adults and peers. Play is creative and encourages children to practise newly acquired skills, to re-enact previous experiences and also to imitate the actions of others.

A lack of imaginative play makes it difficult to interact socially, to develop an understanding of other peoples' feelings and emotions or to share happiness or sorrow with others. The ability to play interactively is an early developmental skill that is difficult for children with autism. Playing games with rules may be considered more developmentally advanced but seems to be an easier skill for these children to acquire. This ties in with the work of Baron-Cohen (1987, 1991, 1995) that explores autistic people's inability to understand other people's thoughts, interests and feelings and that these may differ from their own.

Impairment of imagination, as described by Wing & Gould (1979), focuses on the inability of children with autism to play socially or to create imaginative activities in the same way as typical children. Among the difficulties associated with the development of play and imagination in children with autism is the fact that they do not develop the concept of creative 'let's pretend' play in the way that other children do. Children with autism have a limited range of imaginative activities that are often copied and pursued rigidly and repetitively. Many of the toys and objects they pick up are used purely for physical sensations. Some children do learn to use toys appropriately, such as throwing balls into a bucket, feeding a dolly with a toy bottle or building bridges with wooden blocks, but most children use toys in very limited and rigid ways.

A toy car may be a plaything only to the degree that a child is fascinated and stimulated by the spinning of the wheels, or a bead threading string is used as an object to repetitively flick and flap. Another child may line up wooden blocks into neat rows but never pick up a block and use it as a pretend telephone in an imaginative play activity.

Sally was obsessed with sticks, pencils, straws or any other long thin object that she could flick and flap in front of her eyes. Her interest was very limited, however, and she showed little awareness of how these objects could be used in more functional ways.

Some more able children do learn complex play sequences and so are able to engage in pretend play, however they do not act out imaginative stories but repeat word for word sequences that they have been taught or have rote-learned from TV or videos.

Most of these play sequences are entirely self-directed and do not involve other children, or involve others but only on terms laid down by the child with autism. Some children with autism do reach a stage where they would like to interact or play with other children but do not know how to go about it.

Some people with autism engage in activities that appear to be functional, but close observation indicates that the sequence is usually something rote-learned and repeated over and over again. For example, a child learns the pretend play sequence of bathing, dressing and feeding a dolly and then putting dolly to bed so that he or she knows what to do when presented with a doll at preschool. Another child acts out a sequence of events that he has invented, incorporating scenes from a favourite video. In both examples, difficulties lie in the child's inability to deviate from the learned sequence to incorporate changes or to accommodate other people's needs.

> James has a strong interest in cars and trains. He used to spin the wheels but has learned to drive the cars along the road and the trains along the railway tracks. He is starting to introduce other ways of playing with his cars but he has to be shown what to do first. His play still remains very limited and repetitive because he never wants to play with other toys.

There are a number of people with autism who develop obsessive interests in particular objects or activities such as numbers and letters, makes of cars and trucks, dinosaurs or electrical switches. Usually, they tend to select minor or trivial aspects of things in the environment rather than having an imaginative understanding of the whole scene, or the broader picture. A young adult may have an intense interest in dinosaurs, collect pictures and be able to label the different animals in the species, but have no understanding or interest in the historical aspects of the evolutionary process and how the dinosaur fits in with life on earth today. An adult may be extremely interested in train timetables and obsessively recite times and train numbers, but be unaware of how important and useful timetables are to many everyday commuters.

Children and adults with autism also tend to miss the point of pursuits involving words, such as social conversation, literature, especially fiction, and also subtle verbal humour. Wing (1996, p 45) says 'The pleasures of creative imagination in childhood are denied to autistic people and so are the rewards of adult life. They have limited or no understanding of other people's emotions, so find it hard to share happiness or sorrow. They are impaired in the ability to share ideas with others and to use past and present experiences to plan for the future. Most of the usual sources of satisfaction are a closed book to people with autism. They find their pleasures in their own special interests.'

In addition to the problems associated with a lack of imagination, repetitive behaviour patterns and resistance to change in routine are also notable features associated with autism. People with autism often become obsessed with particular objects or behaviours, focusing on them to the exclusion of everything else.

The Diagnostic and Statistical Manual of Mental Disorders (Fourth Edition), (DSM-IV), established by the American Psychiatric Association (1994) provides a reference of behavioural criteria to assist in the diagnosis of autism. According to the DSM-IV the defining characteristics of autism include:

- Impaired development of reciprocal social interaction: whereby individuals fail to develop normal reciprocal or interactive social relationships with others and are often described as 'living in a world of their own'.
- Impairment in communication and imaginative activity: affects both verbal and non-verbal abilities and pervades every area of development. Impaired imagination refers to the

individual's inability to engage in imaginative or pretend play and frequently limited repertoire of play or leisure behaviours.

- Markedly restricted repertoire of activities and interests: refers to the inability of individuals to relate normally to objects and events in their environment.

Currently, most professionals diagnosing autism use the criteria established by the American Psychiatric Association (DSM-IV) that is slightly different to Wing & Gould's original triad of impairments. There is a direct correspondence between the first two elements of both triads; that is, impairment of communication and social interaction. The minor differences lie in the third element that, in Wing's Triad, is referred to as impairment of imagination but, according to the DSM-IV, is stated as restricted and repetitive behaviours, activities and interests.

The DSM-IV criteria are widely accepted and used by professionals to diagnose autism because the criteria are defined on the basis of a pattern of observable behaviours. The American Psychiatric Association criteria refer to repetitive and restricted interests, activities and behaviours as shown in a range of clearly defined behaviours. Wing's impaired imagination refers to aspects such as difficulty understanding that others may have a different point of view and inflexibility of thought. These are psychological concepts rather than observable behaviours.

What are repetitive and restricted patterns of behaviour or interests?

The rigid patterns of behaviour and/or interests that are so commonly seen in children and adults with autism vary greatly from one person to another. What is obvious in one child may be quite different from the behaviours observed in another child. According to Wing (1996, p 45), the repetitive and stereotypic patterns of behaviour begin to make more sense when they are seen as 'the other side of the coin of impairment of imagination'. She feels that the limited imaginative abilities of the person with autism precludes them from enjoying social interaction with others, stops them from enjoying many activities that require creative thought and does not allow them to integrate past and present experiences to help them to plan for the future. They therefore tend to repeat those activities and experiences that they do find pleasurable.

Among the most commonly observed restricted, repetitive and stereotypic patterns of behaviour, interests and activities are the following:

- repeatedly watching particular videos or video segments;
- lining up and/or ordering objects in a particular way;
- showing a strong attachment to inanimate objects such as a certain toy, piece of string or a particular utensil;
- having a fascination with movement such as spinning fans and wheels, opening and closing doors and drawers;
- pacing or running back and forth or round and round;
- exploring the environment by licking, smelling or touching objects and people;
- showing sensitivity to certain sounds such as people singing, toilets flushing or the noise of a vacuum cleaner;
- difficulty waiting;
- displaying an impaired response to temperature or pain;
- having a fascination for visual patterns, lights or shiny surfaces;
- having a lack of fear or awareness of real danger;
- having an abnormal fear of certain harmless objects or situations such as puppets, dogs and people dressed up as clowns;
- defensiveness to touch that is not self initiated; and
- having a history of eating and/or sleeping problems.

Repetitive behaviours dominate both the social and communication behaviour of children with autism, although they are manifested in so many different ways that it is difficult to list or describe them all. They include body movements such as rocking, flapping and spinning; vocalisations such as squealing, unusual sounds and nonsense babble; and rituals such as opening and closing cupboard doors, drinking or eating from specific utensils or having to have the video tapes lined up in a certain order.

These repetitive actions may be an expression of enjoyment for some children and an expression of stress and anxiety for others.

> James finds waiting difficult and becomes anxious when he has to wait for the video to rewind to the beginning. He begins to rock back and forth, squeals and flaps his hands until the video starts again. The repetitive rocking helps him to remain reasonably calm and also lets his parents know that he is not happy.

One child may enjoy repetitively lining up objects according to shape or colour and feel happy and comfortable when eating from a favourite and familiar bowl, while another child may engage in repetitive activities more intensively when uncomfortable or feeling stressed. A child may engage in repetitive questioning such as 'What are we doing today?' or 'I go swimming today?' in order to try to make sense of the day ahead. Another child may sit on the lounge and rock back and forth when his favourite program finishes on television because he is distressed that the show has finished and he has not yet learned to wait quietly for the video to rewind.

In more able children and adults, especially those diagnosed with Asperger's syndrome, the repetitive activities and interests may present a little differently and be shown as a fascination for particular topics such as electrical circuits, train timetables, ancient history, cameras and lenses, astronomy or capital cities of the world. The interest is generally in collecting (both objects and facts), memorising, and talking about the particular interest to anyone who will listen. 'Tommy ... is an honour-roll student who likes math and science and video games. He's also a world class expert on Animorph and Transformer toys.' (*Time* Magazine, 6 May 2002)

The special activities may be quite complex. They may centre on completing a sequence of actions in a particular order that are then repeated over and over. One person, for example, who was obsessed with trains and train timetables insisted on travelling by train to a different town each weekend based on a particular starting time according to his train timetable.

A special interest may include a preoccupation with numbers, numerical aspects of objects or complicated calculation. It may involve learning facts and collecting memorabilia about a certain subject. This preoccupation is unusual because of the intensity of interest shown or the narrow focus of the area of interest. One young man, for example, may be fascinated with aeroplanes and collect models, pictures and photographs of aeroplanes, label different aeroplanes with all of their corresponding dimensions and spend many hours observing aeroplanes at different airports.

Children and adults with autism have a strong tendency to be rigid and stereotyped in their behaviour and also to become upset and distressed by any changes that occur to their normal routines. The characteristic 'insistence on sameness' that was first observed in autistic children by Leo Kanner, refers to 'a need for rigid adherence to routines and the maintenance of environmental sameness. A high level of anxiety and distress can result when this sameness is not maintained (e.g., when a different route is taken on the way to school or a piece of furniture is moved from its usual place in the room)' (Grados & McCarthy 2000). Individuals with autism engage in restricted and repetitive behaviours, interests and activities to maintain the status quo. It is well documented that most people with autism do not cope with changes to their environment. They prefer everything to remain the same and will follow routines and rituals very carefully in order to avoid any changes to these routines. They become excessively rigid about many aspects of their daily lives, from morning and bedtime routines, to what clothing they will wear; or from the routes that they travel, to room layouts at home. Some individuals may be overly preoccupied with certain activities or objects and overly fearful of others.

> Charles liked to sit quietly by himself and read the Yellow Pages or the White Pages of the telephone book. He enjoyed turning the pages and was fascinated by the advertisements, especially if they contained pictures of cranes, large trucks or earth moving equipment. He loved to look at real trucks and cranes. However he was afraid of animals and would become distressed and extremely anxious whenever he saw pictures of cats, dogs or other animals.

Changes to routine such as varying the regular route to the shop, moving the furniture around, or changing from shorts to long pants may cause distress and anxiety for some children and adults. This distress and anxiety may manifest in a tendency toward repetitive activities such as spinning or rhythmic body movements such as arm flapping, tapping objects, jumping on the spot or flicking objects in front of the face. Higher functioning children and adults may engage in repetitive questioning when anxious, repeat dialogue from favourite television shows, act out video segments or indulge in complex routines in order to calm themselves and bring about a sense of order.

Because the behaviour of other people appears to be so unpredictable and chaotic to the person with autism, they value the predictability of sameness and routine as a means of establishing and maintaining order in a meaningless world. It seems that routine and predictability is much easier to control in the world of objects rather than the world of people. People with autism, therefore, show a marked preference for activities involving objects rather than social activities requiring interaction with other people.

According to Attwood (1998, p 99), 'routine appears to be imposed to make life predictable and to impose order, as novelty, chaos and uncertainty are intolerable. It also acts as a means of reducing anxiety'.

Both Temple Grandin (1995) and Donna Williams (1992), in their respective autobiographies, discussed their need for routines and rituals to help regulate their environment and reduce stress and anxiety. Sean Barron (1992, p 20), in his autobiography, described his childhood experience and dependence on rituals: 'I loved repetition. Every time I turned on a light I knew what would happen. When I flipped a switch, the light went on. It gave me a wonderful feeling of security because it was exactly the same each time.'

The rituals employed to help create order and maintain sameness in a confusing social environment are too numerous to list. One child may insist that he is the first person to approach the front door and ring the doorbell a certain number of times on returning home after an outing. Another child may become extremely upset if the car pulls out of the driveway and turns left instead of right because he knows he has to turn right to go to Grandma's. One adult may insist on only wearing a certain shirt or clothing that is red while another adult may refuse to try new foods or eat any food that is green.

Resistance to change is also commonly seen in the individual diets of both children and adults with autism. So many people with autism have limited diets and will not try new or different foods. Not only is the diet limited but also the way food is prepared and presented can be a nightmare for parents and carers. Children may insist that sandwiches are cut in perfect triangles or in squares and be buttered on one side or not buttered at all. Other children may only eat food of a certain colour, or food that is soft and mushy, or food that is hard and salty. One young man will only eat a particular brand of bread and it must be toasted exactly right and cut into four equal strips. Another young adult is obsessed with food from McDonald's fast food outlets and insists on having a hamburger and fries although he only eats the pickle from the hamburger and a few fries.

The difference between the obsessive interests or the repetitive behaviours and rituals of a person with autism and the hobbies or special interests of people who do not have autism may be seen in the extent to which the obsessions and rituals dominate the person's time and conversation and the limited nature of the interest. A child may be totally obsessed with numbers and letters and stand in front of the microwave or digital clock and count the numbers as they appear. That same child may repeat all the house numbers, love to observe speed signs and collect miniature road signs, 'read' the telephone directory and the Yellow Pages and be able to count to one thousand when he is 4 years old.

Le is obsessed with the solar system. He can name all of the planets and knows where they are placed in relation to the sun. He knows details about each of the individual planets and can talk at length about their composition. He collects information from magazines, watches videos and loves to visit the Observatory to observe the stars.

People with autism tend to focus purely on their interest and have little, or no awareness that others may not share the same interest. In most cases, the obsessive interest of a person with autism is a solitary pursuit that can be carried out alone and in isolation. For example, a boy may have an overriding interest in the different makes and models of cars. He may talk continually about cars, ask everyone what make of car they drive, read car magazines and collect general information, models and photographs of cars and car insignias and love to visit car museums. He is quite happy to pursue these activities alone and, if anyone else is included, it tends to be on his terms.

Children and adults with autism tend to be more interested in objects than people. In young children this may be observed in the way that they play. Most play tends to be repetitive and non-social. Play usually involves repetitive and ritualistic actions (lining up objects or spinning wheels of cars) rather than the social actions of sharing toys and information and playing interactively with peers and familiar adults.

Freddy is obsessed with Buzz Lightyear and always carries around his two toy Buzz dolls. He becomes extremely distressed if they are taken from him and refuses to let them go even to eat or play. He takes them to bed with him at night.

Many children and adults may also be preoccupied with parts of an object or the movement of objects. A child may sit with a toy car and repetitively open and close the doors rather than pretending to drive the car along an imaginary road. Another child may sit at home and watch the blades of the ceiling fan rotate or stand very close to the television and focus on the move-ments on the screen. An adult may be very attached to a piece of string or even a long blade of grass. This can be waved in front of the face repetitively and must always be present either in the hand, in the pocket, on the desk or worktable. Some individuals with autism end up with an extensive collection of objects that are important to them.

Objects are often used in restricted and repetitive ways to help calm and provide a feeling of security to a person that helps to limit their stress and anxiety.

Why engage in repetitive behaviours?

Repetitive and ritualistic behaviours occur in every area of learning, socialisation, communication and behaviour. There are different schools of thought about why people with autism engage in these unusual behaviours. Some professionals feel that repetitive and stereotypic behaviours are a means of regulating sensory stimulation by helping to tune out visual, auditory, tactile and kinaesthetic stimulation that is overwhelming and uncomfortable. These behaviours can also be used, on the other hand, to repeat pleasurable sensory stimulation.

Other practitioners claim that children and adults with autism engage in repetitive behaviours to help create order amid chaos. Repetitive behaviours provide a means of expressing anxiety and help the individual to remain calm and block out unwanted stimuli or unpleasant sensations.

Ozonoff (1995) suggested that ritualised patterns of behaviour are the by-product of impaired cognitive function. Cognitive functions including attention, information processing, social understanding and executive control are impaired and make it difficult for the individual to be spontaneous, creative and flexible. 'The cognitive inability to shift mental focus and generate novel patterns of behaviour results in the child becoming locked in routinized patterns' (Quill 2000, p 20).

According to Temple Grandin (1996), an intense interest in moving objects is part of the sensory impairment seen in autism. However, she also concluded that while some sights and sounds attract people with autism, other sights and sounds may be terrifying and should be avoided. It is therefore necessary to observe and assess individuals to understand what attracts and what repels them. In her book *Emergence Labelled Autistic* she talks about her childhood (p 22–3):

> Spinning was another favourite activity. I'd sit on the floor and twirl around. The room spun with me. This self-stimulatory behaviour made me feel powerful, in control of things ... I enjoyed twirling myself around or spinning coins or lids round and round and round. Intensely preoccupied with the movement of the spinning coin or lid, I saw nothing or heard nothing ... But when I was in the world of people, I was extremely sensitive to noises ... What was exciting and adventuresome to Mother and my younger sisters and brother was a nightmare of sound to me, violating my ears and soul.

Janice Janzen (1996) also suggested that a preoccupation with the movement of objects and other narrow interests are related to sensory sensitivities. She felt that people with autism use sensory fixations to help them to cope in overwhelming situations where they are not comfortable or are unable to understand what is going on around them. Focusing on a small part of an object or a particular movement, allows them to block out the environment and what is happening around them. The repetitive movement or extreme focus blocks out unwanted stimuli and calms them down. According to Attwood (1993), people with autism use fixations as a form of 'self-hypnosis' to help them screen out unpleasant sensations.

Many of the repetitive actions and movements are also 'self-stimulating' and provide the means of stimulating a person who may not be particularly interested in, or stimulated by, their environment.

The notion of a theory of autism — that is, one explanation for the myriad of communication, social and behavioural problems associated with the disorder — is still some way in the future. It is more likely that most of the theories proposed to date have some merit and serve to provide information about the evolving and widening spectrum of disorders and patterns of behaviour that come under the general classification of autism.

Summary

Individuals with autism display a number of narrow interests and repetitive behaviours and rituals. These interests encompass the third element of Wing's triad that she refers to as impairment of social imagination and understanding. This impairment ties in with the DSM-IV criteria of restricted and repetitive behaviours, activities and interests.

Individuals with autism are frequently seen as obsessive about the state of their environment, requiring certain elements to always remain the same, from the positions of objects to the order of routines. Even slight disruptions to a routine, such as a drink being offered in a different coloured cup, or minimal adjustments in an object's position, such as the chair being moved out of the corner, can result in temper tantrums or other extreme emotional reactions until the problem is rectified and the routine is resumed. Such inflexibility can lead to a very rigid lifestyle for the person with autism and for family and friends around them. Similarly, people with autism may develop bizarre attachments to certain objects.

The repetitive behaviours of autism are related to people's resistance to change. Individuals with autism engage in rituals and repetitive behaviours in order to maintain the status quo and to bring order and routine into their lives. Repetitive behaviours are a way of expressing anxiety and stress and help people with autism to remain calm and block out unpleasant and unwanted stimuli. They frequently engage in stereotypical motor movements such as spinning, rocking, handflapping and head banging. They may become absorbed in watching moving objects for hours, such as spinning fans, flashing lights or cars driving past a window. Their reaction to sensory stimulation may vary from total indifference to over-sensitivity. Individuals with autism may experience a profoundly restricted range of interests and a preoccupation with one narrow interest.

There are a number of popular explanations about why individuals engage in repetitive behaviours. These include a link with sensory sensitivities and a form of self-stimulation.

7

Sensory Impairments

Our senses give us the information we need to function in the world.

Kranowitz 1998, p 38

In order to respond appropriately in different situations, a person has to integrate the information that he or she receives from all of the senses and then respond to that information automatically and without conscious thought. Individuals respond to sensory information from their environment in unique ways that help to determine their overall behaviour. If a person's perception of the stimulation they receive from their environment is distorted, then learning may be affected.

An abnormal response to sensory stimuli is one of the characteristics commonly associated with autism. Abnormal responses affect a person's body, co-ordination, organisation and development of perceptual and cognitive functions (Lowdon 1991).

How do the senses work?

Sensation, or what we see, hear, feel, smell and taste, provides information about the environment around us and also about ourselves. The information that is received through the senses helps us to understand our environment and how to act within that environment. The senses receive information from both outside and inside our body. They then provide that information to our central nervous system (CNS), which locates, sorts, and organises the sensations. The CNS sends messages to the rest of the body, enabling us to interact with the environment and with other people.

Myles et al (2000, p 98) explains:

Our central nervous system or brain helps us to regard, disregard, seek out, or avoid sensation to maintain or increase feelings of comfort, excitement, rest and positive interactions with objects and people. It also influences how we try to avoid that which is painful, uncomfortable, or stressful.

The central nervous system (CNS) consists of the cerebral hemispheres (including the cortex), cerebellum, brain stem and spinal cord. Within the cerebral hemispheres it is necessary for both sides to cooperate in order to perform the more complicated functions of the brain.

The brain is divided into two halves called hemispheres. At the base of the dividing fissure is the corpus callosum, which provides a communication link between the two hemispheres. The left hemisphere controls the right half of the body, and vice-versa. Although the right and left hemispheres appear to be mirror images of one another, there are important functional distinctions. In most people, the areas that control speech are located in the left hemisphere, while areas that govern spatial perceptions reside in the right hemisphere. Figures 7.1 and 7.2 illustrate the hemispheres of the brain and the central nervous system.

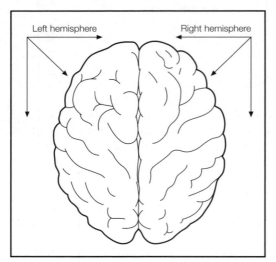

Figure 7.1 *Top view of the left and right hemispheres of the brain*

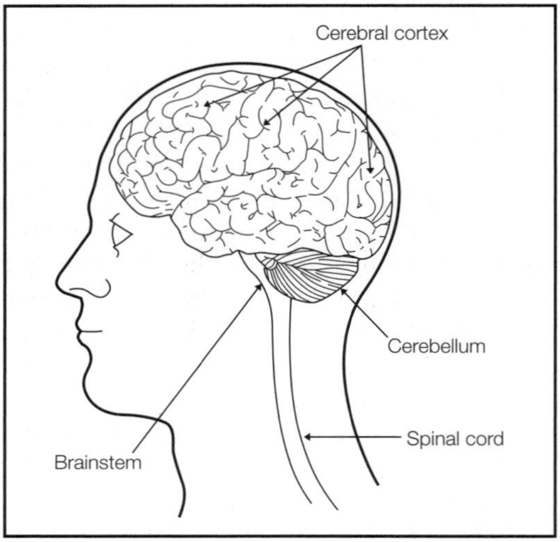

Figure 7.2 *Cross-sectional view of the cerebral cortex, cerebellum, brain stem and spinal cord*

The various parts have the following functions:

- The cerebral cortex processes sensory input from the eyes, ears and body. It executes fine, voluntary body movements and speech and is involved in developing thoughts and goals.
- The cerebellum filters all sensory input and organises gravity and movement as well as muscle and joint sensations for controlled body movements.
- The brain stem encases the reticular formation that contains fibres connecting it to the sensory systems, to motor neurons, and to many other parts of the brain.
- The spinal cord contains large bundles of nerve fibres that carry sensory information to the brain and motor messages via the nerves to the entire body.

The results of the actions we take and the feelings we generate in response to information received through the senses contribute to our sense of wellbeing.

Each person's interpretation of sensation is individual. Reactions to sensory stimuli differ among individuals, even though they may be receiving the same information through their senses. One person may like the scent of a particular perfume, while another may prefer to smell the more subtle scent of fresh flowers. One person may feel the cold and be wearing a heavy coat, while another may be dressed more lightly in a shirt and trousers. While each person interprets information differently, much of this is done at an automatic level, without cognitive awareness or conscious thought about what is taking place.

According to School Therapy Services (2002, p 18):

> Most of the interpretation of our internal and external environments occurs automatically and instantly. This allows us to focus on the specifics of the task at hand and not spend all our time processing or interpreting masses of incoming information.

Sensory processing is the ability to organise and interpret information we receive through our senses. Efficient sensory integration is required for the occurrence of effective sensory processing. Sensory integration refers to the process of creating efficient sensory pathways and connections in the central nervous system (CNS).

Dr Jean Ayres (1972, 1979), had a significant impact on the practice of occupational therapy through her works on the theory of sensory integration. Her published works provide a framework for the understanding of factors that can interfere with a person's ability to participate in a range of different activities. Dr Ayres (1979) defined sensory integration as 'the organisation of sensation for use. She concluded that the central nervous system involves the ongoing, dynamic interplay and comparison of information from all of the sensory systems. People's responses to different situations reflect how they process and integrate the information they receive from their senses.

While the integration of sensory information occurs naturally in most people, individuals with autism experience problems with sensory processing and modulation. Learning is dependent upon taking in information from the environment and from the movements that the body makes. According to current theory, the senses do not work in isolation so that the interaction between the senses also has to be considered. Carol Kranowitz in her book *The Out-of-Sync Child* (1998) claims that the individual senses must be understood before it is possible to understand sensory integration. According to Kranowitz, our senses give us the information that we require to function in our environment. The senses receive information from stimuli both outside and inside our bodies. Every move we make, every bite we eat, every object we touch, produces sensations. In order to ensure appropriate responses, the senses must all work together to provide the right information to the brain.

Both internal and external stimuli contribute to the information that is collected by all of the bodily senses (Kranowitz 1998). This information enables people to function in everyday life and helps them to make decisions about what to do in different situations.

The sensory systems are classified into the following areas:
- auditory — provides information about hearing;
- visual — provides information about seeing or vision;
- vestibular — provides information about movement;
- tactile — provides information about touch;
- proprioception and kinaesthesia — provide information about body position; and
- olfactory and gustatory: provide information about smell and taste.

These senses are divided into two groups that receive information from outside our body (far senses) and inside our body (near senses).

The senses of smell, touch, hearing, sight and taste are the five senses, described as the far senses, that respond to stimuli from outside the body, while three other sensory systems, the tactile, vestibular and proprioceptive systems respond to stimuli from inside the body and are often described as the near senses. The tactile system processes information about touch from the whole body; the vestibular system processes balance, movement and gravity information; and the proprioceptive system processes information about the body's position in space.

The far senses
The far senses involve the environment acting upon the body; that is, they respond to external stimuli from outside the body. The far senses include hearing, seeing, taste smell and touch.

The near senses
The near senses are more refined and relate to how the body perceives itself. They are often referred to as the 'hidden' senses because they respond to what is happening inside the body

and so cannot be directly observed or controlled. The near senses include touch, vestibular and proprioceptive. These senses are fundamental, usually operate automatically and lay the foundation for overall development.

Even prior to birth, the brain is working to organise and integrate sensory information. This sensory organisation is illustrated in Figure 7.3.

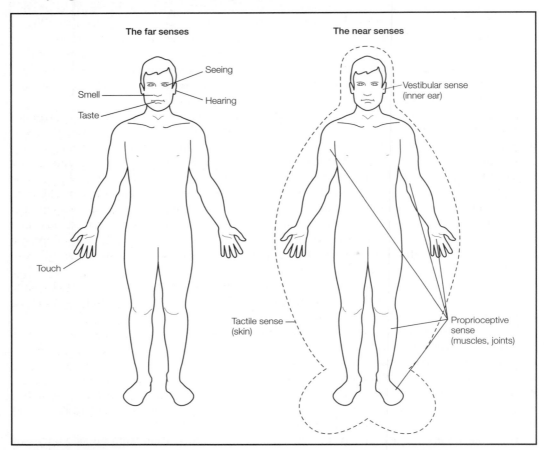

Figure 7.3 *The sensory systems detailing the near and the far senses of the human body (Kranowitz, C, 1998)*

What is sensory integration?

> Our bodies and the environment send our brains information through our senses. We process and organise this information so that we feel comfortable and secure. We are then able to respond appropriately to particular situations and environmental demands. This is sensory integration. (Yack et al 2002, p 21)

Sensory integration is the ability of the brain or central nervous system to organise, integrate and interpret sensory stimulation from the environment to produce purposeful goal-directed responses. It determines how effectively and efficiently a person can process and integrate sensory information from the tactile (touch), vestibular (balance), proprioceptive (position and movement), visual (sight), auditory (sound), olfactory (smell) and gustatory (taste) systems. More than one sense operates at any one time and processing this information usually takes place at an unconscious level. Sensory integration enables people to respond automatically, efficiently and comfortably to the sensations that they receive through their different senses. The ability to process and integrate information through the senses affects many different skills including speech and language, play, eye–hand coordination, motor skills, balance, attention and concentration, organisation, learning and self-esteem.

> Imagine that you are at work and get up to go to the kitchen to get a drink. As you walk into the kitchen you bump into someone leaving the kitchen with a hot cup of coffee. Automatically you adjust your body to maintain your balance and put out a hand to grab the drink. You then step back and remove your hand as you realise that the coffee is hot. This is an example of sensory integration.

In the example above, a person receives information from various sensory channels as soon as they bump into the other person. Their sense of touch tells them that there is an obstacle in their way. The proprioceptive system tells them the position of their muscles and joints, and the vestibular system tells them that their centre of gravity has moved and that they are likely to fall over. The visual system tells them that the other person is holding a cup; their sense of smell tells them that the cup contains coffee; and the sense of touch tells them that the coffee is hot. All of these senses work together to provide information that enables the person to make an appropriate response to the situation.

With good sensory integration, these processes occur automatically and allow individuals to make unconscious adjustments to rectify a given situation.

Williamson & Anzalone, in 1997, identified a number of interrelated components that define the sensory integration process. They claimed that the first step in the process is to register a sensation and the second step is to orient the sensation. The third step was to interpret the sensation and then organise a response. The final step is the execution of a response:

- Sensory registration occurs when a person first becomes aware of a sensory event such as touching, feeling, smelling or seeing something. Children with autism may over-register or are hyper-responsive to sensory stimulation. For example, some children can hear a video playing in the next room or hear the sound of an aeroplane long before it can be seen. Others may complain about the feel of certain textures on their skin. Children with autism may also under-register sensory information. They may not respond when their name is called or they may not feel pain when they fall over.
- Orientation enables a person to pay attention to new sensory information once it is registered. This enables them to determine what information is important and what can be ignored through sensory modulation and the functions of inhibition and facilitation. Children with autism may have poor sensory modulation and may focus on minor sensations rather than attending to what is important. A child, for example, may not attend to what is being said by the teacher because he is focusing on the sound of an air conditioner humming in the next room.
- Interpretation of sensory information allows a person to determine what to respond to and whether or not it is threatening. Interpretation of information enables people to use their accumulated knowledge and relate past experiences to what is happening at present. These experiences may include emotions, memories and past conversations. Atypical language, memory and emotional development in people with autism may interfere with their ability to interpret sensory information. For example, a child may react negatively to change because he is unable to interpret the information he receives through his senses and integrate it with past experiences. Every situation therefore appears as something new and unfamiliar and the child constantly strives for predictability in a world that appears disorganised and changing.

- Organisation of a response occurs when a person determines whether a response to a given event is necessary and what, if any, response they will make. Children with autism who have atypical cognitive and emotional development have difficulty organising appropriate responses. Their emotional responses may be exaggerated or minimised and they can experience difficulties maintaining attention, formulating and comparing choices, and initiating action plans.
- Execution of a response may be a motor, cognitive or emotional action to the sensory message that has been received. The ability to execute a response is dependent on the previous steps and also adequate motor planning abilities (praxis). Children with autism have impaired motor planning abilities (dyspraxia) that significantly interfere with their ability to plan and execute motor responses. An individual, for example, who engages in self-stimulatory behaviours such as rocking, spinning or flapping may do so because he has difficulty switching, regulating or stopping motor acts.

'Sensory integration contributes to the development of self-regulation, comfort, motor planning, motor skills, attention and readiness to learn.' (Yack et al 1998, 2002, p 28)

What is dyspraxia?

Children and adults who have efficient sensory integration usually have good motor planning skills (praxia). Praxia is what enables people to organise, plan and execute a wide range of skills in a refined and efficient manner. This enables them to tie their shoelaces, put things together or pull them apart, follow sequences, understand how parts relate to a whole and how to initiate motor tasks. 'Motor planning (praxia) requires automatically anticipating what the next step is and what strength or speed is needed for performing it, such as bringing a cup of soup to the mouth or riding a bike.' (Arkwright 1995, p 15).

Children and adults with autism may have difficulty with *motor planning (dyspraxia)*. There are several components of praxia that require accurate information from the tactile, vestibular, proprioceptive, auditory and visual systems. The components are:

- Imitation — the early ability to organise facial expression and body language leads to the later ability to use gesture, facial expression and so forth.
- Ideation — the ability to base interactions not only on imitation of others, but also on the ideas that have been generated and communicated.
- Initiation — the ability to initiate activities and an understanding of how to begin the activity.
- Construction — the ability to put objects together in new and different ways and organise self and the local environment.
- Feedback — the ability to process the information received from proprioception that enables the refinement of motor skills. It creates a memory of how things are done and encourages generalisation.
- Feed forward — enables the unconscious anticipation of the next step, strength or speed required to perform a certain motor act.
- Grading — the ability to vary the intensity of what we do. It enables individuals to catch balls of different sizes and climb stairs of different heights.
- Timing and sequencing — the performance of motor tasks at the appropriate time and in the correct order.
- Motor planning — the ability to create, use and combine various motor skills to perform new, more complex acts.

In summary, Arkwright (1995, p 16) says:

If you had a van and then bought a small car, you would need to re-learn how to turn and park, how hard to turn the steering wheel, and how hard to brake. After driving for a while, you learn to make these adjustments and driving becomes automatic. In contrast, a child with dyspraxia continues to do something as though it was the first time — each time. Tasks do not become readily or completely automatic for the child with dyspraxia.

What is a sensory impairment?

As outlined in the previous section, sensory impairment is the inability of a person to 'make sense' of all of the sensations that are experienced; that is, to integrate them. Each individual sensory system within a person also operates in a similar way. The first step in the process is to *register* that the sensation is happening and then to *orient* or pay attention to it. After that, the individual has to *interpret* the possible meaning of the sensation and *organise* an appropriate response to the sensation. The final step is to execute the selected response.

Some people, however, are unable to deal with all of the sensory input they receive. They have difficulty organising and processing the information necessary to perform even the simplest of tasks. Individuals with autism vary greatly in their ability to take in information from their senses, integrate that information with knowledge already stored and then respond with organised behaviour (Prizant & Rubin 1999).

A perspective from Aarons & Gittens (1992, pp 42–3) is:

Sensory abnormalities may take the form of visual or auditory perceptual disturbances, lack or partial lack of body image and position in space, abnormal use of touch, smell, taste, and over- or under- sensitivity to pain, heat and cold. Some children appear to over- or under-react to the stimuli of light and noise. Other children show distress at being touched while others positively seek it out. It is a frequent observation that some autistic children persist in using their proximal senses well past infancy, when such behaviours *would* have been developmentally appropriate.

Temple Grandin puts it this way (1995, p 39):

Problems caused by noise sensitivity, over-sensitivity to touch, and difficulties with rhythm all cause many behaviour problems. These sensory sensitivities influence learning, communication and social abilities.

Unusual sensory experience is a phenomenon that has been observed in individuals with autism for many years and is listed as an associated feature of autism in the American Diagnostic and Statistical Manual (DSM-IV). Recent publications by adults diagnosed with autism have provided information about their sensory deficits. Temple Grandin (*Emergence: Labelled Autistic*, 1986), Sean Barron (*There's a Boy in Here*, 1992), Donna Williams (*Nobody Nowhere*, 1992) and Darren White (*Autism from the Inside*, 1987) have all discussed their sensory problems and provided insights into their extreme reactions to certain sensory stimuli. In *A is for Autism*, a short film about sensory issues and autism, Temple Grandin states:

I was intensely preoccupied with the movement of the spinning coin or lid and I saw nothing or heard nothing. I did it because it shut out sound that hurt my ears. No sound intruded in my fixation. It was like being deaf, even a sudden noise didn't startle me out of my world.

The way that the sensory systems and the brain work together is very complex. People with autism respond to sensory stimuli in many different ways and they also respond differently across the senses. A person with autism may present as over-sensitive or under-sensitive to sensory stimuli and these sensitivities may impact on one or more of their senses. For example, one person with autism may have a limited diet and eat only food that is coloured yellow, be sensitive to certain sounds and like to look at ceiling fans or lights flicking on and off. Another person may eat inedible substances such as soap, cigarette butts, paper or rocks, dislike being touched, wear only cotton clothing and smell everything. One person may be sensitive to certain sounds such as high-pitched noises while someone else may crave sounds and constantly squeal or hum loudly.

What is meant by sensory sensitivities?

Sensory processing difficulties are commonly seen in many children and adults with autism. These difficulties impair their overall ability to function and to perform daily activities. Sensory processing difficulties cause tremendous disruption to people's lives in a number of areas including looking and listening, academic learning, remembering, coordination, social interaction and motor development. Sensory processing difficulties cause many individuals with autism to be under-sensitive or over-sensitive to certain sensory experiences, leading to either seeking or avoidance behaviours. According to School Therapy Services (2002, p 21):

> At a cell level it is the balance between the excitatory transmitters and the inhibitory transmitters at the synapse, that allow the electrical impulses to be passed along the CNS to the brain.

Changes that occur in the balance between the transmitters enable us to focus on the important information that is received and also to screen out information that is not needed. Children with autism are unable to 'dampen' sensory input so that there are too many excitatory transmitters, or they are unable to 'increase the sensitivity' to the sensory input they receive and so end up with an imbalance of inhibitory transmitters. These children fall into two broad categories: either being over-sensitive (hyper-sensitivity), or being under-sensitive (hypo-sensitivity). These sensory responses may fluctuate from day to day so that there appears to be a lack of consistency in a person's response to particular stimuli.

Hyper-sensitivity

Hyper- or over-sensitive response indicates a heightened response to a particular sensory experience as the sensations are registered too intensely. In other words, the nervous system becomes highly stimulated by even a small amount of sensation.

The over-sensitive individual may avoid touching or being touched by objects or people, become overexcited by too much visual stimulation (perhaps in large shopping malls), become distressed and cover the ears to block out certain sounds or voices and may object to certain textures or even temperatures of foods or gag when made to eat.

A person who is over-sensitive responds to stimulation in one of two ways in order to cope with the information he or she receives:

1. The person who has *sensitivity to stimulation* tends to be distractible and has difficulty blocking out incoming information in order to focus on the task at hand.

> Radar is hypersensitive to sounds and whenever he hears an aeroplane in the distance (he can usually hear it long before anyone else is aware of a plane overhead) he becomes very distressed and covers his ears and will lash out at anyone standing near him.

2. The person who is a sensory avoider actively engages in reducing the frequency and intensity of sensory stimulation, is resistant to change and develops rigid rituals to create a predictable environment.

> Josh is hypersensitive to certain tastes and textures. He has a very limited diet of rice and white bread and occasionally eats chicken. He will not try new foods and even refuses to eat the bread if it is the wrong brand.

Hypo-sensitivity

Hypo- or under-sensitive response indicates a dampened response to a particular sensory experience, because the sensations are registered less intensely than normal. In other words, a greater amount of sensation is required to stimulate the nervous system.

The under-sensitive individual registers sensations less intensely than another person and may not receive enough sensory information from everyday events. Subsequently, an increased amount of stimulation is needed to achieve optimal alertness levels. The under-sensitive person may have a high tolerance to pain or temperature, crave fast and spinning movements such as swinging, jumping and rocking, may sniff unpleasant odours, lick or taste inedible objects, touch different textures and study visual patterns.

A person who is under-sensitive may respond to stimulation in two different ways in an attempt to cope with the information.

1. The person who is a *sensory seeker* actively pursues sensory input to stimulate their system. They tend to be active, fidgety and excitable and need sensory stimulation incorporated into daily programs to meet their sensory needs.

> Robert is under-sensitive to different tastes and textures. He is constantly mouthing objects and will eat sand and dirt and things he finds in the garden. He also chews and sucks the sleeves of his t-shirt and bites the furniture at home.

2. The person who has *poor registration* accepts the dampened sensory state and does not really attempt to engage in the environment. They tend to lack initiative and have poor motor control due to reduced sensory feedback.

> Mark is under-sensitive to touch and has poor co-ordination and balance. He is a very passive child who sits around and appears quite self-absorbed. He tends to bump himself and falls over if he attempts to run but does not appear to feel pain.

A person's response to a particular sensory experience may fluctuate from one day to the next. Some days they may actively seek out certain sensory experiences and at other times may avoid them. Abnormal responses to sensory stimuli are indications of sensory dysfunction.

According to Kranowitz (1998), it is important to keep in mind that people with sensory dysfunction do not necessarily show problems in all sensory areas; that they may fluctuate from day to day in their responses to sensory stimuli; that they may show signs of a particular sensory dysfunction but not necessarily have a dysfunction in the particular area; that an individual may be hyper-sensitive in some areas and hypo-sensitive in others and that we all exhibit some sensory integration problems occasionally.

What is sensory dysfunction?

Sensory dysfunction describes an inability to process sensory input. Dysfunction may occur with a specific sensory system or with many systems. A person may have vestibular dysfunction and have difficulty processing information from the vestibular receptors within the ears; another person may have difficulties processing tactile stimulation coming from the skin; or a person may have global sensory dysfunction and be unable to integrate the stimulation from a number of different sensory systems.

In general, dysfunction within the tactile, vestibular and proprioceptive systems may manifest itself in a number of different ways. Arkwright (1995, p 1) says:

> Input from the three basic senses (touch, movement, position) combined with the auditory and visual senses are critical to the development of mature motor planning, coordinated use of both sides of the body, balance, eye–hand coordination, body awareness, language, visual perception and emotional stability.

Activity levels may be either unusually high or unusually low so that individuals may be overly active or extremely passive. Gross motor and fine motor coordination problems are also common when these systems are dysfunctional and may result in speech/language delays and poor academic achievement. Behaviourally, a person may become impulsive, distractible and show a general lack of planning. Some children and adults may have difficulty adjusting to new situations and may react with frustration, aggression or withdrawal. People with sensory integration problems may be overly sensitive (hyper-sensitive) or under-reactive (hypo-sensitive) to sensory input such as touch, movement, sight or sound. For example, wearing certain clothing, lights flashing or loud noises may cause sensory problems in some individuals with autism.

Among the observable signs of sensory dysfunction in individuals with autism are:

■ either hyper-sensitivity or hypo-sensitivity or even mixed sensitivities to sensory stimulation;
■ either seeking or avoiding sensory input;
■ poor motor planning;
■ either over-arousal or under-arousal to stimulation that leads to a person presenting as hyperactive or self-absorbed and passive;
■ poor attending skills; and
■ poor coordination and difficulty learning and remembering new tasks.

When sensory information is not processed adequately, the individual reacts to it in unusual ways and requires assistance to learn more appropriate responses. Because sensory dysfunction can occur within a particular sensory system or within a number of different systems, it is important to have a basic understanding of the different senses and how they impact on a person's behaviour and wellbeing.

What are the sensory systems?

Initially, sensory integration focused primarily on three basic senses — tactile, vestibular and proprioceptive. According to Dr A Jean Ayres (1982), these three senses are not only interconnected but are also connected to other systems in the brain. These senses allow us to interpret and respond to different stimuli in the environment. Current research into sensory problems, however, has found that all of the senses may be affected in some way in people with autism.

The tactile sense

The tactile system provides us with our sense of touch. It is the first sensory system to operate in the uterus, and it is important that it works efficiently from birth.

The tactile system receives information through the receptors in the skin. It receives information about pressure, vibration, movement, temperature and pain. The tactile sense provides essential information that enables us to participate in a range of everyday activities. The tactile system is closely linked to the part of the brain vital for survival and responsible for our 'fight' or 'flight' reactions. This close connection with survival mechanisms means that the tactile system is closely associated with our emotional state. Children and adults with touch processing deficits often have emotional and behavioural difficulties.

As with all sensory systems, the tactile system has both protective and discriminative abilities that complement each other throughout life. The protective system is more primitive and alerts us to danger. It triggers the 'fight' or 'flight' response and is associated with pain, temperature and crude touch. The discriminative system provides information about the quality of the item being touched. It tells you where and what is being touched and is associated with vibration, pressure, proprioception, fine touch and adaptive behaviour.

The two types of responses must be balanced and interact appropriately in an adaptive manner to ongoing sensations from the skin. When the sensory integrative processes of registration, orientation, interpretation, and sensory modulation are intact, we are able to work out which touch is pleasurable, which touch is alarming, which touch can be ignored and which touch needs to be explored further.

What is tactile dysfunction?

Inefficient processing of tactile sensations is described as tactile dysfunction. Children with autism may present with dysfunction in the tactile system. This dysfunction disrupts a child's fine motor skills, motor planning, body awareness and visual perception.

Children may be hyper-sensitive or hypo-sensitive to touch. Children who are hyper-sensitive, or over-sensitive may be described as being tactile defensive. Clothing labels, stitching or wearing constricting clothes (particularly around the neck, wrists, ankles and waist) may cause problems. This may account for a preference for particular clothing. Children may also overreact to being touched by others and resist, or avoid, touching others. Many children also tolerate a narrow range of food, having a limited diet that may include only certain food 'textures'. They may refuse to have their face washed or hair washed, brushed and cut.

Children who are tactile defensive are extremely sensitive to light touch and will avoid touching certain materials, avoid getting their hands dirty (refuse to touch playdough, sand or paint), and will tend to use their fingertips to manipulate objects rather than their whole hands.

It is important to never force a child who is tactile defensive to touch certain substances or materials.

Children who are hypo-sensitive, or under-sensitive, to touch may be described as having a poor response to tactile stimulation. An under-sensitive person requires more tactile stimulation and will often seek out activities that will provide this. A child may constantly touch and feel objects with different textures and love to play with messy substances such as sand, rice or mud. Another person may like to squeeze into tight places, enjoy being held tightly and prefer to wear tight clothing.

Sometimes children with autism appear to be insensitive or overly sensitive to pain. They may not react immediately to an injury or they may carry on for hours over the slightest bump.

The vestibular sense

The vestibular system refers to structures within the inner ear that detect movement, gravity and changes to the position of the head. The system relates to balance and determines the direction and speed of movement in the body. Kranowitz (1998, p 98) explains: 'The vestibular system takes in sensory messages about balance and movement from the neck, eyes and body.'

Just as the tactile system is our sense of touch through which relationships are developed with others, the vestibular system is our sense of movement and gravity. The vestibular system helps to keep people in touch with the world around them. It is through the vestibular system that a relationship with the earth is developed; that is, knowing what is right side up, upside down, left, right, horizontal and vertical. Vestibular input tells us whether or not we are moving, how quickly we are moving, and in what direction we are moving. It provides a physical reference that helps to make sense of visual information, particularly where we and other things are in our environment, in relation to each other. Children and adults with vestibular system dysfunction are likely to have problems in many aspects of daily life. They often appear to be uncoordinated and unable to perform tasks requiring sequencing and timing.

The different types of vestibular movement can have a calming or excitatory effect on a person. Back and forth, side to side, or up and down linear movements, such as rocking or swinging, can be calming. On the other hand, circular movements, such as spinning or twirling, tend to excite the vestibular system.

The vestibular system has both protective and discriminative functions. In young children, movement can stimulate reflexes designed to prevent falling. As the brain develops, more mature reactions also develop in order to help protect the body from harm. According to Yack et al (2002, p 46):

> The vestibular system can discriminate between acceleration, deceleration, and rotary movements. It can detect movements that are slow, fast and rhythmic. Some vestibular sensations, such as slow rocking, can be calming. Other vestibular sensations, like quick movements, can excite the nervous system.

What is vestibular dysfunction?

Inefficient processing of the information about movement, space, gravity and balance is referred to as vestibular dysfunction. Children with autism may present with dysfunction in the vestibular system. This dysfunction disrupts a child's movement and balance, muscle tone, motor planning and bilateral coordination.

Children who are hyper-sensitive may be afraid of movement activities such as swings, slides, ramps and inclines and appear fearful in space. They may have difficulty learning to climb stairs or walk up/down hills and be afraid of walking or crawling on uneven or unstable surfaces. In general they appear quite physically clumsy.

Children who are hypo-sensitive may actively seek intense sensory experiences by spinning, jumping and rocking to stimulate their vestibular systems. They are constantly on the go and do not seem able to sit still. They may not register movement appropriately, or their nervous system may crave excessive amounts of movement to stay alert and organised. These children may not recognise the demands of gravity or adequately register the qualities of movement and may need intensive supervision to prevent them from hurting themselves.

The proprioceptive sense

Proprioception is the conscious and unconscious awareness of body position and movement. The proprioceptive system refers to components of muscles, joints and tendons that provide a person with a body scheme, a sense of his or her own body. Proprioception is stimulation of the sensory receptors inside the joints and muscles. It contributes to body awareness, motor planning and motor control and it tells the brain when and how the muscles are contracting and stretching; when and how the joints are flexing, extending or being pulled or pushed; where one's body parts are in space and what they are doing; the rate and timing of movements; how much force muscles are exerting and how the vestibular system can be modulated.

When proprioception is functioning efficiently, body position in space is automatically adjusted; for example, sitting properly in a chair, stepping off the footpath on to the road and climbing a ladder. It is also responsible for fine motor movements such as writing with a pencil, using a spoon to eat soup, buttoning a shirt and cutting with scissors. Proprioception is responsible for more than pulling, pushing, stretching and pressing. It enables the information from the joints, muscles and tendons to help adjust the body position for smooth movements with the right amount of pressure.

While there are children with autism who display normal or even precocious development in this area, others may lack or have an underdeveloped awareness of their own body image and position in space. For example, Temple Grandin in her book *Thinking in Pictures* (1996, p 62) describes how as a child, 'I would wrap myself up in blankets and get under sofa cushions, because the pressure was relaxing. I used to daydream for hours in elementary school about constructing a device that would apply pressure to my body.'

What is proprioceptive dysfunction?

Some people do not adequately receive or process information from their muscles, joints, tendons, ligaments or connective tissue. Poor proprioception disrupts a person's body position and movement, coordination, motor planning, posture, balance and self-esteem. Poor proprioception is usually associated with tactile and/or vestibular difficulties.

Among the possible signs of proprioceptive dysfunction in a child or adult are:

- stiff and uncoordinated movements;
- clumsiness and a tendency to knock things over or bump into things;
- craving for deep pressure against the body such as tight hugs, climbing into small spaces and being wrapped in a blanket;
- difficulty coordinating muscles to get in and out of a chair or climb up or down stairs; and
- writing or drawing with a pen or pencil and knowing how hard to press down on the pencil.

Children and adults with proprioceptive dysfunction usually display clumsiness, a tendency to fall, a lack of awareness of body position in space, odd body posturing, minimal crawling, difficulty manipulating small objects, difficulty eating independently and resistance to engaging in motor activities.

The visual sense

According to Kranowitz (1998), vision may be described as the process whereby the eyes take in information visually and then organise an appropriate response.

Visual processing is the ability to interpret information received through the eyes.

The visual receptors located in the eyes receive masses of information about the surrounding visual environment including contrast between light and dark, colour and movement. They help us to detect light and to create visual images.

The visual sense delivers information about colour, contrast, line, shape, form and movement. This information impacts on how individuals perceive the world and is important in the development of hand–eye coordination, fine motor skills such as writing, and cognitive skills such as reading. The visual sense helps to determine what to pay attention to and what to ignore as well as helping to direct our actions and movements.

Children with autism commonly show ability in tasks involving visual perception; for example, recognising and matching shapes, letters and numbers, and completing formboards and jigsaw puzzles. The visual characteristics of children with autism include:

- problems shifting attention from one person or object to another;
- difficulty processing visual stimuli such as recognising expressions and feelings in other people;
- difficulty giving and maintaining eye contact with another person;
- a tendency to engage in visual stimulatory actions such as spinning, rocking, handflapping and a fascination with certain parts of objects; and
- problems with depth perception leading to a fear of heights, stairs, elevators or tunnels.

A child who has deficits in visual processing may have good vision but be unable to respond accurately or consistently to visual information.

What is visual dysfunction?

Children with autism who are hyper-sensitive to visual stimuli will often squint, look out of the corners of their eyes or look through their hands and actively avoid experiences that provide visual stimulation. They will stare at certain objects or patterns and flap their hands or flick objects in front of their eyes. Many children appear sensitive to light and are confused by a change of floor pattern or stairways and appear clumsy by bumping into objects. Some children do not appear to notice other people and will walk over the top of another child but at the same time may be fascinated by lights, ceiling fans or shadows on a wall or floor.

The child who is hypo-sensitive to visual stimuli will seek visual sensations and may engage in behaviours such as flicking lights on and off; watching repetitive movements such as turning pages of a book, opening and closing doors, watching fans spin; lining up objects; looking at things out of the corner of his or her eyes and looking at things from unusual angles.

The processing of visual information requires competence in a number of skills including visual tracking (the ability to track one's eyes from left to right in an efficient manner to ensure the quick completion of a task), visual discrimination (the ability to discern similarities and differences visually), visual memory (the ability to store and retrieve information that has been given with a visual stimulus), and visual figure ground perception (the ability to visually attend to the designated stimulus and not be distracted by the background). Children with visual dysfunction have deficits in at least one, or more, of these skills and may need direct or indirect programming support to develop them.

The auditory sense

According to Kranowitz (1998), auditory perception may be described as the process whereby a person receives, identifies, discriminates and then responds to different sounds from their environment. The auditory system uses the outer and middle ear to receive noise and sound information while the hearing receptors are located in the inner ear. It receives information about volume, pitch and rhythm but its primary function is to detect sound. The system processes and organises information and enables us to distinguish between similar sounds, remember what we hear and develop communication and literacy skills.

This system is closely linked to the vestibular sense. As a result, vestibular dysfunction can impact on a person's ability to process information that is heard. Inefficient processing of information related to sound is known as auditory dysfunction.

What is auditory dysfunction?

Children with autism may be indifferent to, distressed by, or even fascinated by, sound. Commonly, children's indifference to speech and lack of alerting behaviour to the human voice often leads to a mistaken diagnosis of hearing impairment. The first step for parents then is to have children's hearing checked to rule out a hearing loss. Careful observation of the child's auditory behaviour will usually reveal a pattern of inconsistency that is incompatible with deafness. A child, while ignoring speech and loud noises, will speedily respond to the slightest sound if it relates to something of interest, such as the opening of the fridge door or the rustle of a chocolate wrapper. Children with autism will often cover their ears to shut out certain sounds that distress them. They may be sensitive to certain pitch or sounds such as a toilet flushing, vacuum cleaner or a person singing.

Some children are hyper-sensitive to certain sound frequencies and are able to hear an aeroplane passing overhead or a siren several seconds before anyone else. The same child may cover his or her ears to block out sounds; cry at certain sounds such as vacuum cleaners, hair dryers or lawn mowers; prefer people to use a soft voice when talking and dislike being sung to.

The child who is hypo-sensitive to sound does not appear to hear what people say; likes music and certain sounds; likes toys that make sounds; prefers people to talk in an animated way and does not notice loud noises such as vacuum cleaners, lawn mowers, or car sirens.

Sound sensitivities often fluctuate from day to day and behaviour problems commonly occur because people may be overly sensitive to certain sounds and anticipate them in different situations.

The olfactory sense and gustatory sense

The sense of smell is very sensitive and is closely linked to the sense of taste. Taste depends heavily on the stimulation of olfactory receptors. In fact, taste is 80% smell. This explains why many children with autism will smell food before they eat it. The temperature and texture of foods can also enhance or detract from their taste.

What is olfactory and gustatory dysfunction?

As with other sensory areas, children with autism may have a hypo- or hyper-impairment to any or all of the factors involved in the gustatory process. For example, they may have a heightened or lowered sense of one of the basic taste qualities, such as sweet or bitter, or have a heightened or lowered sense of the temperature of food. This is also likely to be closely linked with smell.

Taste, however, is different from other sensory impairments because children are not constantly bombarded with taste sensations from their environment (such as sounds and sights). Children also have control over taste to some extent by limiting the type of food that they eat. A sensory impairment in this area is likely to be a problem only when a person has a restricted diet that is not adequate to provide sustainable nourishment for them, when a person places non-food items in the mouth or licks non-food items, or displays inappropriate social behaviours such as sniffing people.

For individuals with autism, the sense of smell may be highly attuned. Their perception of certain smells may inhibit their concentration on the task at hand. It is also possible that certain smells will evoke memories that trigger a particular behaviour.

The person who is hyper-sensitive to taste and/or smell usually prefers bland foods, reacts negatively to certain smells such as perfume, has a very limited diet and only eats foods of a certain texture.

The person who is hypo-sensitive to taste and/or smell usually enjoys highly seasoned food, explores things by licking and/or smelling them and will eat things he or she should not eat.

REMEMBER

- Some people may be under-responsive to sensory input and not fully register information from the senses.
- Other people may overreact to certain stimuli and experience a sensory overload.
- Being aware of a person's difficulty in processing sensory information is an important step in assisting that person to manage it.
- Sensory fluctuations occur so that a person's ability to process information from the senses may vary from day to day.

Once parents or therapists have identified that a child or adult has unusual responses to sensory stimuli, they should observe the individual, make notes and complete an interview with relevant adults. This is the first step in establishing a sensory history and profile. The profile can be completed from published questionnaires or informal checklists.

How are an individual's sensory needs and strengths assessed?

If a child or adult has sensory problems, it may be beneficial to complete a sensory screening questionnaire. A number of sensory questionnaires have been published and provide valuable information about sensory processing. Screening measures can be categorised as either formal or informal. Formal assessments include standardised instruments that compare an individual's profile to those of typically developing peers. Some therapists prefer to use more informal checklists and questionnaires and to observe the child or adult in a number of different settings. Informal assessments consist of reviews of records, inventories, checklists, interviews and observations.

Among the most commonly used formal assessments are:

- The *Sensory Profile* (Dunn 1999) has a number of behavioural statements that are organised into all the sensory systems and includes observations about activity level and social and emotional behaviours.
- The *Short Sensory Profile* (Dunn 1999) is an abbreviated 38-item form of the Sensory Profile and is appropriate for children aged 3–7 years.
- The *Sensory Integration and Praxis Test* (Ayres 1989) is designed to identify patterns of function and dysfunction in sensory integration and motor planning.

Among the informal assessments are the following:

- *Building Bridges Through Sensory Integration* (Yack et al 2002) considers a child's behaviours across sensory areas within the context of specific daily tasks.
- *Motivation Assessment Scale* (Durand & Crimmins 1992) is useful in determining whether a specific behaviour has a sensory function or not.

The interpretation of results of sensory screening assessments is usually completed by occupational therapists or other professionals trained in sensory integration. A skilled interpretation provides parents with comprehensive information about a child's needs and strengths across environments, in a variety of settings, with different adults and peers.

The sensory profile should include recommendations that are detailed enough to be implemented by all of the professionals and parents who have regular contact with the child. The sensory information helps in the development of programming strategies that will support the child through a number of different environments.

It is also important to maintain close collaboration among all of the therapists involved to ensure that the recommendations are effective and address the child's particular needs.

The sensory questionnaire and sensory profile should indicate specific problems associated with the person's ability to process sensory information. One of the most common problems associated with autism is a difficulty with motor planning (dyspraxia).

What is a sensory diet?

A sensory diet is a planned and scheduled activity program designed to meet specific sensory needs. Wilbarger & Wilbarger (1991) developed the approach to provide the correct amount of sensory input to achieve and maintain optimal levels of arousal and performance in the nervous system and said, 'The ability to appropriately orient and respond to sensations can be enhanced by a proper sensory diet.'

In order to balance a dysfunctional sensory system, children require a certain amount of activity and sensation to be organised, alert and adaptable. A calming integrating response may be achieved through a 'sensory diet' of different strategies. A sensory diet however does not involve simply increasing the amount of sensory experiences that a child is exposed to on a daily basis. The most successful sensory diets are individualised and take into account the individual needs of the person. Each person has unique sensory needs and the diet must reflect these needs and be customised to meet these individual needs and responses.

A sensory diet should be developed by an occupational therapist. The occupational therapist will conduct an extensive evaluation and complete an individual sensory profile to assess sensory processing abilities and determine what types of sensory activities would be most beneficial. Engaging children in sensory experiences on a regular basis can assist them to focus, attend and interact more easily. A sensory diet may include:

- Calming strategies — these strategies help children who are anxious and who are sensory defensive because they help to relax the nervous system and reduce exaggerated responses to sensory input.

- Organising strategies — these strategies help children who are either over- or under-active to become more focused, alert and attentive.
- Alerting strategies — these strategies can help a child who is under-reactive to sensory input, passive or lethargic become more focused and attentive. They should be closely monitored to prevent over stimulation.

Learning and interaction with others is maximised when children's bodies are calm and relaxed and they are attentive to the task ahead.

Summary

Many children and adults with autism have a dysfunctional sensory system. One or more senses are either over- or under-reactive to stimulation. Sensory issues are, therefore, relevant for children and adults with autism. Sensory impairment is listed as an associated feature of autism in the DSM-IV and is now confirmed as a major problem for many individuals with autism.

The different senses work to provide essential information to the central nervous system and brain to enable us to function in different settings and situations. Here I've provided an explanation about how the central nervous system registers, orients, interprets and organises sensory information and then executes appropriate responses. This process is known as sensory integration. Sensory integration contributes to the development of many of the skills that we need to learn in order to be able to live independently.

Sensory integration focuses primarily on three basic senses — tactile, vestibular, and pro-prioceptive. Their interconnections start forming before birth and continue to develop as the person matures and interacts with the environment. The three senses are not only interconn-ected but are also connected with other systems in the brain. The inter-relationship among these three senses is complex. Basically, they allow us to experience, interpret, and respond to different stimuli in our environment.

Sensory impairment in autism is most notable in the extreme reactions to sensory stimuli. These reactions have been documented in publications and descriptions written by individuals with autism. The way that the sensory systems and the brain work together is very complex. People with autism respond to sensory stimuli in many different ways and they also respond differently across the senses. A person with autism may present as over-sensitive or under-sensitive to sensory stimuli and these sensitivities may impact on one or more of their senses. Some individuals fluctuate between these extremes.

Parents and therapists need to be aware of the sensory sensitivities commonly seen in autism and understand the different senses and the results of dysfunction within these senses.

The ability to plan and execute different motor tasks is called praxis. In order for this system to work properly, it must rely on obtaining accurate information from the sensory systems and then organising and interpreting this information efficiently and effectively.

Evaluation and treatment of basic sensory integrative processes is performed by occupa-tional therapists and/or physical therapists. The therapist's general goals are:

- to provide the child with sensory information which helps organise the central nervous system;
- to assist the child in inhibiting and/or modulating sensory information; and
- to assist the child in processing a more organised response to sensory stimuli.

8

Diagnosis and Assessment

There are no tests yet developed that can be used to make the diagnosis of autism nor any that can tell the difference between sub-groups within autistic disorders ... There is reason to hope that useful tests will be found but we do not have them at the present time.

Wing 1996, p 27

Autism is a lifelong disability of biological origin. In order for a diagnosis to be given, a person must present with deficits in communication and social skills, imitation and problem-solving abilities, and a distinctive pattern of repetitive and ritualistic behaviours.

There may also be evidence of abnormal sensory responses. Individuals with these deficits are classified autistic according to the DSM-IV (Diagnostic and Statistical Manual of Mental Disorders from the American Psychiatric Association) or the ICD-10 (International Classification of Diseases, Version 10). These classification systems divide the general category of pervasive developmental disorders (PDD) into several subcategories that include:

- autistic disorder;
- pervasive developmental disorder not otherwise specified (PDD-NOS);
- Asperger's disorder;
- Rett's disorder; and
- childhood disintegrative disorder.

The term PDD, however, is considered by many diagnosticians to be too general. It does not cover the diversity of conditions that are associated with the label and fails to adequately describe them. Many professionals have moved away from using PDD and prefer to use the term, introduced by Wing & Gould (1979), 'autistic spectrum disorders' (ASD) to describe and label the group of conditions outlined in the DSM-IV and ICD-10.

What are autism spectrum disorders?

As outlined earlier in Chapter 1, autism or autistic spectrum disorders refers to the traditional form as identified by Leo Kanner in 1943 and originally labelled as 'early infantile autism'. According to the DSM-IV, a diagnosis of autism is dependent on a person having six out of a possible twelve diagnostic criteria with at least two from the area of qualitative impairment in social interaction and at least one each from the areas of qualitative impairment in communication and restricted, repetitive and stereotyped patterns of behaviour, interest and activities.

Asperger's syndrome was first recognised by an Austrian physician Hans Asperger in 1944. He observed a group of children with similar characteristics to those described by Kanner, but he also recognised a number of differences including an odd use of language, poor social skills and a lack of humour. It was not until the publication of the DSM-IV in the mid 1990s that Asperger's syndrome was widely recognised and acknowledged. There are eight diagnostic criteria for Asperger's syndrome. In order for a diagnosis to be given, a person must have at least two impairments in social relating and at least one in behaviour/interests. According to the diagnostic criteria for Asperger's syndrome, there should be no significant delays in either language or cognitive development.

The diagnosis of pervasive developmental disorder-not otherwise specified (PDD-NOS) is made when there is a severe and pervasive impairment in the development of reciprocal social interaction or verbal and non-verbal communication skills; or when stereotyped behaviour, interests and activities are present, but the criteria is not met for a specific pervasive developmental disorder, schizophrenia, schizotypal personality disorder, or avoidant personality disorder. This category includes 'atypical autism' where the criteria for autistic disorder are not met because of late age of onset, atypical symptomatology, or sub-threshold symptomatology, or all of these.

Although autism is probably present at birth, it may not be noted until infants fail to develop appropriate communication skills at 18–36 months of age. It is important to identify children with autism and begin appropriate interventions as soon as possible. Early intervention will help to improve a child's overall development, reduce inappropriate behaviours and lead to better long-term functional outcomes.

There are several ways that children with autism can be identified. Parents are usually the first to question their child's development when, for example, the child fails to respond when they are called or fails to develop speech to communicate basic needs. The initial reaction of many parents and professionals is often to question whether the child has a hearing impairment and to request a hearing assessment. Children are then usually referred to a paediatrician who begins to explore alternative possible diagnoses. Health care workers or other professionals may be concerned about a child's development either at the time of a periodic health examination or when a child is being evaluated for some other health problem (such as a possible hearing loss) or developmental problem (such as poor sleeping patterns, eating problems or delayed speech).

Although autism is considered a medical condition, and should be diagnosed by a medical practitioner, it is a condition that neither presents, nor can be tested for, medically. Despite numerous medical research projects into a diagnosis of autism, there are currently no genetic markers, blood tests, urine tests, scans or other medical tests to diagnose the condition. A number of tests may be recommended by a paediatrician to rule out other possible conditions rather than to confirm a diagnosis of autism. Among the tests commonly completed for young children with suspected autism are hearing tests to check for a possible hearing impairment, blood tests to check for chromosome abnormalities such as Fragile X syndrome or other gene abnormalities, brain scans to check for neurological conditions or EEGs to rule out possible seizure disorders or Landau-Kleffner syndrome. The most effective approach to identifying children for possible autism is to look for clinical clues of autism. These possible clues can then be followed-up with appropriate screening tests and further assessment if heightened concerns or clinical clues are identified.

There is no specific test to diagnose autism. The diagnosis is subjective and based on the presence of a number of behaviours and descriptive characteristics. The diagnostician uses observation and a detailed parent interview to ascertain a particular pattern of behaviours and developmental characteristics. The diagnostic procedure should also include a full family and child history, a number of standardised tests to assess current abilities and autism specific questionnaires and rating scales, as well as observation of the child in a number of relevant settings, and parent interviews. This then leads to a provisional diagnosis of autism based on the child meeting the criteria set down in the diagnostic manuals (DSM-IV or ICD-10). The assessments and questionnaires are subjective and not a scientific/objective process. This makes it much harder for a definite and accurate diagnosis, especially if a child is very young.

An experienced paediatrician, clinical psychologist or child psychiatrist may diagnose a young child with an autism spectrum disorder as early as 2 years of age. However, many children are not diagnosed until 3 years and children with good language skills may not receive a diagnosis until age 5 or older. Some paediatricians prefer not to diagnose autism at an early age but to give a tentative diagnosis of 'autistic features or tendencies'. As children develop and mature, the autistic features become more obvious and therefore easier to diagnose definitively. A diagnosis of autism may be obtained at any time during a person's lifetime although most children with significant autistic features are diagnosed either before they start school or soon after.

Some more able individuals with autism are not diagnosed until late childhood. There are a number of adults who, never having been diagnosed with an autism spectrum disorder during childhood, are diagnosed with the condition as adults. Many of these people were misdiagnosed or labelled in childhood either mentally retarded, eccentric, attention deficit disordered, emotionally disturbed or learning disordered. Some people with Asperger's syndrome may never receive a diagnosis.

What are some of the early signs of autism?

As discussed briefly in Chapter 1, there are a number of early signs in a young child that suggest to parents the need to seek professional advice and a possible assessment for autism. These early flags for parents may be categorised into a number of key developmental areas that reflect the established autistic deficits. Both receptive and expressive language skills are delayed and disordered in children with autism. A child with autism:

- may not respond to his/her name when called at 12 months of age;
- presents with a language delay with no functional speech by 24 months or a loss of words after 12 months;
- appears to have hearing loss or selective hearing where child responds only to certain sounds such as TV advertisements or the fridge door but ignores the human voice;
- does not use spontaneous phrases to communicate by 24 months;
- has no babbling by 12 months;
- is not pointing to indicate needs or wants and no waving to indicate social interaction by 12 months; and
- is unable to follow simple directions or instructions.

The social relating skills of children with autism are delayed and disordered. A child with autism:

- may show a lack of awareness of other children;
- avoids contact with other children;
- does not smile socially or look directly at another person;
- appears to tune-out or switch-off from other people;
- tries to become independent to avoid social contact with others; and
- does not share objects or information with another person.

A number of behavioural indicators are also usually present in children with autism. A child with autism:

- has a number of unusual preoccupations and attachments;

- may appear over-active and uncooperative;
- uses tantrum behaviour to communicate;
- has very limited and repetitive play behaviour;
- may line up or spin objects;
- has very short attention span;
- has a preference for TV or videos; and
- has difficulty coping with changes to normal routine.

Most children with autism have some form of sensory impairment. A child with autism:
- may walk on tiptoe;
- may have unusual sensory reactions or preoccupations;
- may be afraid of certain sounds;
- will only wear certain clothing;
- may have a very limited diet and refuse to try new foods;
- may be unable to touch certain textures without gagging; and
- uses peripheral vision to look at objects.

Children with autism have impaired imagination, which is reflected in the way they play. A child with autism:
- prefers to watch TV or play alone rather than play interactively;
- will not share toys;
- will not take turns in play;
- has limited interest in playing with a range of toys;
- may carry around one or two objects;
- does not engage in pretend play activities; and
- tends to wander aimlessly rather than engage in play activities.

The above indicators are examples of autistic-like behaviours. All children will engage in some of these behaviours at different times. It is only when a child engages in a number of these behaviours persistently and over a period of time that the alarm bells may sound and further investigation is warranted.

Even though autism may be diagnosed at any time, it is an early onset disorder and the symptoms are present, even if not readily observable, before the age of three. Some of the early indicators such as a lack of eye contact to initiate joint attention, emotionally distant behaviour or dislike of affection, failure to alert to mother's voice, lack of imitation or social reciprocity, inability to settle, lack of functional use of non-verbal communication, and preoccupation with certain objects or movements, may be observed within the first 12 months of life. Screening for autism is also recommended if a sibling or other family member has a diagnosis within the autism spectrum. Unfortunately, it is not usually until after a child has been diagnosed that parents, in hindsight, recognise that there were early signs of the disability.

What is the step-by-step process for diagnosis and assessment?

Once parents have read the information about how children are diagnosed and assessed for autism things may appear somewhat clearer. Breaking the process down into small steps may take away some of the anxiety and enable parents to feel that they have addressed and explored all possible avenues.

Step 1: Parents have concerns about their young child or a close friend or professional indicates possible concerns.

Step 2: Parents should contact their local general practitioner to discuss their concerns.

Step 3: If the doctor also has concerns about the child's development, the doctor will provide a referral to a developmental paediatrician or refer the family for diagnosis and assessment through local disability services.

Step 4: If parents are referred to a developmental paediatrician, the doctor will complete a child and family history, examine the child and discuss parental concerns. The paediatrician may give a diagnosis of autism or autism spectrum disorder if warranted. The paediatrician will then refer the family to a psychologist or to local disability services for a more detailed diagnosis and assessment. The paediatrician may take a blood sample from the child and recommend other medical procedures. These procedures are to help rule out similar disorders.

Step 5: Parents attend a multidisciplinary team assessment with their child for in-depth testing and assessment. This assessment will provide detailed information about the child's autistic characteristics, degree of disability and perceived functional abilities. The information is helpful for both parents and professionals to assist in determining most effective and appropriate interventions. Parents will be assigned a case manager from the assessment team who will provide ongoing support and assistance. The case manager will assist parents to refer the child to specialist services.

What tests are used to help diagnose autism?

Among the rating scales commonly used to detect a pattern of behaviours indicating autism are:
- Autism Behaviour Checklist (ABC);
- Autism Diagnostic Interview – Revised (ADI-R);
- Childhood Autism Rating Scale (CAR);
- Checklist for Autism in Toddlers (CHAT);
- Pre-Linguistic Autism Diagnostic Observation Schedule (PL-ADOS);
- Gilliam Autism Rating Scale (GARS);
- Diagnostic Interview Schedule and Childhood Observation (DISCO); and
- The Asperger Syndrome Diagnostic Scale (ASDS).

Particular skills, including communication, sensory impairments, social skills, attending skills as well as cognitive and motor skills should also be assessed for deficits.

These assessment instruments can be used in various ways in assessing children with possible autism. Sometimes the instruments may be used to determine whether autism is likely, so that a decision can be made to seek a more formal diagnosis. At other times, some of the assessment instruments may be used as part of the formal diagnostic procedure. In addition, some of the assessment instruments may be used to rate the severity of symptoms in order to determine particular intervention programs, help monitor individual progress and assess possible outcomes. The main assessment tools are outlined below in more detail.

Autism Behaviour Checklist (ABC)

This consists of a list of questions about a child's behaviour. It was first published in 1980 and may be completed independently by a parent or a teacher familiar with the child. The ABC has 57 questions divided into five categories: sensory, relating, body and object use, language and social and self-help.

Autism Diagnostic Interview – Revised (ADI-R)

This is a semi-structured interview for clinicians to use with a child's parent or principal caregiver. The ADI-R focuses on obtaining maximum information from a parent in three key areas: reciprocal social interaction, communication and language, and repetitive, stereotyped behaviours.

Childhood Autism Rating Scale (CARS)

This is the most widely used standardised instrument specifically designed to aid in the diagnosis of autism with children as young as two. Published in 1980, it is a direct observational tool used by a trained clinician. The 15 items on the CARS include: imitation, affect, use of body, verbal and non-verbal communication and visual and auditory responsiveness.

Checklist for Autism in Toddlers (CHAT)

This is a brief screening instrument to detect possible autism in toddlers. The CHAT was first published in 1992 and takes only five or ten minutes to administer and score. The CHAT is designed for use with children as young as 18 months. It consists of nine yes/no questions to be answered by a child's parents. Specific questions are designed to assess children's behaviour. The questions address issues such as social play, interest in other children, pretend play, joint attention and rough and tumble play.

Pre-Linguistic Autism Diagnostic Observation Schedule (PL-ADOS)

This consists of eight tasks, four focusing on social behaviours and four on communicative behaviours. The test was intended for older, higher-functioning, verbal autistic children. It is a semi-structured assessment of play, interaction and social communication and takes approximately 30 minutes for a trained clinician to administer.

Gilliam Autism Rating Scale (GARS)

This helps to identify and diagnose autism in individuals between the ages 3 to 22 years and to estimate the severity of the problem. Items are based on the definitions of autism adopted by the DSM-IV and are grouped into four sub-tests: stereotyped behaviours, communication, social interaction, and developmental disturbances. Behaviours are assessed using objective, frequency-based ratings. A person familiar with a child's behaviour can complete the scales in approximately 5–10 minutes.

Diagnostic Interview Schedule and Childhood Observation (DISCO)

This is a semi-structured interview schedule that elicits information relevant to the whole autism spectrum and to conditions such as obsessive-compulsive disorder, Tourette's syndrome and catatonia, that overlap with autistic disorders. The schedule consists of eight parts divided into sections that record developmental changes and can be used with individuals of any age and ability. Parts 1 and 2 cover general information and early development. Part 3 looks at developmental skills in line with the triad of impairments and part 4 covers repetitive activities and responses to sensory stimuli. Behavioural disturbances including sleeping problems and emotional issues are covered in parts 5 and 6 while part 7 rates the individual's social interaction. Part 8 covers issues of behaviour related to the law including sexual behaviour and psychiatric disorders. While the DISCO is primarily a clinical instrument, it can also be used for research purposes.

Asperger Syndrome Diagnostic Scale (ASDS)

This scale (Myles, Bock, & Simpson 2001) is appropriate to use with individuals aged 5–18 years who possess characteristics associated with Asperger's syndrome. A person who knows the individual well, such as a teacher, a family member, or other caregiver, completes it.

What tests are used to assess children's cognitive abilities?

In addition to the tests outlined above to help professionals diagnose autism, a number of standardised tools are available to psychologists and paediatricians to enable them to assess children's developmental levels and cognitive abilities. Among the most commonly used assessment instruments are:

- Bayley Scales of Infant Development;
- Griffiths Mental Developmental Scale;
- Psychoeducational Profile-Revised;
- Vineland Adaptive Behaviour Scale;

- Stanford-Binet; and
- Wechsler Intelligence Scale.

The Bayley Scales of Infant Development

The Bayley Scales of Infant Development allows diagnostic assessment at an earlier age and is designed to identify children with cognitive or motor delay. The Mental Scale evaluates a variety of abilities, including sensory-perceptual acuities, learning, problem solving, vocalisation, and beginning verbal communication. The Motor Scale assesses degree of body control, large-muscle coordination, fine motor manipulative skills and motor quality. The Behaviour Rating Scale provides information to supplement the Mental and Motor Scales and measures attention, arousal, orientation, engagement and emotional regulation.

The Griffith Mental Development Scale

The Griffith Mental Development Scale is a standardised test that examines a child's mastery of a number of different skills. The test is divided into five subscales that measure a child's performance and provide developmental age-equivalent levels that give an indication of what a child can do or has achieved. The descriptive classification of the scores also takes into account how a child's test performance deviates from the average for their age. The Griffith scales test children's locomotor skills, personal–social skills, hearing and speech, eye and hand coordination and performance.

Psychoeducational Profile-Revised

Psychoeducational Profile-Revised (Pep-R) offers a developmental approach to the assessment of children with autism and related developmental disorders. It is an inventory of behaviours and skills designed to identify uneven and idiosyncratic learning patterns. The test is most appropriately used with children within the chronological age range of 6 months to 7 years. The PEP-R provides information on developmental functioning in imitation, perception, fine motor, gross motor, eye–hand integration, cognitive performance and cognitive verbal areas. The test also identifies behavioural abnormality in relating and affect, play and interest in materials, sensory responses and language. The test usually takes approximately an hour to administer and score.

Vineland Adaptive Behaviour Scales

Vineland Adaptive Behaviour Scales comes in three forms varying in degree of detail and proposed setting. There is the Survey Form, the Expanded Form and the Classroom Edition. In the Vineland, parents, teachers or carers are interviewed about a child. The scales range in age from birth to 19 years. The scales measure communication, daily living skills, socialisation, motor skills and maladaptive behaviours. The Adaptive Behaviour composite score includes the domains noted above and reflects overall adaptive behaviour.

Stanford-Binet Intelligence Scale, Fourth Edition

This is a standardised test that assesses intelligence and cognitive abilities in children and adults aged 2 years to 23 years. It is used as a tool in school placement, in determining the presence of a learning disability or a developmental delay, and in tracking intellectual development. It is sometimes included in neuropsychological testing to assess the brain function of individuals with neurological impairments. The scale tests intelligence across four major areas: verbal reasoning, quantitative reasoning, abstract/visual reasoning and short-term memory. The areas are covered by fifteen subtests, including vocabulary, comprehension, verbal absurdities, pattern analysis, matrices, number series, memory for sentences, memory for digits, memory for objects, and bead memory. Total testing time is 45–90 minutes, depending on the subject's age and number of subtests administered.

Wechsler Intelligence Scales

These are the most frequently used tests for the assessment of general intellectual ability. There are three separate versions of these scales developed for different age groups:

- the Wechsler Preschool and Primary Scale of Intelligence-Revised (WPPSI-R) used for children between the ages of 3 and 7;
- the Wechsler Intelligence Scale for Children-Third Edition (WISC-III) used for children between the ages of 8 and 17; and
- the Wechsler Adult Intelligence Scale-Third Edition (WAIS-III) used with subjects 18 years and over.

Each of the Wechsler scales reports three IQ scores: verbal, performance IQ and full scale IQ. The verbal scale measures expressive language and comprehension. The performance scale measures the non-verbal areas of spatial perceptual abilities, such as completing puzzles and ability to transfer visual information rapidly. The three IQ scores and the specific pattern of strengths and weaknesses indicate how well the subject is able to learn and whether there are any specific learning disabilities.

What is a multidisciplinary team assessment?

Partly because there is no way to diagnose autism definitively through established medical procedures, it is recommended that the diagnosis of autism be made after a thorough multidisciplinary assessment. The diagnostic team should include a paediatrician or child psychiatrist, psychologist and speech pathologist as well as other allied health professionals. The assessment process should include:

- a full medical assessment;
- a developmental assessment;
- a speech and language assessment;
- observation of behaviour and social skills;
- cognitive skills assessment using standardised tests;
- hearing assessment; and
- autism checklist, such as those listed above, across a number of settings.

Step 1: The first step in the assessment process is to consider the purpose of the evaluation. The purpose of the assessment will likely depend on the referral question, source of referral (e.g. parent, teacher, other professionals), and setting (e.g. preschool, school, clinic, residential placement). Among the most common reasons for an assessment are:

- to screen for early indicators of autism spectrum disorder;
- to provide information to clarify a diagnosis of autism (assessment for the purpose of diagnosis typically occurs in clinics or private practices and is led by psychiatrists, psychologists, or physicians.);
- to establish a child's eligibility for special education services;
- to measure a child's cognitive and academic strengths and weaknesses, and/or emotional health. The information received is important for intervention and curriculum planning; and
- to evaluate intervention efficacy or for research purposes.

Step 2: Once the purpose of the assessment has been clarified, the next step is to interview the parents/caregivers to obtain a social and developmental history and other information about the child's current level of functioning. The interviewer will ask questions to determine the age of onset of the disability, to find out information about family history of illness or psychopathology and, if appropriate, to find out about the child's academic history and current educational performance.

Step 3: The next step in the assessment process is to assess the degree of autism. A number of rating scales that are consistent with current DSM-IV criteria are available as outlined above.

Step 4: After the initial parent/caregiver interviews, the next step in the assessment process is usually to administer behavioural checklists to caregivers, teachers, and any other professionals involved with the child. There are many rating scales available that measure a wide-range of behaviours. The Achenbach Child Behaviour Checklist (ACBC), for example, developed for children aged 4–18 years and completed by a parent or caregiver, looks at both internalising and externalising behaviours.

Step 5: Standardised measures of intellectual ability and academic achievement are also an important part of the assessment process, but using such tests with individuals with autism spectrum disorders may not yield conclusive results. In brief, standardised intellectual and achievement tests may not yield accurate results or provide useful information for treatment or educational planning because they are heavily reliant on verbal ability, auditory processing, and the ability to follow sequential directions. These are areas of particular difficulty for individuals on the spectrum. In addition, the testing environment can be problematic; for example, an unfamiliar room and examiner, a break in typical routine. Standardised procedures may be near impossible, especially if the child possesses behaviours that interfere with the testing process. The Wechsler tests and the Stanford-Binet-IV are commonly used for school-aged verbal children. The Stanford-Binet may be more appropriate to use with individuals with autism spectrum disorders because it has a lower floor; that is, a greater number of items meant for a lower developmental age and it also includes more non-verbal options and subtests that measure memory. For individuals who are non-verbal, the Griffiths Mental Development Scales Assessment and the Leiter International Performance Scale-Revised are options with good reliability and validity that do not require verbal responses.

Step 6: The adaptive behaviour of the individual is another area that may be assessed as part of the evaluation process. According to Sattler (1992, Chapter 15), adaptive behavior assessment considers two issues:

(a) the degree to which individuals are able to function and maintain themselves independently and (b) the degree to which they meet satisfactorily the culturally imposed demands of personal and social responsibility.

The Vineland Adaptive Behaviour Scales (VABS) (Sparrow, Balla, & Cicchetti 1984) is an example of a reliable and valid measure of adaptive behaviour.

Step 7: Finally, speech and language pathologists, occupational therapists, and/or physical therapists should evaluate the individual to determine difficulties in related areas. The speech evaluations should measure not only receptive and expressive language, but also the social and pragmatic aspects of communication. Fine and gross motor skills and sensory processing are evaluated, usually by an occupational therapist and/or physical therapist.

Recently there has been increased awareness of emotional difficulties, particularly anxiety and depression, experienced by high-functioning individuals with autism. Therefore, it is recommended that measures of social–emotional wellbeing are used in the evaluation process, especially when intervention planning. There are many reliable and valid tests for anxiety and depression available for use with children, adolescents, and adults that are easy to administer and score, adding little additional time to the overall evaluation process.

What conditions co-exist with autism?

There are a number of other conditions that may co-exist with autism and that make any diagnosis more complex and less clear. Among the most commonly occurring co-existing conditions are intellectual impairment, epilepsy, attention deficit disorders (ADD, ADHD), obsessive compulsive disorder, sensory integration disorders, Tourette's syndrome and auditory processing disorders.

It is important to complete a thorough health evaluation for each child suspected of having autism. A health evaluation will provide a general assessment of the child's health status, identify any co-existing conditions that are sometimes confused with autism, and identify and assess medical conditions or genetic syndromes that are associated with autism. An important purpose of a comprehensive health evaluation for children with suspected autism is to identify possible associated medical conditions that are seen more commonly in children with autism than in the general population. These may include a variety of neurological problems (such as seizure disorders), genetic syndromes (such as Fragile X syndrome) and metabolic disorders.

Another more controversial use of health assessment methods is the application of specific immune, allergic or metabolic tests to identify subgroups of children with autism who may respond to specific medication or dietary interventions.

The justifications for such testing are based on various controversial theories about the cause of autism. The theory behind the use of these medical tests maintains that in some children autism may be caused by certain immune, allergic, or metabolic processes related to diet, yeast infections, prior viral infections, or other causes. These theories however, are not generally accepted in the scientific community. While some of the assessment methods, such as allergy testing, are well established as general diagnostic tools for specific health conditions, the use of these methods in children with autism is considered controversial. For some of these assessment methods, extensive research literature exists, while for others, very little published scientific research is available. There is, however, anecdotal evidence from parents and others in the community to support the use of these methods.

After the multidisciplinary assessment, what next?

These are the first steps that families go through on the journey towards achieving some degree of independence for their child with autism. The journey will take most families through awareness, denial, understanding and finally acceptance of their child's limitations and also, ultimately, pride in their child's idiosyncrasies and achievements.

The steps may vary a little from family to family. However, the ultimate aim of the diagnostic and assessment process is to clarify what the problem is and to provide families with the information they need to move forward. The next chapter will provide suggestions for families about what they can do next on their journey forward.

Summary

The evaluation of individuals with autism spectrum disorders can best be described as multidimensional. There are a number of reasons why an assessment is initiated. The assessment procedures will depend on the purpose of the evaluation, the referral question, the source of referral, and the setting of service provision. It involves thorough diagnostic testing and evaluation of individual strengths and needs. The accurate identification and assessment of autism spectrum disorders is dependent on the assessment process, not the results of a single measure or procedure. As such, collaboration between professionals, parents, and teachers is a necessary component of an effective assessment process and an accurate interpretation of information gathered.

In most cases, the diagnostic and assessment process involves a multidisciplinary team of paediatrician, psychologist, speech pathologist, social worker and other therapists as required.

Once a multidisciplinary team has completed an assessment, a detailed report is prepared outlining the child's strengths and individual needs. The report should also contain recommendations for management and appropriate program options.

The involvement of parents in the assessment process is vital. They are able to provide valuable information and insight into their child's development and behaviour to assist the process and they are also responsible for ensuring that all of their child's needs are met. Autism can co-exist with other conditions, most commonly intellectual impairments and epilepsy. Other co-existing conditions include visual and hearing impairments.

Autism is a life-long disability that affects the person's communication and social interaction skills throughout their adulthood. Some adults with autism are able to live independently but most individuals require some degree of support within their structured community setting. The diagnosis and assessment is the first step on the journey towards awareness, understanding and acceptance for most family members.

CHAPTER

9

After Diagnosis — What Next?

As a parent of a child with an autism spectrum disorder there are many new things to learn. At times it will be challenging to balance routines, schedules and plans so that all family members feel accepted, supported and valued. Establish time for all family members to revitalize and gain perspective. Maintain your sense of humor. Laugh together to relieve tension. You can and will have your ups and downs. Keeping things in perspective and taking time for yourself are vital in reducing the stress that is common when parenting any child, including your child with an autism spectrum disorder.

Wheeler & Pratt 2001, p 1

After a child has been diagnosed with autism, parents continue their journey of discovery — what lies ahead for them and their child, what services and support are available and how can they become the most effective advocate for their child.

However, immediately after their child has been diagnosed with autism is not the best time for parents to be making major and even life-changing decisions about therapies, moving house to be closer to specialist services, flying overseas for second opinions and radical 'cures', moving closer to extended family members, or signing up for intensive interventions that are recommended as the only real and successful 'fix' for autism.

This is a time when parents are anxious, confused, vulnerable and often angry. The best advice is to take a little time, even though time is of the essence. It is worth taking a few days to come to terms with the diagnosis, discuss feelings and concerns, calm down and look at things in a proper perspective. During this period, it is also advisable to talk with a friend, someone who can remain objective but still provide comfort and support and a sympathetic ear.

Once parents are over the initial shock, a little research into the disorder is recommended. Even though the disability of autism may have been explained in some detail during the diagnostic and assessment meeting, chances are that parents were in shock and did not hear much of what was covered during the session. Probably the only word that registered was 'autism'.

Most diagnostic services provide a follow-up session with families: to ensure that they are OK, that they have understood the diagnosis and to answer any of the questions that the parents could not articulate at earlier meetings. This follow-up visit by the family provides an opportunity for them to obtain written information about the disorder and also contact details of specialist services.

Once parents have had time to digest the fact that their child has autism they can then work out what to do next. It must be emphasised however that where parents have concerns about their child's development, it is imperative that they seek professional advice and diagnosis. To embark upon the next steps (as outlined below) before obtaining professional consultation and a diagnosis may be foolhardy, even if well meaning.

The next steps?

Once parents have been given a diagnosis of autism, or 'autistic features' or 'autism spectrum disorder' for their child, it is time to make some important decisions fairly quickly. Parents need to decide about intervention services, family support and how to understand and address the needs of their child. They also have to begin to consider the needs of other family members and the impact of the disorder on them.

Step 1

The first step for parents is to take a brief period to consider their child's diagnosis before making any definite decisions about future interventions.

Parents need time to overcome the initial shock and distress at the diagnosis; a few days of discussion with close family and friends usually provides an effective platform for making plans for their immediate future. Once parents have had time to think things through and discuss the diagnosis, they can start collecting relevant information about the disorder and about specialist services. This information will assist them to make informed decisions about what to do next. Parents also need to organise a follow-up visit with the diagnostic service, their paediatrician or contact local disability services.

Step 2

The second step is to make a return visit to the assessment service armed with lots of questions and a request for referrals to specialist organisations.

The follow-up visit will enable parents to clarify the diagnosis and to ask any questions that they did not ask during the initial consultation. The follow-up visit should take place no later than two weeks after the original consultation. During the follow-up visit, parents may request written information and the names of relevant specialist services. At this time, a referral may also be made to the nearest Autism Association for ongoing consultation, information, services and support. Parents will also be encouraged to begin to find out more about the disorder and how it affects their child.

There is an Autism Association in each state of Australia (see Appendix 3) as well as local and national bodies in most other countries. The Autism Association will provide families with information, intervention, parent training, resources and access to other families. Some Autism Associations provide specialist school services, outreach school support and supported employment and residential services for adults with autism. They will also be able to provide information and contact numbers for a range of alternative specialist autism services.

Step 3

By this time, most parents are anxious to find out more about autism and how it will impact on their family in the future. The next step is for parents to begin their research into autism, especially research into information that is relevant to their situation.

If parents obtain information about autism they can then begin to understand their child better and to work out what their child needs in terms of individual support and intervention. Once parents have a general understanding of the core characteristics of the disorder they can make informed decisions about services for their child; they are also in a better position to discuss their options with professionals. There are a number of books and articles on autism that parents can read (see Appendix 5) that will provide essential background information and also provide practical intervention strategies.

Step 4

In addition to reading about the disorder, parents can contact their nearest Autism Association and receive information and support as well as access to relevant early intervention services.

The Autism Association will provide a package of information about the disorder as well as information about local specialist services. The organisation may offer to come to the home to discuss concerns, specific issues or behaviours and service options. If the association has an early intervention service, request information about the service and apply for any recommended programs. Ask for information about other specialist services.

Step 5

In addition to accessing information through specialist organisations, parents may also use the Internet and other means to carry out further research.

Information is available about specialised intervention services in autism that provide ongoing intervention and support. The Internet is an effective starting point. Local and state government authorities will also provide details of service providers. Parents may collect information about many different services for children of similar age to their child. It is recommended that parents look for services that are available locally. Some programs may be home-based, especially early intervention programs for behavioural issues including eating, sleeping and toileting as well as the core deficits of autism. Most home-based programs offer a collaborative approach with a strong parent-training component.

Some programs provide individualised or small group centre-based services. Other programs offer intensive intervention based on a particular service model. Some programs are government funded or subsidised while other programs are private and may be more expensive.

Parents should look at cost, intensity, programs that are well established and extensively evaluated, particular service models and philosophies, location and availability when searching for interventions. Parents can collect information about a number of different service options and make appointments to visit those programs that address their particular child and family needs. It is only by observing different intervention approaches and talking with the teachers and therapists involved that parents are able to make the right decisions for their child. It is often beneficial to talk with other parents of children with autism but remember that 'to know one child with autism is not to know autism'. What works for one family may not suit another family. Parents should make decisions for their child based on their knowledge of their child's needs, not what has worked for someone else. The decisions are then based on parental knowledge, up-to-date information and professional recommendations. Once parents have reached a decision about specialised services, they should enrol their child in the program. If they are not happy or they do not feel that their child is progressing or having his/her needs met, they can always change to another service. It is important to remember that no one intervention works for all children. Most established intervention services, if structured, intensive and attempting to address the core deficits of autism, will be of huge benefit. There is no cure for autism so don't fall for the program that offers 'magic answers' or 'cures'.

Step 6

The next step for parents is to check out local services that may provide both intervention and family support.

Parents should not dismiss generic services that cater to the needs of children with different disabilities. These services provide essential intervention and address a range of children's particular needs. They include speech therapy to address communication impairments, occupational therapy to address motor and sensory impairments, physiotherapy to address motor impairments, and educational programs that place children in small groups and address social impairments and teach social play skills. Parents may also access other programs such as kindy gym, swimming lessons and music therapy. In addition, one of the most effective programs for children with autism is to attend a regular preschool with their peers for at least one or two days per week.

Step 7

One of the most important local services for children is access to a structured day care or preschool program. Once a child is accessing individualised intervention, parents should consider enrolling their child in a local preschool or day care program. Parents may consult with family members and professionals to determine which program is most appropriate.

Parents may need to shop around to find an appropriate centre that will provide support for their child and address the child's particular learning needs. Most centres are eligible to apply for additional government funding if they have a special needs child enrolled in their program. This additional funding enables them to employ extra staff members. Most centres willingly take children with disabilities and welcome support from other agencies. Depending on the age of the child, parents may look at childcare/daycare centres (for children 0–5 years), long day-care centres (extended hours for children 0–5), or preschools (for children 3–5 years). Preschool centres tend to offer a more structured program as they prepare children for school. (See Appendix 6 for what to look for in a childcare/preschool centre.)

Step 8

Once their child is settled and is receiving a range of appropriate services, parents can begin to relax and enjoy their child before moving on to the next important decision.

Once parents have completed the first steps — they have contacted relevant services, started appropriate therapy, selected specialist intervention and have either started a program or are on waiting lists, enrolled their child in preschool, and have their week organised to the point that they need a diary to keep tabs on all of their appointments, it is time to take a breath and take stock of the situation. They have come a long way and have learned a lot of information. They have also started to understand the importance of advocacy. The service providers for their child will come and go and the frequency and intensity of the services provided will change over time. The only real constants in each child's life are the parents and family members. They are the people who look after the child, make decisions and become their spokesperson and advocate as they become adults. Parents must, therefore, remain informed and aware of all options and requirements throughout their child's life. As their child's primary advocates, they must feel both able and empowered to make correct decisions.

Before too long, however, parents need to start thinking about the next phase in their child's social and cognitive development.

Step 9

Well before it is time for their child to start school, parents may need to make decisions about the most appropriate schooling for their child. Specialist programs have long waiting lists so parents need to become informed about options early and shop around before choosing a particular school program.

There are a number of options for parents to consider when looking at school placement. Some children with autism may attend a regular school program, requiring some level of support in the classroom and the playground, while other children may need to attend a specialised class in a regular school and still other children may require a specialised school placement.

Parents should begin looking at school options for their child at least a year before their child is due to start school (see Chapter 16 for information about what to look for in a school).

Choosing an appropriate school is a difficult and stressful time for parents who want the best for their child but who are also aware of the special needs and limitations of their child. Both parents and child should feel comfortable with the choice of school. Once a child starts school, he or she moves into a new environment — an environment with new rules and routines and different teachers and children.

Step 10

Once schooling decisions have been made, parents may start to prepare their child for the transition from preschool to the much larger school environment

Children with autism do not cope well with changes to their regular routines. The enormous change from preschool to school is usually a difficult time for children and transition planning is important.

Once a school placement has been decided and the enrolment process completed, parents can begin to prepare their child for the changes ahead. Parents can help their child to transition from preschool and structured early intervention programs to the new school environment with minimal stress and anxiety. The transition process involves using many of the strategies already introduced in regular teaching sessions, including visual supports, social stories, modelling, planned change and shaping appropriate responses. (For detailed discussion about planning ahead for change and the transition process see Chapter 16.)

Within a few years after the initial diagnosis, most children with autism are enrolled in school, with a level of support that will enable them to enjoy life, achieve some measure of success in class and make friends.

The diagnosis of autism is a traumatic event for parents. Moreover it is the start of a long journey of discovery as parents guide their child through the many stages of life from infancy to adulthood. While every parent embarks on this journey, the journey ahead for parents of a child with autism is usually a difficult and rocky one. However, well-informed and proactive parents are able to provide their child with the security and support that will underpin a successful journey, albeit along a different path to that of children without autism.

What should parents and professionals consider when developing and implementing school-based interventions?

Every child is different and it is important to accept each child as an individual, whether that child has autism, another form of disability or no disability at all. According to Koegal & Koegal (1995), there are a number of clinical factors, however, that may assist both parents and professionals in choosing appropriate interventions and supporting children with autism. Many of the strategies developed for children with autism may be successfully applied to assist all students.

Koegal & Koegal state that:

- all intervention should be individualised because of the variability in the disorder among children;
- it is critical to begin intervention as early as possible in order to minimise or prevent the emergence of severe problems;

- it is important to use the natural environment as much as possible when teaching new skills and encouraging and motivating children to learn;
- it is important for parents to be actively involved in all aspects of their child's program and ensure that there is consistency across different environments. This involves coordinating the individual service providers to enhance their child's progress; and
- the functions of each child's behaviours should be closely analysed and the child's independence encouraged by responding to any attempts to communicate and socialise.

Koegal & Koegal also stress the importance of considering not only the needs of the child with autism but also the needs of the other family members. Parents and professionals have to work together to ensure long-term positive outcomes for the child, while taking into account their individual strengths and needs.

By working closely together, parents and professionals can plan for full school and community inclusion for their child. They can work together to ensure that each and every child with autism has the help and support they need to maximise their potential and be recognised and valued as a member of their community.

Summary

Once a diagnosis of autism has been finalised, there are a number of steps that parents can follow in their quest to access the most appropriate services for their child.

Immediately after the diagnosis, it is important that parents take a little time to come to terms with the label of autism before they start applying for programming support. This is the time when parents are most vulnerable and are also fired-up to fix problems. It may not necessarily be the time when they are able to make the most rational decisions. It is recommended that parents spend a short time talking with family and friends, gathering information, observing different programs and generally collecting their thoughts before they make decisions and choose a particular path to follow.

There are usually a number of options available: some options are for specialist services and other options are for more generalised services. Children may be able to access a combination of different programs that offer a range of different services. Ideally children should access an intensive program that provides one-to-one intervention as well as another program that provides small group intervention. Children should also access a large group, such as preschool, where they have opportunities to practise their skills among their peers.

Once children are settled into early intervention services, parents can turn their attention to their next major decision — school placement.

10

Asperger's Syndrome

Each of us holds our own secret blend of these traits, our own recipe for what makes us tick. Add to this the gene pool, the home environment, one's culture, gender issues and intelligence quotient, and presto ... magic occurs.

Willey 2001

Asperger's syndrome, a neurobiological disorder, is an autism spectrum disorder in which dysfunction of certain parts of the brain and central nervous system significantly impairs the way individuals relate to other people, process information and make sense of their environment. Uta Frith, in her book *Autism and Asperger's Syndrome* (1991) described individuals with Asperger's syndrome as 'having a dash of autism'.

Hans Asperger, a Viennese physician, first published a description of a number of children he had observed with impaired communication and social interactions in 1944. He identified a consistent pattern of different abilities and behaviour that predominantly occurs in boys. According to Attwood (1998, p 11), 'this pattern included a lack of empathy, little ability to form friendships, one-sided conversations, intense absorption in a special interest and clumsy movements'.

Today, the term Asperger's syndrome is used to describe similar children and adults. It was not until 1994, however, that Asperger's work was recognised in America with the publication of the fourth edition of the *Diagnostic and Statistical Manual of Mental Disorders* (DSM-IV). While the formal definition of Asperger's syndrome was not recognised by the American professional community until this time, it has been widely accepted in Europe among professionals diagnosing and assessing children and adults since Asperger's paper was first published in 1944.

Individuals with Asperger's syndrome exhibit a number of different characteristics that range in severity from mild to profound. These characteristics include marked impairments in social and communication skills, unusually strong and narrow interests, difficulties with transitions or changes to routines, a preference for sameness and inflexible and repetitive behaviours. Many individuals have difficulty reading non-verbal cues such as body language and also have difficulty determining appropriate body space. Generally, children and adults with Asperger's syndrome do not show their emotions through their facial expressions, having a rather flat facial affect. Most have excellent rote memory skills and may become intensely interested in one or two subjects rather than having a wide range of interests. This narrow interest leads individuals to talk at length about a particular topic with no awareness that they may be boring their audience.

Sensory sensitivities, such as problems with touch, taste, smell, and fine and gross motor difficulties (clumsy and poorly coordinated movements and unusual postures), are common among people with Asperger's syndrome. For example, a person with Asperger's syndrome may only wear certain clothing, eat certain foods and become distressed by certain sounds or sights. Like children and adults with autism, individuals with Asperger's perceive the world quite differently from their non-disabled peers.

By definition, persons with Asperger's syndrome have IQ scores within the normal range, with some children and adults showing an exceptional skill or talent in a particular area. Even though individuals with autism present with IQ scores within the normal range, in practice, however, they display unusual and uneven profiles and abilities on most standardised tests of intelligence. Most researchers and practitioners recognise that although the majority of students with Asperger's Syndrome have average to above-average intellectual functioning and are usually included in regular, mainstream classes, they experience difficulties academically. Because of their particular learning styles and interests, they may be perceived as eccentric or odd and are often victims of bullying and teasing by their peers. They find it difficult to become fully integrated and to actively participate in and comprehend the classroom curriculum and the social rules of the playground.

Asperger's syndrome differs from autism in that early speech generally develops within normal limits (single words used by age 2 and phrases by age 3). As children grow, however, their language development may appear, on the surface, to be within the normal range but they tend to have deficits in the pragmatics and prosody of language. Children may have extensive vocabularies but they are also extremely literal and are unable to express themselves very well in social situations.

While there is no cure, many individuals show significant improvement over time, particularly if their learning strengths and individual interests are recognised and nurtured.

How is Asperger's syndrome defined?

In the DSM-IV manual (American Psychological Association, 1994), Asperger's syndrome is defined under the more general category of pervasive developmental disorder along with a number of other related disorders. The other disorders are autistic disorder, Rett's disorder, childhood disintegrative disorder and pervasive developmental disorder not otherwise specified (PDD-NOS). The criteria for a diagnosis of Asperger's syndrome are set out in the DSM IV as shown below.

299.80 Diagnostic Criteria for Asperger's Disorder (DSM IV)
A. *Qualitative impairment in social interaction, as manifested by at least two of the following:*
   1. marked impairment in the use of multiple nonverbal behaviours such as eye-to-eye gaze, facial expression, body postures, and gestures to regulate social interaction;
   2. failure to develop peer relationships appropriate to developmental level;
   3. a lack of spontaneous seeking to share enjoyment, interests or achievements with other people (eg: by a lack of showing, bringing, or pointing out objects of interest to other people);
   4. lack of social or emotional reciprocity.
B. *Restricted repetitive and stereotyped patterns of behaviour, interests, and activities, as manifested by at least one of the following:*
   1. encompassing preoccupation with one or more stereotyped and restricted patterns of interest that is abnormal either in intensity or focus;

2. apparently inflexible adherence to specific, nonfunctional routines or rituals;
3. stereotyped and repetitive motor mannerisms (eg: hand or finger flapping or twisting, or complex whole-body movements);
4. persistent preoccupation with parts of objects.

C. *The disturbance causes clinically significant impairment in social, occupational, or other important areas of functioning.*

D. *There is no clinically significant general delay in language (eg: single words used by age 2 years, communicative phrases used by age 3 years).*

E. *There is no clinically significant delay in cognitive development or in the development of age-appropriate self-help skills, adaptive behaviour (other than social interaction), and curiosity about the environment in childhood.*

F. *Criteria are not met for another specific Pervasive Developmental Disorder or Schizophrenia.*

Dr Christopher Gillberg (2002), a Swedish physician with a particular interest in Asperger's syndrome, proposed six criteria for a diagnosis, elaborating upon the criteria set out in the DSM-IV. His criteria capture the unique characteristics of these children. His criteria included:

1. *Social impairment with extreme egocentricity, that included at least two of the following behaviours:*
   - Inability to interact with peers
   - Lack of desire to interact with peers
   - Poor appreciation of social cues
   - Socially and emotionally inappropriate responses
2. *Limited interests and preoccupations that included at least one of the following:*
   - Rote learning information without necessarily understanding meaning
   - Limited interests
   - Repetitive adherence
3. *Repetitive routines or rituals that were*:
   - Imposed on self, and/or
   - Imposed on others
4. *Speech and language peculiarities, that included:*
   - Possible delayed early development
   - Superficially perfect expressive language
   - Odd prosody, peculiar voice characteristics
   - Impaired comprehension including misinterpretation of literal and implied meanings
5. *Non-verbal communication problems, such as:*
   - Limited use of gesture
   - Clumsy body language
   - Limited or inappropriate facial expression
   - Peculiar 'stiff' gaze
   - Difficulty adjusting physical proximity
6. *Possibility of motor clumsiness*

Asperger's syndrome appears to have a somewhat later onset than autism, or at least tends to be recognised later, with many children not diagnosed until they are at school or even adults. In very young children, motor delays or motor clumsiness may be the first indication of the disorder. Once children attend school, their difficulties with social interaction become more obvious and problematic. During this period many of the children develop particular interests and idiosyncratic behaviours (such as an interest in how machines work, a knowledge of bus or train timetables or a fascination for collecting plastic dinosaurs). As adults, individuals with

Asperger's syndrome have difficulty relating to others, especially in establishing empathy and being able to modulate social interactions. These difficulties impact on their ability to form friendships and other long-term relationships.

Since 1994, Asperger's syndrome has been recognised as a separate disorder, with the introduction of Asperger's in the DSM-IV, but there remains confusion among professionals who diagnose the disorder. It is not at all clear whether Asperger's is a milder form of autism or whether the conditions are linked by nothing more than their broad clinical similarities.

Some professionals feel that Asperger's syndrome is the same as high functioning autism, while others describe it as a non-verbal learning disability. Asperger's syndrome must also be distinguished from obsessive-compulsive disorder and schizoid personality disorder. It is also not uncommon for children who were initially diagnosed with attention deficit disorder (ADD) or attention deficit hyperactive disorder (ADHD) to be later diagnosed with Asperger's syndrome. Additionally, some children originally diagnosed with pervasive developmental disorder-not otherwise specified (PDD-NOS) are later given a diagnosis of Asperger's syndrome while some individuals end up with a dual diagnosis of high functioning autism and Asperger's syndrome.

Many less impaired children, who technically would meet criteria for a diagnosis, actually remain undiagnosed and are merely viewed as 'different', 'odd' or 'unusual'. Some people are even misdiagnosed as ADD or emotionally disturbed. Some children struggle through school and eventually enter the workplace at a huge disadvantage knowing that they are different but unable to access any support. It may not be until they are adults and perhaps even have a child of their own with autism or Asperger's, that they are finally diagnosed and begin to understand and cope with their differences.

Liane Willey in her book *Pretending to be Normal* (1999), describes growing up and living with the disorder. Liane has a daughter with Asperger's syndrome whose diagnosis led to an understanding that she has the same condition. Liane, while different from her peers, remained undiagnosed until adulthood (pp 18, 30):

> By the time I was three years old, my parents knew I was not an average child. My paediatrician suggested they have me evaluated by a psychiatrist. Several conversations and an IQ test later, my diagnosis was decided: gifted and indulged. Smart and spoiled.
>
> ...
>
> Looking back, I can easily see why my parents, my psychiatrist and my paediatrician dismissed my actions as precocious or creative alternatives to the norm. Thoughts of anything related to autism would have been the farthest thing from their consciousness. Children with autism lived in a world of their own. They often hurt themselves, shrieked, raged and never spoke.

Lorna Wing was instrumental in bringing attention to Asperger's syndrome when, in 1981, she first used the term to describe a group of children and adults with a similar profile of abilities and behavioural characteristics to those first described by Hans Asperger in his doctoral thesis published in 1944. In 1983, Burgoine and Wing described the main clinical features of Asperger's syndrome as (p 263):

- lack of empathy;
- naïve, inappropriate, one-sided interaction;
- little or no ability to form friendships;
- pedantic, repetitive speech;
- poor non-verbal communication;
- intense absorption in certain subjects; and
- clumsy and ill-coordinated movements and odd postures.

In the last ten years, it has become the recognised view that Asperger's syndrome is a subgroup within the autism spectrum and a pervasive developmental disorder because the condition affects the development of a wide range of abilities. The evidence also suggests that Asperger's syndrome accounts for the majority of individuals diagnosed with an autism spectrum disorder (see Figure1.3 in Chapter 1).

There are no medical or genetic screening tests that can be used to diagnose Asperger's syndrome. Diagnosis requires a thorough and multidisciplinary approach using various diagnostic questionnaires and rating scales. A diagnosis of Asperger's syndrome involves parents and teachers and includes:

- Comprehensive early developmental history taking — this involves parents and other carers of the client providing background information and completing a questionnaire.
- Observations across a range of settings — this includes observation of the client at home, at school, in the playground and in any other relevant situation where his/her abilities and behaviour may be seen.
- Interactions with client — this involves engaging the client in play and conversation with the clinician but also involves observation of the client's interactions with others including parents, teachers and peers.
- Diagnostic interviews — these should be conducted with parents, teachers and other key professionals involved with the client. A diagnostic assessment takes at least an hour and examines specific aspects of social, language, cognitive and movement skills as well as qualitative aspects of the client's interests. This may include some formal testing using a range of psychological tests and rating scales.
- Comparison between information collected and formal diagnostic criteria as per established international diagnostic manuals (e.g. DSM-IV & ICD-10) — once all of the information has been collected and the client has been observed in a number of settings, a diagnosis is made on the basis of a comparison with the client's abilities and behaviour and those outlined in established international diagnostic manuals.

What causes Asperger's syndrome?

The causes of Asperger's syndrome are not known for certain but the general consensus is that there is no single cause. It is now believed that genetic factors play a major role in conjunction with other biological factors. Research has identified strong evidence of a neuro-developmental basis with differences in the brain structure and functioning of individuals with Asperger's syndrome being identified. As with autism, factors suggested for the differences in brain function of individuals with Asperger's include:

- genetic;
- prenatal;
- physical trauma; and
- metabolic.

Genetic factors

Asperger's syndrome is believed to have a strong genetic basis. This is evidenced in families where there is a history of developmental or behavioural problems, often undiagnosed. Studies have shown that up to 30 per cent of the fathers and 10 per cent of the mothers of children with Asperger's syndrome have similar difficulties. Though single gene abnormalities have been found in a minority of people with Asperger's syndrome, to date there is no indication of a consistent abnormality.

Prenatal factors

Prenatal conditions describe the health of the mother during pregnancy including exposure to viral or bacterial infections such as measles, rubella or mumps or premature birth.

Physical trauma

This may include birth trauma, including lack of oxygen, infantile spasms. Traumatic birth events appear to be more of an associated condition rather than the cause of the developmental difficulties in Asperger's syndrome.

Metabolic factors

These include measles and phenylketonuria. Asperger's syndrome is less commonly associated with other medical conditions than are other autism spectrum disorders. There is slightly increased incidence of epilepsy, neurofibromatosis, tuberous sclerosis and fragile-X syndrome in children with Asperger's syndrome than in the regular population.

Early occurrence

It appears that the predominant known and suspected causes of both autism and Asperger's syndrome occur early in children's lives. Before conception and during pregnancy, the parents' genetic makeup, metabolic disorders, environmental contaminants, diseases and infections, and social conditions, including poverty, substance abuse and inadequate prenatal care, affect reproduction and the development of the foetus.

At birth, birth complications and conditions of the newborn, such as prematurity or low birth weight, are known to affect brain development and increase the risk of impairment.

During early childhood, diseases and illnesses, malnutrition, lead poisoning, abuse and neglect, and injuries may result in autism or Asperger's syndrome.

While it is not known definitively what causes Asperger's syndrome, it is widely understood and acknowledged that the disorder is *not* caused by the way a child is parented.

What is the longer term prognosis for Asperger's syndrome?

Because varying developmental, neurological and genetic factors are considered to contribute to Asperger's syndrome, individuals vary greatly in their presentation. Asperger's syndrome affects the way a person communicates and relates to others but there may be a wide variance in these skills among individuals. The disability is also life-long. Many people diagnosed with Asperger's syndrome, however, are able to lead full and successful lives, following careers of their choice if provided with timely and appropriate support. Unlike autism, children and adults with Asperger's syndrome develop language skills early although they may have difficulty using these skills effectively. In addition, many individuals with Asperger's syndrome are of average to above average intelligence.

As Liane Willey, in her book *Asperger Syndrome in the Family* (2001, p 28) suggests, there is much that the general population can learn from individuals with Asperger syndrome (or Aspies):

I see aspies as books with unusual plots, multi-layered characters and far-out settings. I sit and shake my head in disbelief when I meet up with NTs (neuro-typicals) who aren't interested in turning our pages. If only they knew … if only they knew what they were missing.

People with Asperger's syndrome have a strong moral code that forces them to do what is right. As Liane states (p 29), they are 'rule followers and rule enforcers who can help others to see how much better the world would run if everyone obeyed the letter of the law'.

They also have a different way of seeing and sensing things that provides an unusual perspective to many routine events (p 28): 'We can tell you what intangibles feel like and secret flavours taste like. We can describe for you, in unbelievable depth, the intricate details of our favourite obsessions.'

And many people with Asperger's syndrome also have an uncanny ability to get to the heart of a matter or to pick out the relevant details of an argument and to know the right answer to a question (p 28): 'We can teach you how important it is to follow your instincts, for many of us have very strong gut knowledge, sort of like the way many blind folks have excellent hearing.'

What are the key features of Asperger's syndrome?

Children and adults diagnosed with Asperger's syndrome pose some difficult and specific challenges for the professionals and peers who work with them. These challenges are a result of their unique thinking and learning styles. They are typically seen as eccentric, egocentric and also strange by their peers and, because of this, may become the victims of bullying or become the scapegoat for their peers' inappropriate behaviours. Children with Asperger's syndrome are often described in the research literature as presenting like 'little professors' — very pedantic and driven by facts.

Individuals with Asperger's syndrome have poor motor skills, presenting as clumsy and badly co-ordinated, and not really interested in participating in general sporting activities. Some children and adults however may develop an obsessive interest in obscure topics including sporting achievements such as Australia vs England cricket scores over the past twenty years, the names of all of the winners of the FA Cup soccer competition or the names of the St George Football team players since the team was formed. Other obsessive interests include train arrival and departure times, species of dinosaurs, planets, car models and number plates, lawnmowers and road signs.

Children with Asperger's syndrome have difficulty understanding human relationships and the rules of social convention; they present as naïve and lacking in common sense. They are inflexible and unable to cope with change. This leads to stress and anxiety and makes them extremely emotionally vulnerable.

Children and adults with Asperger's syndrome are usually of average to above-average intelligence and have superior rote memory skills. They excel in certain areas and their obsessive focus on specific interests can lead to great success in adulthood. This is dependent on their thinking and learning styles being understood and their interests channelled into functional skills. Van Krevelen (cited in Frith 1991) stated that the child with autism 'lives in a world of his own', but the child with high functioning autism or Asperger's syndrome 'lives in our world but in his own way'.

Asperger's syndrome is recognised as being on the autism spectrum with characteristic difficulties in a number of key areas. These include a social impairment, communication impairment and repetitive behaviours and restricted interests, cognitive impairments, sensory and motor impairments and emotional vulnerability.

What is the social impairment in Asperger's syndrome?

The person with Asperger's syndrome stands out from peers, not by any distinguishing physical features, but by his or her unusual social and communication skills. For example, a child with Asperger's syndrome may run around after other children at the park thinking that he is playing when in fact the other children do not seem aware of his presence. He may approach another child at school with the greeting 'My Dad drives a red Falcon ute' rather than the more conventional greeting of 'Hi, my name is Adam, do you want to play?' An adult with Asperger's syndrome may appear unaware of other people's boredom and lack of interest when he holds forth about the specifications of the Boeing 737 Jumbo Jet or the Douglas DC10 at a social gathering. He tends to ignore other people's attempts to change the subject or to exit the group.

Children and adults with Asperger's syndrome are unable to understand complex rules of social engagement, are naïve and appear to be extremely egocentric. They may not like physical contact and tend to talk at people rather than to them. They have difficulty understanding jokes, irony or metaphors; they use monotone or stilted, unnatural tone of voice; they use inappropriate gaze and body language and appear insensitive and lacking in tact.

Most individuals misinterpret social cues: they are unable to judge 'social distance' and show limited ability to initiate and sustain conversation. They are easily taken advantage of because they do not perceive that others may trick or lie to them or deliberately set them up to take the blame for wrongdoing. Children and adults usually have a desire to be a part of the social world and to be liked by their peers.

The social impairments commonly found in children and adults with Asperger's syndrome include difficulties in:

- understanding social situations — may become confused or distressed;
- understanding other people's thoughts and feelings (empathy);
- forming and sustaining friendships and other relationships;
- social and imaginative play;
- taking part in 'small talk';
- initiating and sustaining conversations; and
- judging social appropriateness of words and actions.

According to Andron (2001, p 73):

> Many of the difficulties with social interaction that the children experience seem to be because of anxiety and motor planning. We have repeatedly seen evidence that the children do learn certain appropriate rules in an intellectual way ... We have found that unless they can see the situation they cannot relate to it.

Auditory processing and motor planning difficulties make it difficult for children to respond appropriately to ensure smooth social interaction. They become anxious and, even though they may want to interact and make friends with their peers, they are fearful of doing or saying the wrong thing or making a mistake.

Some programming suggestions to assist social integration may include teaching children and adults to respond to social cues and providing them with a number of possible responses to use in different social situations. Sometimes it may be necessary to teach the individual what to say and how to say it. Use lots of modelling and role-playing to teach two-way interactions.

Tony Attwood (2000) suggested that the emphasis should be placed on teaching 'friendship' skills rather than social skills. Because children and adults with Asperger's syndrome have difficulty interpreting and reading other people's body language and facial expression, as well as using those forms of non-verbal communication themselves in regular social situations, he outlined the following skills as important:

- entering — how the child enters a group of children and responds to their welcoming attempts;
- assistance — recognising when and how to provide assistance to others as well as how to obtain help;
- compliments — knowing how to give compliments to others and also how to receive compliments;
- criticism — knowing when criticism is appropriate, how to give constructive criticism and how to tolerate it from others;
- accepting suggestions — allowing others to suggest ideas and then incorporating these ideas into events and activities;
- reciprocity and sharing — sharing of conversation, direction of an activity and resources;
- conflict resolution — managing disagreement, learning to compromise and acknowledging the opinions of others;
- monitoring and listening — regularly observing others, being aware of their contribution and reading body language. Using body language to show interest in others;

- empathy — recognising when appropriate comments and actions are required, recognising the needs and feelings of others; and
- avoiding and ending — the appropriate behaviour and comments to avoid interaction or to end the interaction.

Friendship skills can be taught as part of a broader social skills training program.

Carol Gray (1993) developed the idea of using social stories as a way of providing both guidance and direction to promote self-awareness, self-calming and self-management in responding to social situations for students with autism and Asperger's syndrome. A social story describes social situations specific to individuals and circumstances.

Comic strip conversations were also introduced by Gray (1994) to illustrate and interpret social situations and provide support for 'students who struggle to comprehend the quick exchange of information which occurs in a conversation'. Comic strip conversations promote social understanding by incorporating simple figures and other symbols in a comic strip format.

It is important to foster involvement with others. This may entail encouraging individuals to actively socialise with others and limiting the amount of time spent in isolation or engaged in obsessive interests. Allowing individuals to build on their interests is an effective means of encouraging them to interact with others. For people with autism and Asperger's syndrome, socialisation and interaction is more effective if it is secondary to their interests. Encouraging a child with Asperger's syndrome, who is fascinated with computers and how they work, to join a computer club will provide opportunities to socialise with other members in an interesting and comfortable environment.

Tell her your name

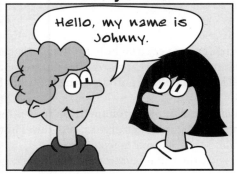

Wait for her answer

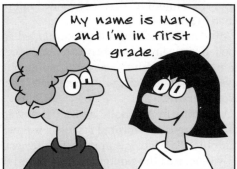

Smile and be friendly

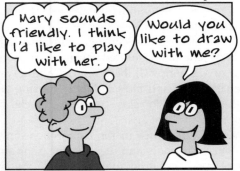

Remember to smile and take turns

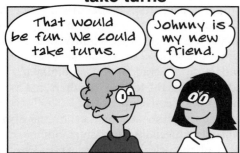

Figure 10.1 *Example of a comic strip conversation to teach social skills*

Linda Andron (2001, pp 67, 79) talks about the myth of social skills:

> Since the primary challenge these children face is social interaction, all those who love and work with them have sought to find a set of rules we can teach them that will allow them to function 'normally'.
>
> ...
>
> We must ask ourselves whether the goal is to teach the children a series of rules and skills that we deem requisite for social interaction. Is it not more important to teach people with HFA (high functioning autism) and AS (Asperger's syndrome) to value themselves for who they are? They must, of course, learn not to be totally egocentric and keep the perspectives of others in mind. But this does not require them to be something that they are not, only to be truly who they can be.

What is the communication impairment in Asperger's syndrome?

Previously, the difficulties of language and behaviour seen in autism and Asperger's syndrome were presumed to be the cause of the social difficulties that children and adults experienced. However, now the difficulties in social interaction and understanding are seen to underpin the difficulties in communication and to cause many of the problems in behaviour.

Impairments in verbal communication occur particularly in the pragmatics or practical and social use of language — often difficulty in initiating and sustaining conversation rather than in the pronunciation and syntax of language. Most individuals with Asperger's syndrome use language to communicate specific information, rather than as a means of social interaction and interactive communication. For example, a child may talk to request a video or talk at length about the content of a favourite video but be unable to tell you how their day was or what happened at school.

Most individuals have well-developed speech but poor communication and are sometimes labelled 'little professor' because their speech is pedantic and very scholarly or literal. There is often difficulty with the semantics of language or understanding that words and phrases may have multiple meanings. For example, the phrase 'it's raining cats and dogs outside' may be taken literally.

According to Attwood (1998), the development of grammar and pronunciation in children with Asperger's syndrome typically follows the same pattern as that of normally developing children. The problems appear in the way children and adults communicate:

- by repeating the same phrase over and over or asking the same question over and over;
- by talking in a monotone or with exaggerated inflexion;
- by talking about a particular topic of conversation that may be of no interest to anyone but themselves; and
- by being unable to sustain a conversation unless they are the dominant party and the topic of the conversation is about their particular narrow interest.

Impairments in non-verbal communication are also reflected in social behaviour, including limited use of gestures; clumsy and awkward body language; limited facial expressions; inappropriate facial expressions; or peculiar, stiff gaze (Gillberg & Gillberg 1989). Children and adults with Asperger's syndrome may also appear detached and have difficulty sensing and understanding the feelings of others, not look at others or stand too close to others in social situations when conversing.

Students with Asperger's syndrome also experience difficulties in the comprehension of language, especially in understanding abstract concepts; understanding the meaning and intent of rhetorical questions; and using figures of speech such as metaphors, idioms and allegories, particularly in written texts.

The communication impairments commonly found in children and adults with Asperger's syndrome include:

- limited understanding and use of non-verbal communication (e.g. limited facial expressions and gestures);
- unusual eye contact;
- unusual and often monotone vocal qualities;
- pedantic, repetitive speech;
- monologue rather than dialogue conversational style;
- tendency to provide too much or not enough information; and
- difficulty with non-literal language (e.g. slang, humour, sarcasm).

Programming ideas to assist the verbal and non-verbal communication skills of the person with Asperger's syndrome may include creating an environment that develops communicative intent, both verbal and non-verbal; develops the ability to initiate and maintain a conversation; and enhances an understanding of meaning. There should be awareness that a person's language level may not represent their communication level — it is important to check the person's understanding of language as well as their ability to use language functionally.

It is necessary to be explicit when giving instructions and not assume that the context will help to clarify meaning. Keep language simple and relevant to the situation and use visual supports to explain difficult concepts. Give one instruction at a time rather than a string of instructions that require advanced processing skills and keep facial expressions and gestures simple and clear.

Remember that it takes time to process information so give the person time to formulate a response and be sensitive to any attempts to communicate. Assess the individual's ability to use language socially, and teach conversation skills such as initiating a dialogue, listening to replies and following-up with an appropriate response.

What are the restricted and repetitive interests and behaviours in Asperger's syndrome?

Children and adults with Asperger's syndrome have eccentric preoccupations or odd, intense fixations. A person may develop an extreme interest in train timetables, dinosaurs, lawnmowers or studying the mechanics of clocks, radios or television sets. They tend to constantly 'lecture' on their specific areas of interest, ask repetitive questions on these topics and find it difficult to discuss other topics because they refuse to learn about anything outside their narrow field of interest. Instead of socialising with their peers, children and adults with Asperger's syndrome typically engage in their solitary interests (Szatmari 1991).

According to Attwood (1998), it is possible that individuals with Asperger's syndrome use these interests because they facilitate conversation, indicate intelligence, provide an enjoyable activity, serve as a means of relaxation or provide order and consistency in their life. As an expert on a particular topic, the individual with Asperger's syndrome may be respected and admired by their peers and also have a means of engaging in conversation in social situations.

Individuals with Asperger's syndrome are typically seen as rigid because they prefer order and sameness in their day-to-day routines, have to complete activities once started, may develop fears and phobias based on a single experience and have a preference for rules and structure.

The restricted and repetitive interests and behaviours commonly found in children and adults with Asperger's syndrome include:

- unusually strong, intense and narrow interests;
- resistance to change;
- preference for routines; and
- repetitive themes in stories, art and play.

Practical suggestions to assist the child or adult with Asperger's syndrome may include providing a predictable and safe environment with a consistent daily routine. Preparing for any change to a normal routine in advance will avoid surprises and allow the individual to understand what is happening.

Discourage any perseveration by not allowing individuals to continually discuss or ask questions about isolated interests. Limit the behaviour by establishing some rules. For example, a child who is fixated on car models and repeatedly asks everyone what make of car their family drives, may be restricted to asking each person once and only at recess. If this is part of the daily routine and the child is taught the rule, he will quickly learn to control the behaviour at other times.

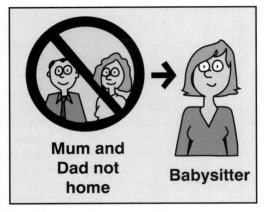

Mum and Dad not home

Babysitter

Figure 10.2 *Ideas for preparing someone for change*

What are the cognitive impairments in Asperger's syndrome?

Individuals with Asperger's syndrome usually are of average to above-average intelligence but lack higher-level thinking and comprehension skills. They tend to be very literal because their thinking is at a concrete level and abstraction is poor. Their pedantic speaking style and impressive vocabularies give the false impression that they understand what they are talking about, when in reality they may be parroting what they have heard or read. The person with Asperger's syndrome typically has an excellent rote memory, but it is mechanical in nature. Some children can recite an entire video or know when the person reading to them skips a page of a book because they have memorised the entire sequence of words.

Problem solving skills are generally poor with these children and adults and they face difficulties in generalising knowledge and skills. In other words, they may have difficulty applying information and skills learned in one setting to different situations and different people.

It is assumed that individuals with Asperger's syndrome possess the ability to process visual and auditory information but they often have difficulty processing both types of information concurrently. In addition, they typically require a longer time to take in and process information presented both orally and visually.

The cognitive and general learning impairments commonly found in children and adults with Asperger's syndrome include:

- specific learning disabilities despite normal IQ;
- poor comprehension relative to vocabulary use;
- difficulty with imaginative story writing;
- poor organisational and problem solving skills;
- problems processing spoken language, especially that which is abstract or complex;
- difficulty selecting important from unimportant information;
- tendency to focus on details; and
- problems seeing the 'big picture'.

Programming ideas to assist cognitive development may include ensuring that learning situations are structured in such a way that they are rewarding and not anxiety-provoking for the individual with Asperger's syndrome.

Ensure that individuals really understand information and instructions rather than assuming that they understand because they are able to parrot back what they have heard. Do

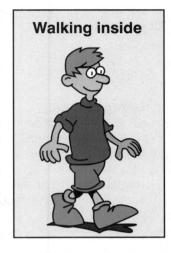

Walking inside

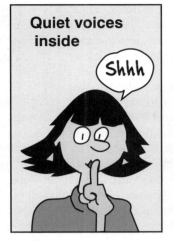

Quiet voices inside

Shhh

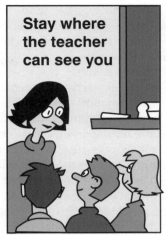

Stay where the teacher can see you

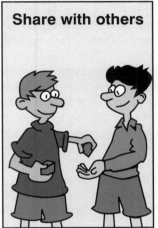

Share with others

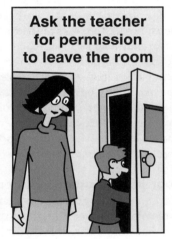

Ask the teacher for permission to leave the room

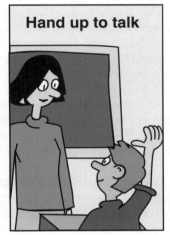

Hand up to talk

Figure 10.3 *Example of a rules board to teach school rules*

not assume that they understand what they so fluently read as this may be an example of their exceptional reading recognition skills rather than their comprehension skills.

Try to simplify any abstract concepts and capitalise on an individual's exceptional memory abilities by offering factual information in a concrete fashion that is easily processed and retained. Use visual supports such as sequence boards, choice boards, rules boards and timetables to assist the individual's understanding of different concepts. The use of visual supports to assist children and adults with an autism spectrum disorder has proven effective over time. For more detailed information about visual supports, see Chapter 12.

What are the sensory and motor problems in Asperger's syndrome?

People with Asperger's syndrome are usually clumsy and awkward, with poor balance and coordination. They are also prone to unusual sensory responses such as hypersensitivity or hyposensitivity to certain sounds, tastes, smells and visual stimuli. Some individuals may be unable to tolerate bright light, flickering light or sunlight and may feel calmer in a darkened room. Other individuals may be overly sensitive to specific sounds such as sirens, vacuum cleaners, flushing toilets or someone singing, or be overly sensitive to certain touch or textures.

The sensory and motor impairments commonly found in children and adults with Asperger's syndrome may include:

- over- or under-sensitivity to taste, touch, sight smell, sound, temperature and pain;
- low muscle tone;
- unusual posture;
- clumsy or awkward movements; and
- repetitive motor movements (e.g. finger flicking, handflapping, rocking and pacing).

Some programming suggestions to assist children to manage their sensory difficulties may include having an understanding of each individual's sensory problems and eliminating any sensory inputs that impinge on their ability to function in the home, classroom or work environment. Probably the most important and effective strategy for dealing with sensory problems is to be aware of them and to also understand some of the resultant behaviours in the individual when sensory overload occurs: 'All the behavioural intervention in the world will not stop a child from becoming distressed if the sound of the bell hurts.' (Quill 1995)

Children and adults should have a safe place to retreat to when sensory overload occurs. This should be a place where the individual can calm down and feel safe and secure. A retreat can be created within the home, the classroom or the workplace and may include a comfortable chair, big pillows, headphones, favourite books and/or a trampoline or swing. For some individuals, deep pressure exercises may also be calming. This may include wrapping up in a blanket or sitting in a large beanbag.

Some children with sensory difficulties may engage in excessive and repetitive behaviours such as rocking, hand flicking or head banging when their sensory system is overloaded or when the system is under-stimulated. Allowing some controlled periods of self-stimulation may act as a 'stress de-activator' or may provide necessary stimulation to the vestibular system. Sensory integration may assist some children and adults to become desensitised to problem areas and to learn to regulate their behaviours.

What emotional issues occur in Asperger's syndrome?

Children and adults with Asperger's syndrome are intelligent enough to cope in society but they often do not have the emotional resources to cope with the ordinary demands of everyday life. They are easily stressed, partly because of their inflexibility. Typically they have poor self-esteem and are self-critical. Individuals with Asperger's syndrome, especially adolescents, are prone to depression and anxiety, and temper outbursts are common in response to any stressful or frustrating situation. A recent study by Tonge, Brereton, Gray & Einfield (1999), indicated that 85% of children with Asperger's syndrome experienced clinically significant levels of behavioural and/or emotional disturbance. This is compared with approx 10–15% of the normative population in the study who experienced behavioural and emotional disturbance.

One suggestion to assist children and adults with Asperger's syndrome to cope is to offer a high level of consistency. Prepare them for changes in daily routines to minimise anxiety and lower stress levels. Individuals with Asperger's syndrome typically become fearful, angry and upset when faced with forced or unexpected changes.

Provide strategies to show individuals how to cope when faced with stressful situations and to prevent behaviour outbursts. Present these strategies in a concrete way that the person can refer to when upset.

A visual strategy may be used in the classroom to explain to a child that a change in the normal routine will occur because it is too wet to play outside after morning tea. Instead of playing outside, all of the children will watch a video.

It is important for professionals and family members to remain calm, predictable and matter-of-fact in interactions. According to Hans Asperger (1991, p 57), 'the teacher who does

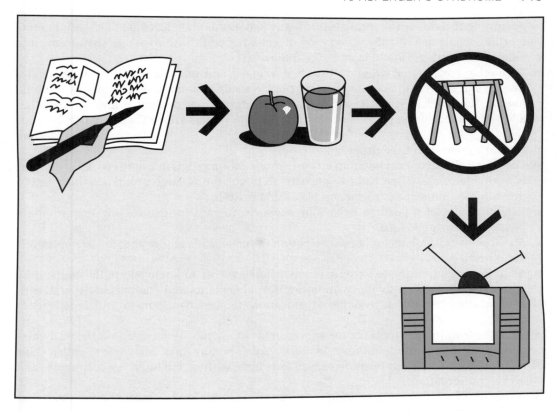

Figure 10.4 *Example of visual strategy to teach and reinforce change to a normal routine*

not understand that it is necessary to teach children seemingly obvious things will feel impatient and irritated'.

Be alert to changes in behaviour that may indicate depression, such as greater levels of disorganisation, inattentiveness and isolation; higher levels of stress; fatigue; crying or talk of suicide. It is important to be aware that adolescents with Asperger's syndrome are especially prone to depression. Social skills are highly valued in adolescence, and those with Asperger's syndrome usually start to notice their differences and the difficulties they have forming relationships during this period of development.

What treatment options are available?

Students diagnosed with Asperger's syndrome usually attend mainstream programs such as early intervention preschool services or school settings. Many children and adults with Asperger's characteristics also remain undiagnosed or are misdiagnosed with either attention deficit disorder (ADD) or attention deficit hyperactive disorder (ADHD). All of these children and adults present particular challenges for their parents, teachers and peers.

For the successful integration of these children and adults into mainstream programs, there needs to be a close working relationship between parents and professionals. Most treatment options include developing a plan that takes into account the particular needs, temperament, strengths and deficits of the individual and also the resources of the family. Any discussions should include parents and professionals as well as the individual with Asperger's syndrome, especially any discussions related to future planning and treatment.

According to Prior & Cumming (2000), any successful plan developed between parents and professionals to assist the integration of a child or adult with Asperger's syndrome into a mainstream setting, should include the following:

- A suitable educational program that is developed and implemented for the particular person and takes into account their particular needs is important. The program should look at the ways in which instructions and materials are presented and also whether additional specialist support is necessary in certain subject areas. There needs to be goals set   and regular evaluation of the program.
- For young children, enrolment in an early intervention program where specialist support is available to assist the child to participate in small and large group activities and to develop communication, social and play skills is vital.
- Establishment of a positive behaviour support program to manage any inappropriate behaviours is a good idea.
- Social skills training including participation in social skills groups that are age appropriate is needed.
- Adaptive skills training to encourage independence both at home and in the community is required. This is particularly important for adolescents and may include special programs to teach skills in hygiene, organisation, money management and independent travel.
- Vocational training, especially for adolescents with a view to focusing on the particular person's strengths and interests is necessary. Training may include specialist skills required for a particular position as well as rèsumè writing, job interview techniques and overall presentation.
- Inclusion of management techniques or treatments for any co-morbid conditions that may impact on the child or adult's behaviour is important. This may include additional therapies such as speech or occupational therapy. Sometimes, pharmacological intervention such as medication to control certain co-morbid conditions, for example ADD or ADHD, may be necessary.
- Recognition of the individual's obsessions or special interests and inclusion of creative management strategies to ensure that these obsessions do not interfere with learning opportunities is a helpful tool.

Do people with Asperger's syndrome have special abilities?

When individuals with Asperger's syndrome are compared to their non-disabled peers, 'one is instantly aware of how different they are and the enormous effort they have to make to live in a world where no concessions are made and where they are expected to conform' (Everard 1976, p 2). However, when one compares these individuals with their non-disabled peers, one is also made aware of some of their special strengths and abilities that allow them to stand out from their peers and to offer a unique perspective on the world around them. Among the particular strengths commonly seen in individuals with Asperger's syndrome is a strong visual learning style that enables the individual to work well in structured, routine environments. Most individuals also have an excellent memory for facts and most develop an expertise in areas of particular interest.

People with Asperger's syndrome are logical thinkers and often excel in computing, maths and the sciences. They also show outstanding strengths in their ability to rote learn information, attention to detail and in their ability to sustain focus over long periods of time in areas of interest. These strengths enable some individuals with autism to obtain and maintain particularly specialised jobs, especially in the mathematic and computer science areas.

Asperger's syndrome is recognised as a disability that affects a person's ability to function in society. As a person diagnosed with Asperger's syndrome, however, Liane Willey (2001, p 139) has a different view:

> I like to say aspies are not defective, but rather that we are simply different; differently able, if you will. Yes, we have learning inefficiencies, but never are we without the ability to learn, grow, cope and progress. Pushed further, I would assert we aspies are fine like we are, or at least we would be, if only society would learn to be more accepting and empathetic toward the a-typical.

Summary

While there are recognisable similarities among individuals with Asperger's syndrome, it still affects each person it touches in unique ways. All people with Asperger's syndrome share a number of common traits such as:

- difficulty making friends — socialisation problems;
- difficulty reading or communicating non-verbal social cues, such as facial expression — communication and socialisation problems;
- difficulty understanding that others may have thoughts or feelings different from his or her own — egocentric perspectives;
- obsessive focus on a narrow interest, such as talking about dinosaurs — perseverations, obsessive interests, rigid thinking;
- awkward motor skills — odd fine and large motor clumsiness;
- inflexibility about routines, especially when changes occur spontaneously — literal mindedness; and
- mechanical, almost robotic patterns of speech — semantic/pragmatic misunderstandings.

However, while children and adults with Asperger's syndrome have broad characteristics in common, the individual key features present in many different ways in each person. The characteristics of autism include the core deficits as well as emotional problems, sensory and cognitive impairments that affect individuals with Asperger's syndrome. A number of strategies that may assist individuals with Asperger's syndrome to cope have been recommended.

It is important to recognise and understand the particular difficulties faced by individuals with Asperger's syndrome and it is also essential to recognise and acknowledge the particular strengths of these individuals and to acknowledge the unique contributions that they can and do make to society.

Does autism start as a glitch in one area of the brain — the brainstem, perhaps — and then radiate out to affect others? Or is it a widespread problem that becomes more pronounced as the brain is called upon to set up and utilize increasingly complex circuitry? Either scenario is plausible, and experts disagree as to which is more probable. But one thing is clear: very early on, children with autism have brains that are anatomically different on both microscopic and macroscopic scales.

Time Magazine 6 May 2002

Any attempt to understand autism should include knowledge of how people with autism think and learn; that is, an understanding of the unique ways in which they obtain and process information from their environment. Major differences in the learning styles of people with autism tend to be noticed early, usually in the play of young children when they fail to develop appropriate social play skills.

This chapter will put into perspective much of the information, previously discussed, about the characteristics of autism and how these characteristics affect individuals with autism. The characteristics or core deficits of autism are responsible for the unique ways that these individuals think and learn; the differences are most evident in their communication, social relating, general behaviour and the way they process information from the senses.

Observations of children with autism have shown differences in the ways they explore objects and relate to others. They have difficulties with eye gaze and listening. They also appear unable to focus on what is happening around them, leading to many problems associated with attending. Their play tends to be limited and focused more on the use of particular objects rather than an interest in, or an awareness of, other people. They may appear almost obsessively interested in certain objects such as trains, blocks or cars but only to line them up or spin the wheels. There is little attempt to study different ways of playing with the objects/toys or of playing socially with someone else.

Young children with autism tend to fear change. They often engage in ritualistic self-stimulatory behaviour, such as spinning or lining up objects, to assist them to cope in new and unfamiliar situations. These problems indicate that there are differences in the way that they select stimuli, process the information collected, and then give the appropriate responses. According to Trevarthen et al (1996, p 25):

> Abnormalities of perception, attention and exploration undoubtedly handicap the learning and thinking of autistic children, leading to an accumulation of disability. Those (children) that appear to develop high intelligence usually do so in narrow or specialized areas that seem to be practiced through the child's unusual capacity to become absorbed over and over again in a preferred activity in isolation from other people.

This observation ties in with Kanner's early emphasis on 'autistic aloneness' as the basis for a diagnosis of autism — aloneness that has nothing to do with being alone physically, but rather with being alone mentally and emotionally. The second feature of prime importance to Kanner was termed 'obsessive insistence on sameness'. It suggested repetitiveness, rigidity, single-mindedness, pedantry and inability to judge the significance of subtle differences. Examples of these behaviours include simple repetitive movements, utterances and thoughts as well as elaborate routines, often without any purpose. There is also a pursuit of extremely narrow topics of interest, a preoccupation to the exclusion of almost everything else. Both Kanner (1943) and Asperger (1944) were impressed with the 'strikingly intelligent physiognomy' of the children with autism and by their unusual skills and interests. The behaviour of children with autism will often hint at capabilities out of the ordinary, occasionally even rare talents.

Even though Kanner's research was conducted in 1943, the patterns of behaviour he described are still recognised and accepted today. They still form the basis of our understanding about how children and adults with autism think and learn. In order to understand the differences that people with autism show in their thinking and learning styles, it is necessary to look at how they take in, analyse, store and then retrieve and use information.

Janice E. Janzen (1996) likens the central nervous system to a computer that does all of these tasks simultaneously:

- the input system takes in information from the environment;
- the information processing system analyses the information and extracts meaning from it; and
- the output system integrates the information, stores it and then formulates a response.

In most people, these systems function and interact simultaneously to organise and integrate information from new experiences with relevant information from past experiences. People's natural curiosity encourages these systems to work constantly to take in, analyse, store and retrieve information from the many natural sources that occur through interaction with the environment. This curiosity supports the notion that most of what is learned comes through incidental learning — observation, imitation and trial-and-error practice.

Children and adults with autism have input, processing and output systems that 'cannot interact and function simultaneously and automatically' (Janzen 1996). These irregularities lead to some differences in behaviour that can only be explained and understood when the learning style is clarified.

What is the learning style of people with autism?

The individual learning styles of children and adults with autism vary from person to person but there are a number of core characteristics that form/make up the cognitive thinking patterns of all individuals with autism.

These core characteristics include difficulties with eye gaze, attending, understanding meaning, generalising, auditory processing, sensory processing, sequencing and higher order cognitive abilities. The strengths of people with autism include rote memory abilities, visual spatial abilities, compartmentalised chunk learning abilities and preference for structured routines and rules.

As discussed earlier, there are individual differences to be considered along the autism continuum. Not all people with autism will experience the same problems and difficulties in each of the core characteristics, nor will they experience the same level of difficulty. Some people will have strengths and weaknesses in certain areas while someone else may have learning strengths and weaknesses in other areas. Uneven profiles of skills and deficits (strengths and weaknesses) are common characteristics of children and adults with autism. A person with autism may have a superior ability to see spatial relationships or understand numerical concepts but be unable to achieve in these areas because of the difficulties they have organising and communicating effectively. This supports the hypothesis that to know one person with autism is not necessarily to know autism.

Many of the core differences associated with autism have been discussed in previous chapters but will be revisited here in order to develop an overall picture of how individuals with autism think and function on a day-to-day basis. This knowledge will assist parents and professionals to better understand and assist any individuals with autism that they know and work with. Among the core differences in autism are the following:

- poor eye contact;
- difficulties attending;
- difficulties processing information;
- poor listening skills;
- sensory sensitivities;
- difficulties empathising;
- concrete, literal thinking;
- unusual rote memory abilities;
- visual spatial abilities; and
- compartmentalised chunk learning style.

Poor eye contact

Over the years, the importance of eye gaze or eye contact and children with autism has been blown out of all proportion. Some doctors have even based a diagnosis of autism on whether or not a child 'will look at you'. Most parents are told of the importance of having their child look at them and are required to 'encourage eye contact' in their child in many different situations throughout the day. Children are therefore required to look at a person before they are acknowledged, given objects or played with.

In reality, limited eye gaze is just one of the unique learning characteristics of children with autism and the degree of eye contact will vary enormously from person to person. Some children with autism actively avoid looking directly at another person and may become distressed and anxious when required to look at, or attend to others. Some children appear to make eye contact relatively easily but may actually be focusing on something else or looking right through the other person so that it is not a true communicative or social exchange.

There has, to date, been no indication among people with autism that eye contact serves any useful purpose for them; that it provides a means of either receiving or sharing mutually understood messages. It is important to consider the possible purposes for requiring eye contact and the assumptions underlying the need for it then before parents are pressured to continue to prioritise developing eye contact in their young children over other skills. Eye gaze is usually seen as a way of obtaining a child's attention, for example the cue 'Look at me'. Eye gaze is also a way of gauging a child's ongoing attention to the task at hand. The assumption is that when a child is giving eye contact, or looking at a person, they are attending, and those failing to conform to the request cannot be paying attention. If a child fails to respond to a verbal cue to 'look at me!' it may be also seen as non-compliance. Eye contact then becomes a means of measuring compliance.

Every child is different, and requiring eye contact in order to obtain, focus and maintain attention depends on the individual child and the circumstances surrounding the expectation. It becomes necessary to consider whether insisting on eye contact in a particular situation helps children to attend, or whether it actually hinders what the parent or teacher is attempting to achieve.

A number of adults with autism have described the difficulties they have making eye contact. These difficulties are summed up by Jean-Paul Bovee (1999, p 19) an adult with high functioning autism who wrote:

> Eye contact is something that I have always had trouble with. It does not come naturally to me and I do not appreciate having to give it all of the time, especially to people that I do not know. All of the stress that is put on doing it makes me more nervous, tense and scared ... I can look at a person's eyes and not be able to tell what they are saying to me ... I can concentrate better not having to keep eye contact at the same time.

It may be difficult for people with autism to attend to more than one source of sensory input at a time. Therefore if people insist that children give eye contact, especially during structured play sessions, chances are they will be concentrating on complying with that request and will fail to attend to what is actually being said or shown to them.

Emily found it difficult to interact with other people, even close family members, and rarely gave eye contact. She would actively avoid looking directly at another person but tended to use her peripheral vision to provide her with the visual information she required. Emily became distressed if she was forced to give eye contact. Eventually her teachers found it was more effective to encourage Emily to concentrate on the activity she was doing rather than to look at another person. Emily was happier and less distressed and her schoolwork improved dramatically.

When developing strategies to encourage children with autism to focus and attend to particular activities, recognise that conventional social expectations might in fact, interfere with their learning. It is more beneficial to guide individual children to focus on the task at hand rather than to force them to give eye contact and then have to shift their attention from the person back to the activity.

Another interesting point is made by Andron (2000, p 71):

> We must remember that in some cultures eye contact is actually seen as rude. Moreover, it is equally important to break eye contact intermittently, so that the other person does not think that you are staring. However, there are no specific rules we can teach for when this should happen — It is far better to teach the concept of shared attention (Sigman & Capps 1997). Thus the goal is to help the children learn to look at what they or the other person are talking about.

The important issue is to determine what is to be achieved in a particular situation before insisting on eye contact. If the goal is to teach children to interact with others, encourage them to look at the person as a means of acknowledging their presence. However, if trying to show children how to play with a particular toy (how to build a block tower, pop bubbles or put shapes into a shape sorter) or complete a particular activity (such as a puzzle, a drawing, a bead threading sequence) it is much more important that they are able to focus on, and attend to, the actual task at hand. In this situation, it may therefore hinder their ability to attend and focus on the task if they are forced to look at the other person first.

Difficulties attending

Attention is the ability to focus selectively on a desired stimulus or task. According to Williamson & Anzalone (1997), the two components of attention are known as selection and allocation.

Selection enables a person to choose what to attend to and to shift between several different options. It is like going into a bookstore and scanning the shelves for the topics that are of interest and then choosing one or two books from that section to look at in more detail.

Allocation determines how long a person can attend to a stimulus as well as how much effort it takes to maintain that focus. If a particular book is really interesting, it may take little effort to become engrossed in the story for a long period of time whereas another book may take more effort to read and be hard to maintain interest for very long.

Children and adults with autism tend to have difficulty attending to auditory and tactile input and may prefer visual and vestibular channels (Kientz & Dunn, 1997). According to Sigman & Capps (1997), children also tend to avoid eye contact and joint attention and generally favour attending to inanimate objects rather than to other people.

Some individuals have a narrow focus of attention so that they focus on minute details and are oblivious to the bigger picture; others have problems shifting attention either within or between modalities. Another common problem occurs when a person appears withdrawn and unable to focus on particular stimuli. Some people with autism may focus on stereotypic activities such as spinning, rocking or handflapping in order to exclude environmental input. They will then tend to avoid multi-sensory experiences that are uncomfortable or confusing.

> Joshua is a 4-year-old boy who will happily spend hours spinning the wheels of his toy cars. He also enjoys lying on the ground driving them back and forth past his eyes so that he can watch the wheels rotate. He enjoys the visual stimulation but becomes distressed if anyone else tries to join in his activity, especially if they talk to him, introduce additional toys and try to change the way that he plays. He does not appear able to attend to more than one variable at a time and becomes confused and distressed at the additional information to be processed.

As outlined in Chapter 2, children and adults with autism have difficulties with many aspects of attending. Common attention problems associated with autism include:

- switching on attention, especially when people are required to attend to something that is not of particular interest to them;
- selecting what to attend to, so that the important details are selected and any irrelevant information is discarded;
- shifting attention from one activity or person to another without losing the focus of what is important;
- sustaining attention over a longer period of time in order to take in any relevant information;
- sharing a focus of attention with others and developing the idea of shared meaning; and
- attending to multi-sensory information that comes from a number of different sensory sources rather than rely on information from only one sense at a time.

It is often difficult for children and adults with autism to pay attention to what is going on around them because they tend to focus their attention on those things that appear most interesting and relevant to them. They also tend to shift focus quite rapidly from one sensation to another. When this occurs, it is unlikely that they are actually taking in any of the relevant information.

According to Mesibov (1997), children with autism are easily distracted from paying attention by things that appear to be motivating or stimulating for them, such as a desire for a particular video, object or food, as well as the need to engage in repetitive questioning, counting or reciting facts.

Children and adults with autism are sensitive to certain stimuli and may be distracted by different sounds, smells, visual patterns or small parts of objects.

These may include flashing lights, sounds of a particular frequency, repetitive movement of objects such as spinning fans or certain scents or textures. People may be interested in different stimuli so they do not find many everyday activities or objects stimulating enough to maintain their attention for long periods. Frith says (1989, p 108): 'One of the recurrent themes in biographical accounts of autistic people is that certain stimuli seem to hold some inexplicable fascination for them while other stimuli, normally interesting and salient, apparently leave them untouched.'

> Selene is sensitive to smell, touch and different textures. She goes to a special school and she is doing well in class. However, in the playground, she tends to ignore the other children and does not join in the activities the teacher introduces. She prefers to walk around the playground touching the wooden fence and rubbing her hands over the brickwork. She also likes to stand close to the teachers and sniff their shoulders to see if they are wearing perfume. Selene knows that she is not allowed to do this.

Temple Grandin (1986, p 22), in her autobiographical account of her life as a child with autism, discusses her preoccupation with things that would be of little interest to most people. 'I also liked to sit for hours humming to myself and twirling objects or dribbling sand through my hands at the beach ... My mind was actively engaged in these activities. I was fixated on them and ignored everything else.'

People with autism do not focus on the big picture but tend to focus on minor details within their environment. They pay attention to those things that they perceive as important, meaningful and relevant to themselves. They are able to sustain attention for long periods of time, but only for certain activities, when anyone else would have lost interest. They are able to concentrate on things that would be of little interest to other people. One child will watch a particular video, or part of a video, over and over again with great enjoyment while another person will sit and read the Yellow Pages of the telephone directory for hours at a time. A person with autism may be content to focus on a narrow topic that is of particular interest for a long period of time, whereas most people would attend to it briefly and find it interesting or relevant only as one part of a larger pattern.

People with autism have difficulty interpreting and prioritising external stimulation as well as the many internal thoughts that bombard them. Some people are constantly moving and exploring as if all sensations are equally exciting. Other people ignore or shut out most of the external sensations and become preoccupied with a small number of objects or with a limited activity. A young adult may be more interested in the credits scrolling across the screen at the end of a television show than the content of the show itself. Another child may become totally focused on the leaves on the trees moving in the wind rather than what the teacher is saying at preschool.

> Bella loves to play outside where she can run around and chase the leaves that blow along the grass. She does not notice that it is getting dark and has started to rain. She is totally focused on watching the movement of the leaves and does not feel cold or wet.

Difficulties processing information

As people develop and learn through exposure to different experiences, they memorise information and then recall it whenever they need to, perhaps in a similar situation. New experiences impinge on what they remember, changing and adapting the information to redefine all related knowledge and modifying their responses. In contrast, people with autism have unusual memory and processing skills characterised by concrete perceptual abilities and poor generalising skills. Most individuals with autism are very concrete thinkers with little ability to understand abstract concepts — they see the world in black and white rather than shades of grey. They also experience difficulties in generalising skills from one situation to other settings and people.

There is evidence to suggest that children and adults with autism have abnormal ways of processing information, ways that involve less attention to overall pattern, structure and meaning, and more attention to small elements of structure or finer details. It has been suggested that individuals with autism do not process information in a methodical way. Information does not tend to be independently organised and analysed in such a way as to store relevant details and discard the clutter, to elicit meaning from the information or to combine new and previously stored information to develop meaning.

Children and adults with autism have a tendency to focus on one aspect of a situation or on small details such as the letters on the side of the cereal box or the numbers on the gate of a house. They focus on the small details and miss important elements in the larger setting. They often miss the big picture that provides the information required to make sense of what is happening around them. Because they miss most of the information that is normally provided by looking at the big picture, people with autism do not accurately read their environment or understand the purpose of many actions or events.

As typical children grow and develop, they learn to reason and infer from the information

---

Olivia attends a special school where she has been taught to line up at the door when the bell rings before going out into the playground with the other children for recess and lunch. At home, Olivia usually goes and stands at the back door and waits for a prompt from her mother whenever she wants to go outside and play, even if the door is open and other people are already in the yard.

---

they take in and process. They are able to integrate all aspects of a situation and make response decisions based on a choice of possible meanings and explanations. They learn to predict, to take an overall view, to sequence and to generalise.

Children with autism, however, find higher cognitive abilities difficult because they are unable to make sense of the people and the world around them. They have difficulty remembering the precise order of tasks because they focus concretely on specific details and often do not see relationships between them. The use of visual supports to show individual steps and an overall sequence compensate for these difficulties. A visual sequence can highlight the sequence of events and indicate the correct order to follow (see Figure 11.1).

Children and adults with autism seem unable to generalise skills and activities from one setting to another. This inability to generalise has implications for both educational practices and situations at home. Children and adults frequently do not apply what they have learned in one situation to other similar settings. According to Mesibov (1998, p 320), 'appropriate generalization requires an understanding of the central principles in learned sequences and the subtle ways in which they are applicable to other situations'. Because they tend to focus on specific details, people with autism will often miss these central principles and

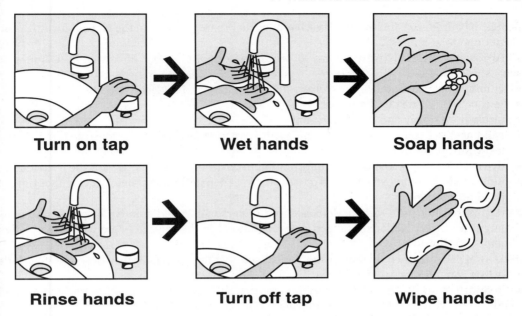

| Turn on tap | Wet hands | Soap hands |

| Rinse hands | Turn off tap | Wipe hands |

Figure 11.1 *Example of a visual hand-washing sequence for children and adults with autism*

how to apply them generally. They have difficulty processing information and formulating appropriate responses.

The work of Hermelin & O'Connor (1970) was innovative in information processing research. They carried out systematic research into the cognitive abilities of children with autism in comparison with younger normal children and intellectually impaired children. They introduced the idea that input is separated from output, and both are separated from central processes where information is received, stored and analysed. Hermelin (1976) also concluded that autistic children have a central deficiency in the processing of incoming and outgoing information. She found that children with autism found it difficult to code and categorise information and have an 'echo-box' memory store as demonstrated in the prevalence of echolalic speech.

Donna Williams, a woman with Asperger's syndrome, in her book *Autism and Sensing — The Unlost Instinct* (1998) explains many of her difficulties in terms of general information processing problems. She explains information processing as taking in information from the senses and then organising it for meaning and personal significance. Individuals need to monitor their own actions and feelings and also monitor what is being expressed for intention and meaning. Information processing is also about accessing previous experiences and knowledge to relate to new information and then formulating a response. According to Williams, people have to maintain a grip on their thoughts, feelings and experiences to formulate meaningful responses to current situations. For individuals with autism, the ability to maintain a grip on the present while accessing stored information and monitoring expression can be overwhelming. For most people, this happens unconsciously and without consideration of what is being done.

According to Frith (1989, p 74), people with autism are unable 'to draw together information so as to derive coherent and meaningful ideas. There is a fault in the predisposition of the mind to make sense of the world.' The work of Francesca Happe (1994), looking at cognitive learning style in autism, has supported this theory. Happe suggests that people with autism are not global thinkers and have 'weak central coherence'. As a result of weak central coherence, people may produce what they hear verbatim, rather than understand the global meaning of an event or action.

To assist individuals with autism to process information more effectively, the following suggestions may help:

- simplify language and use key words rather than long and involved speeches;
- be concise and stick to the point;
- speak more slowly and clarify meaning;
- avoid abstract concepts and keep things at a concrete level so that things are tangible and easily interpreted;
- give clear messages and present information in whatever format works for the individual;
- allow the individual extra time to process information and remain quiet during that time to avoid distractions;
- keep communication formal, detached and impersonal. Avoid emotive language and body language. Direct explanations and demonstrations to the objects or items related to that demonstration;
- be aware that many individuals with autism suffer chronic stress and anxiety and that these factors can influence behaviour;
- be aware of an individual's sensory preferences and sensory sensitivities, and understand how the environment influences information processing;
- cut down on irrelevant, excessive and distracting sensory information; and
- individual health issues also impact on a person's ability to function, so ensure that any general health problems are appropriately addressed.

Poor listening skills

In most learning environments, instructions — information, directions, rules, requests, prompts and reinforcements — are traditionally presented verbally. This can create enormous difficulties for children and adults with autism who generally have poor auditory processing abilities and poor listening skills. Children with autism perform better in spatial, perceptual and matching tests than in verbal tests that require auditory processing abilities (Prior 1979). People with autism are visual learners. They are generally described as being 90% visual and 10% auditory learners (Hodgdon 1995).

Many young children with autism are initially thought to be deaf because they fail to respond to the sound of the human voice. They fail to respond when parents call their name or ask them to complete a simple task. According to Janzen (1996), one of the common problems associated with autism is a perception of hearing loss. However, people with autism can hear. Unfortunately, they have problems processing the information that is presented verbally.

Other auditory processing problems associated with autism include:

- Sensory impairments that lead to distortions in what is being heard — children who are hypersensitive to certain sounds may be overwhelmed by the painful quality of auditory stimulation. They focus on avoiding the sounds rather than concentrating on processing the relevant information.
- The amount of time it takes for people with autism to take in, analyse and respond to auditory stimuli — there may be a significant delay between an initial verbal request and the production of a meaningful response. Response time may be anywhere from 20 to 60 seconds, or longer. Most people are not used to waiting that long so either give up or repeat the request, usually in a different way. This often leads to confusion or anxiety for the person with autism.
- The transience of verbal information does not lend itself to long response times — the information is presented and then is gone, often before the person with autism has had time to take it in.

■ Because people with autism tend to process information in chunks and their attention is inconsistent, some parts of information that are presented verbally may be missed and remain unprocessed. This ensures that the meaning is lost.

Sensory sensitivities

Children and adults with autism may have sensory impairments that affect the way they register, store and process information from their environment. They may show unusual responses to different sensory experiences, especially sounds or touch, but also taste, vision, smell and pain. People with autism may over-react (hyper-sensitivity) or under-react (hypo-sensitivity) to these different sensory stimuli, often perceiving ordinary sensations as weak or intense.

Many people have problems maintaining optimal arousal and focused attention. They also fail to orient, process and respond to new and unpredictable stimuli or events in the same way as their peers.

Kanner, in his initial paper (1943), did not specifically mention sensory impairment as an important feature in the diagnosis of autism. He noted that loud noises were disturbing for some children with autism but he felt that this was part of their desire to withdraw from the world. According to the psychodynamic theorists of the 1950s, children with autism were born with unusual sensitivities that allowed them to cut themselves off from the world because their mothers did not appropriately regulate the input they received. This caused stress and forced them to build protective barriers to help them to cope.

Once the psychodynamic theories were rejected, it was not until Ornitz (1973) proposed that functional disturbance in sensory modulation was a core characteristic of autism, that interest in sensory modulation and sensory processing were revived.

Sensory modulation may be defined as the capacity to internally regulate the amount and intensity of sensory input (Huebner 2001; Dunn 2001).

Sensory processing includes an ability to register, decode, comprehend and categorise sensory input and sensory patterns from a number of different sources.

Sensory integration is the ability to organise input from multiple senses for use in adaptive responses.

At least 90% of children with autism experience sensory processing difficulties (Eaves et al 1994; Kientz & Dunn 1997).

A number of autobiographical works have described individual childhoods. These included descriptions of sensory problems encountered trying to function in a world where it was impossible to filter out irrelevant background noise and where many of the environmental sounds were magnified and distorted. However, it has only been in the last few years that interest in sensory processing, as an important part of the learning and thinking style of people with autism, has evolved and grown.

Research to date on the importance of sensory processing has supported the work of early neuroscientists who claimed a relationship between the way the nervous system receives, interprets and uses sensory information and the way the person experiences and reacts to daily life. Once the sensory processing style of people with autism is understood, the meaning of their behaviours can be interpreted and more effective management interventions introduced. The sensory systems provide the means of communicating with the brain. When the sensory systems operate differently (e.g. by processing in a distorted way, too slowly, too intensely), then the output systems produce unusual responses (e.g. maladaptive or ineffective behavioural responses).

Recent research, summarised by Huebner (2001), provides information on the sensory processing and integration problems associated with autism. Failure to process and integrate new or unpredictable stimuli may be related to difficulties in arousal regulation. Arousal is defined as a physiological state of readiness elicited by an organism's perception of its environment or as the general state of nervous system excitation that affects behaviour (Belser & Sudhalter 1995). On the attention continuum, low arousal may be associated with drowsiness and mental lethargy; high arousal may be associated more with distractibility, hyperactivity and manic behaviour. On the affective continuum, low arousal may be associated with boredom and higher arousal with increasing levels of excitement, anxiety and fear.

Typically, people have a wide range of optimal arousal and can function adequately throughout a number of different circumstances. In contrast, children with autism seem to have a very narrow range of optimal arousal (Klinger & Dawson 1992; Royeen & Lane 1991). Clinical observations and reports from people with autism suggest that many people with autism experience sensations differently than others, including exaggerated perceptions of sensory input and arousal disorders.

Assuming that these hypotheses are correct, it appears likely that people with autism are in an almost constant state of over-arousal where they are continually bombarded with different stimuli from a range of new, changing and often unpredictable situations. These stimuli may include any number of different sounds, sights, tastes or textures. Most children and adults learn to avoid these situations because they are unable to self-regulate to receive just enough stimulation to maintain arousal and attention.

Matt is a 4-year-old child with autism who becomes extremely distressed and covers his ears whenever his mother switches on the vacuum cleaner.

Sarah always finds it difficult at the beginning of a new season to adapt to wearing different clothing. She just gets used to wearing shorts and t-shirts or dresses in summer then the weather becomes cooler and her mother tries to put her in long trousers and sweaters. Initially she will scream and try to remove her clothing because she does not like the feel of the different fabrics on her skin.

It is therefore critical to maintain a balance between new and unpredictable stimulations and things that are familiar and predictable when planning new instruction and when teaching new skills to children with autism.

Difficulties empathising

In autism, all behaviour is learned, and social behaviour, because it does not follow a predictable pattern, is the most difficult behaviour to learn. People with autism often have little self-consciousness so rarely feel shame or guilt over their actions. They rarely feel the need to change or worry about what they say or do when out socially. They really do not understand other people. Their minds simply cannot effectively or efficiently grasp, analyse and interpret a range of social information in a coherent and flexible manner. Without an understanding of how others are the same or different from themselves, they have little understanding of how to interact or to conform.

Perhaps the greatest problem that individuals with autism must cope with socially is their inherent lack of empathy. Empathy requires the ability to know what another person thinks and feels despite the fact that this is different from one's own mental state at the time. Empathy presupposes recognition of different mental states.

The social difficulties of children with autism are exacerbated or caused by their deficits of empathy. Social behaviour is driven by complex feelings rather than logic, and individuals with autism have a limited understanding of complex emotions. As well as an inability to empathise with others, individuals with autism also have difficulty expressing emotions. It has been well documented that children with autism have difficulty recognising emotional states in others. Uta Frith (1989) postulated that the fundamental difficulty in autism is that people with autism have little understanding of their own and others' mental states. It is not just that they cannot understand what people are thinking and feeling, but that they cannot understand that other people do think and feel; that is, that people have minds. They are unable to work out the meaning of other people's behaviour and have difficulty empathising with others. Frith (1989) and Baron-Cohen (1995) found that people with autism have difficulty understanding that other people may feel different emotions, think and believe differently from themselves.

Baron-Cohen & Bolton (1993), stated that 'in autism there is a failure to develop a normal understanding that people have minds and mental states and that mental states relate to behaviour'.

Imagine how hard it would be to get through a whole day without an ability to read minds. People, whether consciously or unconsciously, do it all of the time. Most people base their behaviour, thoughts and feelings, on the behaviour, thoughts and feelings of those around them. Individuals with autism, who lack this innate ability to intuit or interpret the minds of others, are at a loss to understand how to react or conduct themselves in many situations. It just does not occur to them to alter or adjust their behaviour in response to its effect on others, because they have no idea what others are thinking about them. They fail to intuit social expectations or pick up the social cues that would enable them to fit in and participate socially.

The inability to conceptualise states of mind, to make sense of what motivates people to do and say and feel, provides no basis for comparing or reflecting on their own mental state. With little understanding or confidence in themselves, it becomes even more difficult to relate to others in any meaningful way.

Concrete, literal thinking

People with autism are very concrete and literal in the way that they use and understand language. Even the most able children and adults with autism have difficulties interpreting abstract concepts and expressions that are a common part of the English language. For example, to tell a person with autism that he 'is over the hill' would not be interpreted as getting older, but would be understood literally; that is, that he is on the other side of a hill and can not be seen.

Interpreting language in a literal fashion has an impact on how people with autism function and cope in different situations. Confusion caused by their literal interpretation of information is a major cause of problem behaviour and non-compliance at school, in the workplace and at home for people with autism. A child with autism who is told to 'pull up your socks' or to 'shake a leg' is unlikely to understand that these phrases have multiple meanings depending on context. The child is likely to interpret the phrases literally, regardless of context, and bend over and pull up the socks or shake a leg. This literal interpretation is often mistaken for rudeness or non-compliance.

Another difficulty associated with the interpretation of language is the fact that people with autism do not understand that some words have multiple meanings. One word may be used to label objects, feelings, ideas and actions. The word ball may mean a round object or a large formal dance; it may also mean to have fun and is also used in the colloquial phrase 'the ball is in your court' (it is up to you to make the next move). The meaning of a word may change depending on the context. Intonation and inflexion, as in humour or sarcasm, may also change the meaning.

In addition to multiple meanings, people with autism also find it hard to understand that some objects may have more than one name or label. Many commonly used objects may be

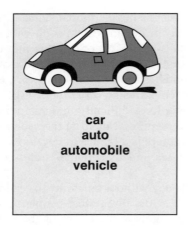 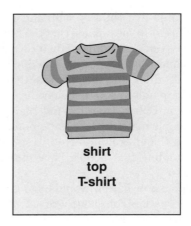

Figure 11.2   *Examples of illustrations with multiple labels*

labelled in any number of different ways. This adds to the confusion surrounding speech and language that individuals with autism are faced with on a daily basis. For example, the two objects in Figure 11.2 may be described in different words but still retain the same meaning.

Unusual rote memory abilities

As people develop and learn, they tend to memorise certain experiences so that they can be recalled whenever necessary in a similar situation. As they have further experiences, these will alter and shape what is remembered, enabling them to develop new concepts and modify their ideas.

People with autism have unusual memory abilities including excellent rote memory skills. Rote memory is the ability to remember things without consciously thinking about the meaning. People with autism are often able to recall a list of facts, repeat verbatim a favourite video and echo complete conversations, but their memory tends to store information without any idea of meaning or ability to discard what is irrelevant, so that they have to repeat an entire sequence from the beginning.

> Justin is a 6-year-old boy with autism who is obsessed with cars. He is able to recognise most makes of cars and tends to know people by the car that they drive. Whenever he sees someone he recognises, he always greets them in the same way by stating what car they currently drive. 'Sue drives a red Toyota Camry' or 'Bill drives a black Ford station-wagon'. He is able to remember people he has not seen for months and also recall the colour and model of their cars.

Apart from acknowledging that children and adults with autism have good rote memory abilities, it is also important to know which aspects of memory skills are responsible for these abilities, and which aspects are responsible for the fact that they apparently derive little benefit from these skills in everyday life.

According to Frith (1989), children with autism may be able to recall all of the details of a train timetable without being a train enthusiast or wanting to travel by train. This is an example of rote memory as opposed to memory that is meaningful. Kanner, in 1943, mentioned the phenomenal memory of these children that allowed them to recall complex 'nonsense' patterns exactly, no matter how disorganised they are. This, however, should not necessarily be regarded as an achievement, as the ability to recall nonsense is far less useful than the ability to recall facts for meaning. Children with autism may have excellent rote memory abilities, but unless the information remembered is meaningful, the isolated feats of rote memory could be seen as a sign of dysfunction, rather than a particular ability.

Although people with autism may have good rote memory abilities, they find it hard to remember personal details and do not appear to remember things associated with particular emotions or feelings. Most memories are likely to be prompted by certain external cues. These cues then serve to trigger the recall of a memory or routine that then interferes with other current activities.

Visual spatial abilities

Children and adults with autism are visual learners. It can therefore be helpful to modify the environment and to use visual strategies to assist children and adults to understand and use communication. At least 90% of the information that is processed successfully by individuals with autism comes through visual means while only approximately 10% of information presented verbally is successfully integrated.

Although most people with autism are visual learners and possess remarkable abilities to remember things that they see, there is often no meaning attached to the things they see or the chunks of visually presented information they appear to take in. Some individuals have remarkable visual memories as shown by their ability to complete complex jigsaw puzzles, recognise letters, numbers, shapes and colours as well as to remember when objects in a room are moved around.

It is possible to harness this visual ability to assist individuals to learn and think more effectively. When information is organised and presented in a clear and consistent visual format that emphasises the critical elements of the information, people with autism are more able to process it and then use it meaningfully.

> Timmy does not respond to verbal directions. He does not appear to comprehend what is being said and so ignores any verbal requests. However, when the teacher uses visual cues to augment her language, Timmy is more compliant. He needs to look at the picture cue for a few seconds before he responds.

Compartmentalised chunk learning style

The gestalt style of learning refers to the ways in which individuals take in information, store it, process it and retrieve it for use in different situations. As has already been discussed, most people with autism take in chunks (or whole pieces) of information, then store and eventually retrieve these, in their entirety, without analysing the interrelated meaning of the different parts.

Over the past few years, great strides have been made in understanding the unique learning patterns associated with autism. People with autism demonstrate a learning style that is grounded in holistic, gestalt processing. This processing strength is well suited to the comprehension of spatially organised, non-transient information (information that is presented in a visual format).

Weaknesses with gestalt learning lie in the processing of analytic, sequential information that results in difficulties understanding transient information such as verbal information (Prizant & Schuler 1987).

It has been estimated that many children with autism may not develop functional language. Those children who do develop language present with major difficulties; in particular, speech that is largely echolalic or stereotypic. Most of the speech produced by individuals with autism consists of 'the immediate or delayed literal repetition of the speech of others, often without an appreciation of the conventional meaning of the utterances involved' (Quill 1995, p 17). These speech patterns are consistent with a gestalt style of learning.

> Seven-year-old Mary has begun to realise the importance of conversation as a way of social-ising with other children. She does not always understand the meaning of the words she hears. For example when another child approaches her in the school playground and says 'Hello Mary, would you like to play?' she usually replies 'Would you like to play?' If the child corrects her and says 'No, Mary, say "Yes, please"', Mary answers 'Mary say yes please.'

Prizant (1983), discussed the impact of the gestalt language learning style with particular relevance to echolalia and overall communicative behaviour in autism. Echolalia may serve a variety of communicative and cognitive functions (Prizant & Rydell 1984) and, like imitation for normally developing children, it may be a productive learning strategy for many children with autism. Children who use echolalia initially repeat phrases associated with particular sit-uations or emotional states and eventually learn their meanings by finding out how they work. Over time, many children learn to use these 'gestalt forms' purposefully, eventually even break-ing down the echolalic chunks into smaller meaningful units as part of the development of a functional communication system.

As we have seen, the particular characteristics of autism impact greatly on how individuals with autism function generally. Autism affects everything that they do, how they feel, how they think and how they take in and process information from all of the senses. Individuals with autism look like everyone else. They do not learn the same as everyone else.

Because the problems that define autism are not reversible, it is not possible to normalise children and adults with autism. The goal of any intervention is, rather, to understand their strengths and limitations and develop procedures that will assist each individual to fit as well as possible into society as an adult. It is important to respect the differences that autism creates in each individual and to work within the boundaries set by each person's individual thinking and learning style. Until it is widely recognised, acknowledged and understood that people with autism think and learn differently, they will continue to struggle as they attempt, in their own ways, to make sense of the world they live in.

Summary

The major difficulty that characterises the thinking and learning style of children and adults with autism is the inability to derive meaning from their experiences. They can learn skills, they can respond to routines and structure, some can learn to use language but they do not understand what many of their experiences mean. Children and adults with autism have difficulty processing information for meaning, especially information that is presented verbally. They do not understand the relationships between ideas, actions or events. Their world appears to consist of a series of unrelated experiences, while the underlying themes, concepts, reasons or principles remain unclear. The difficulties associated with an inability to generate meaning play a major role in the overall cognitive, communicative and social functioning of all people with autism.

Among the most commonly recognised problems that affect how individuals with autism function and learn are difficulties processing information and poor listening skills, sensory sensitivities and lack of empathy. However, individuals with autism also show remarkable visual spatial abilities, unusual rote memory skills and ability to pick up the fine details.

An understanding of the learning styles of people with autism will provide direction for teachers and parents to structure intervention and recognise and solve problems. A thorough assessment of individual functioning is important prior to developing individual programs and should include learning styles, social and communicative functioning, independent skills as well as academic abilities and anything else likely to impact on the learning situation.

Rather than focus on the limitations of each individual, the focus should be upon individual learning strengths. These strengths include the ability to take in chunks of information quickly and remember that information for a long period of time, the ability to take in and understand information presented visually, the ability to respond appropriately to rules and routines as long as these are presented visually and are implemented consistently, and the ability to concentrate on topics of special interest.

12

Visual Supports

Effective communication does not just happen. It takes considerable effort from both the sender and the receiver of information to ensure that communication attempts accomplish their intent. Those who experience communication disorders encounter exceptional difficulty participating in the communication process. Fortunately, employing visual aids to support the communication process can significantly improve their successful participation.

Hodgdon 1995, p 7

As previously discussed, the triad of impairments that underpins autism includes an inability to communicate socially. Communication consists of exchanging messages between people and being able to express individual needs and share thoughts, ideas and feelings. Usually communication involves the use of language, either spoken or written, and often involves the social activity of conversation. Children and adults with autism miss out on the pleasures involved in social communication because they do not tend to engage in social exchanges and are slow to develop language.

Many studies have shown that the strength of behaviour is determined by the consequences that immediately follow it. That is, if behaviour is followed by a pleasant consequence, that particular behaviour will be more likely to occur in the future. Alternatively, if behaviour is followed by unpleasant consequences, that behaviour will be less likely to occur again. By applying pleasant consequences to desirable behaviour, we increase the likelihood that a particular behaviour will occur more often in the future. The same principle may be applied to communication. By rewarding people's attempts to communicate, by providing adequate supports to assist their attempts to communicate and by encouraging communication during fun and motivating activities, children and adults are more likely to develop a desire to want to communicate. It is important to ensure that any responses to a person's communicative attempts are in fact rewarding for them.

Children and adults with autism have problems processing information that is presented verbally. Over the past ten to fifteen years, increasing emphasis has been placed upon studying the unique learning styles and strengths of people with autism in order to find the most effective and successful intervention procedures. It has become increasingly obvious that the vast majority of people with autism are 'visual learners'; they understand and respond more effectively to visual stimuli than to auditory stimuli. Visual supports help them to understand and use the process of communication. Visual supports also encourage the development of spoken language and appropriate social communication. Visual supports help people with autism to make sense of the world and of other people, and to foster the communication process.

Parents and teachers generally find that information presented verbally may need to be repeated a number of times before a response is initiated. If the verbal instructions do not work after being repeated, it becomes necessary to add gestures or physical prompts, or even to model what is requested, in order to get the message across. Unconsciously, many parents and teachers start moving away from verbal instructions to increasingly more visual methods of providing information and instruction to people with autism.

Visual supports and visual strategies are used interchangeably here to describe the visual tools that enhance communication, support behaviour and assist children and adults to learn. Alternative terms are used widely in the literature and include:

- augmentative and alternative communication (AAC);
- visual systems;
- visual tools; and
- visual aids.

Visual supports are portable and easily understood by people in general. The introduction of visuals provides a basis for a communication system that is functional for people who may never develop speech. They are used to assist the development of skills in a number of areas apart from communication including social skills, living skills, self-help skills and leisure skills. Visual supports are also used to teach rules, establish routines, indicate change and provide positive behaviour support.

What are the most effective visual supports?

As mentioned in Chapter 4, visual supports may include:

- *Non-verbal communication* such as body language (including facial expression, natural gestures and tone of voice); for example, pointing, smiling or frowning, shouting, and standing with hands on hips are non-verbal means of communicating information.

> Whenever Jordan is angry because his brother borrows his mobile phone, his backpack or his favourite shirt, he doesn't have to say anything. He just stomps around the house, frowning and muttering to himself until his brother returns the borrowed items. It is obvious to everyone that Jordan is not happy.

- *Cues from the environment*; for example, black clouds that indicate thunderstorms, flashing lights that indicate accident ahead, are natural cues in the environment that are presented visually.
- *Specially designed materials to provide information to meet an individual's specific needs.* These materials include choice boards, transition guides, photographic sequences, individualised calendars and timetables, shopping lists and menus (see Figure 12.1).

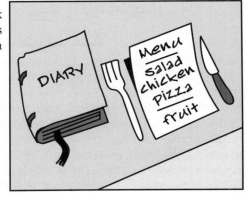

Figure 12.1 *Examples of individual information*

Most of these visual supports are designed for a particular individual and will vary considerably depending on the person's abilities and requirements.

■ *Generic materials that provide information about the general community*; for example, bus and train timetables, calendars, shopping lists, road signs, menus and advertisements are visual means of communication that assist people to be organised and understand rules and routines (see Figure 12.2).

When introducing visual systems into the home, preschool, school or the workplace for children and adults with autism, it is important to remember that they will be functioning at

Figure 12.2 *Examples of community information*

different cognitive levels and will therefore require different levels of visual representation. It is important to use visual symbols that are understood by the individual who will be using them. The visual symbols should therefore be pitched to the level that the person is currently functioning at. The recognised hierarchy of visual representation is shown in Figure 12.3.

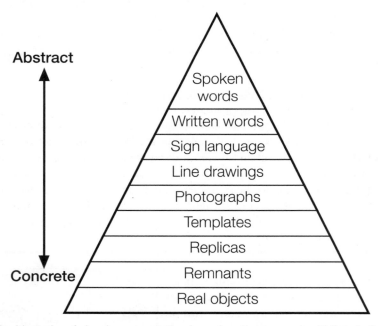

Figure 12.3 *The hierarchy of visual representation based on the research of Mirenda & Musselwhite*

Objects, photographs, line drawings and written words can all be used to augment language and the choice will depend on the needs of the individual. Traditionally, objects were used with children at an early developmental stage, followed by the use of photographs and, only later, the use of line drawings. However in autism, as with many other aspects of development, the normally developing progression from object to photograph to line drawing may not necessarily be appropriate. Sometimes people with autism may find a simple line drawing less confusing than a detailed photograph. This may be due to the fact that most individuals with autism tend to perceive and focus upon details rather than the whole picture. They become overwhelmed by the detail in the photo or may be confused if the photo used in a particular situation does not exactly match the real life object or place to which it refers.

Some individuals with autism may recognise and 'read' written words, but not necessarily understand the meaning behind the words (hyperlexia). Because of the visual strengths of people with autism, it is often beneficial to pair written words (in the more commonly used and easily recognised lower case), with a more concrete visual support such as a photograph or line drawing to assist with meaning.

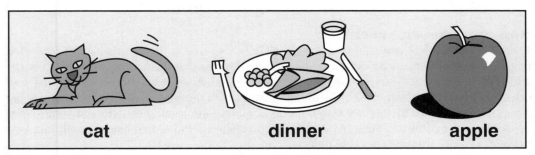

cat   **dinner**   **apple**

Figure 12.4 *Examples of visual supports that show the picture but also present the written word to assist people with hyperlexia*

Although some children and adults have the cognitive skills to cope with high-level representation, the use of a variety of different types of support helps to motivate and maintain interest levels. It is therefore not only possible but often recommended that a variety of different levels of visual supports (such as remnants, photos and line drawings) are combined in one example as long as the individual understands and relates to the level of representation used.

When developing a series of visual supports for a particular individual, the first step in the process is to look at the hierarchy of visual representation and decide what type of visual supports will be most effective. Remember, it is important to determine what types of supports the person will understand and relate to and then to use supports at that level or lower on the hierarchy of representation.

Once the types of supports have been chosen, it may then be determined how they should be used. The way they are used will, to some extent, depend on the type of visual support.

How are real objects used?

Real objects are the most concrete and easily recognised form of visual support. Using real objects includes showing children the actual milk and juice containers when encouraging them to make a choice about what they would like to drink. At this time, verbal communication should involve merely labelling the objects 'milk', 'juice' as each object is shown.

Other examples include showing a young child a nappy when it is time to be changed, showing the car keys when it is time to go out in the car or presenting a bar of soap, wash cloth, towel and pyjamas in the correct sequential order at bath time when teaching a bathing sequence. Show children a choice of fruit when you want them to indicate their preference. Figure 12.5 gives some examples.

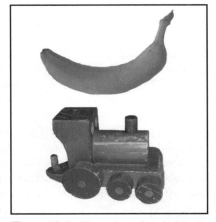

Figure 12.5 *Examples of real objects*

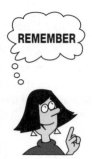

REMEMBER

■ It is very important to label each object as it is presented. For example say 'apple' (as you show the apple) and 'mandarin' (as you show the mandarin).

How are remnants used?

Remnants are parts of real objects or the packaging they come in. Remnants may be presented instead of real objects once children have mastered the idea that the packaging 'represents' the real object. Remnants refer to the empty packaging, labels or logos from food, drinks, and other materials or objects. An empty potato crisp packet, muesli bar wrapper, label from the front of a milk/juice carton or empty yoghurt container are remnants commonly recognised by children and adults. Remnants may be used on choice boards when teaching children how to make a choice from two or more objects

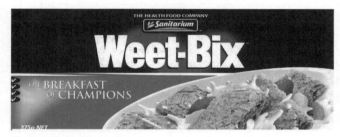 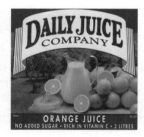

Figure 12.6   *Examples of remnants of real objects*

How are replicas used?

Replicas of real objects may be introduced when the actual objects are too big, heavy, dangerous or inappropriate to be included in a visual sequence. For example, a replica of a toilet may be used during toilet training to remind a child that it is time to go to the toilet or as a part of a bedtime sequence.

How are templates used?

The outline of real objects may be used to assist children and adults to learn new skills such as packing away objects, setting the table, setting up a complex play activity, setting out railway tracks to play trains or creating specific playdough shapes. Most individuals with autism are very good at sorting and matching activities and have little difficulty understanding and using templates as visual learning tools (see Figure 12.7). In the workplace, templates are used to assist individuals through the different steps of a complex task, such as folding and stuffing envelopes, sorting and packing objects into different bags or to keep tools in their proper place.

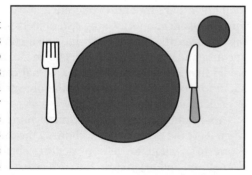

Figure 12.7   *Example of how a template is used to teach a child to set the table or to show where eating/drinking utensils should be placed*

How are photographs used?

Photographs are realistic representations of objects. They may be used with children and adults who are concrete thinkers and who already respond to real objects as a means of communicating basic needs. The aim is to gradually move children towards more abstract (and portable) visual supports. When photographs are first introduced they should be in colour, clearly show the subject matter and, initially, be paired with the real object (see Figure 12.8.)

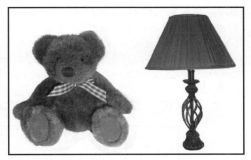

Figure 12.8 *Examples of photographs of real objects*

How are line drawings used?

Line drawings are commonly used with children and adults with autism at school, home and in the community to augment communication, encourage social interaction and support behaviour. Line drawings are more readily available than photographs, less expensive and more portable. Commercial programs are available including Bliss Symbols, Compic, Picture Communication System (PCS) (see Figure 12.9).

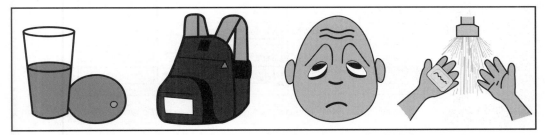

Figure 12.9 *Examples of line drawings from the commercial PCS (Boardmaker) program*

Line drawings may vary in their level of abstraction from detailed drawing to abstract outlines. Less realistic, more abstract, representations of objects may be used with more able children and adults. Individuals may use a variety of line drawings from different commercial programs quite successfully as long as the symbols are meaningful for that person.

When children are moving from photographs to line drawings, it is a good idea to pair the line drawing with the photograph to begin with and then gradually fade the photograph as the child understands that the drawing represents the real object. For example, a rule may be shown as: 'complete your homework and then you can play on the computer' as shown in Figure 12.10.

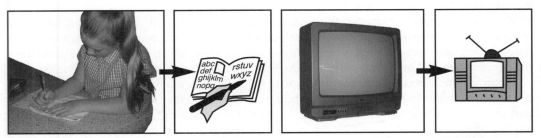

Figure 12.10 *Example of how to move from photographs to line drawings to ensure that children understand the level of representation*

How are written words used?

Written words are the most abstract form of visual support and the most difficult to understand for many people with autism.

Written words may be used in visual timetables for more able students to assist them to be organised and to organise their thoughts as shown in Figure 12.11.

DAY:	TUESDAY				
Period	● Subject	● Room	● Teacher		Changes
1	History	H5	Miss Booth		
2	Art	A3	Miss Jones		
3	English	G12	~~Miss Cross~~	→	Mr Hayden
Recess					
4	Maths	M8	Mrs Elliott		
5	Maths	M8	Mrs Elliott		
Lunch					
6	Geography	G4	Mr McGraw		
7	Science	S11	~~Miss Nairn~~	→	Mrs Arthur
8	Science	S11	~~Miss Nairn~~	→	Mrs Arthur

Figure 12.11 *Example of a visual timetable for high school students showing staff changes using written words*

What is the function of visual supports?

Visual supports are designed to help people to understand what is happening around them and to assist them to participate more fully in society. Visual supports are especially useful for individuals with autism because research has already indicated that these people are visual learners and have difficulty processing information that is presented verbally.

Visual supports (Ulliana 2001):

- facilitate comprehension and assist individuals to understand their social and physical environments;
- support speech;
- teach people to manage their own behaviour through positive behaviour supports;
- assist with the development of functional skills; and
- support emotional development.

Visually augmented communication systems (that is, a system that is used in addition to any naturally acquired speech, gestures or vocalisations currently in place) should emphasise the development of a strong communicative foundation for these skills; that is, the desire to want to communicate and the social aspects of the communication process.

According to Mirenda & Erickson (2000), symbolic systems such as manual signing or pictures are often introduced with young children even though they may not have mastered the basic social and communicative functions of joint attention, turn taking and sharing or even developed an awareness of, or interest in, the whole communication process. In most young children, early forms of communication include gestures, facial expression and vocalisations. These forms eventually expand to include more complex gestures and speech.

In young children with a severe communication delay, interventions that promote the use of natural gestures and vocalisations in a variety of natural contexts, and encourage the development of social play skills, are the first steps in mastering basic communicative functions. Obviously, the goal of such interventions is the development of natural speech and language. If this does not occur, then augmentative systems, such as visual supports, may be introduced to encourage interest in communicating with others.

It is not enough to teach individuals with 'limited interest in communication how to say or sign something, or how to point to or show a picture or another visual display. Instead, attempts should be made to extend the current nonverbal means and to diversify the existing communicative functions across contexts' (Mirenda & Schuler 1989, p 29).

Visual supports are introduced to children with autism to augment, or support, language, not as an alternative to speech. By always pairing the visual support with the spoken word, the aim is that eventually children will come to rely less on the visual and be able to respond appropriately, and use the spoken words in isolation. The visual supports may then be faded in situations where they are no longer required to augment language.

Many parents feel that once their children 'learn to talk', the autism will be far less of a problem, or less noticeable, and the children will be able to attend mainstream school programs. A common concern for parents, when the issue of using visual supports is first raised, is how the technique will affect their children's natural speech development. They feel that if children are provided with an alternative form of communication, then the desire or need to communicate verbally will decrease, making it less likely that their children will ever develop natural speech patterns.

According to Mirenda & Erickson (2000), research has demonstrated that using augmentative systems of communication such as signing actually encourages the use of the spoken words after approximately 200 signs have been mastered and children are starting to use two or more signs together. However, there is also evidence that some individuals never speak or use many signs functionally even after intensive instruction in the use of manual signs. It appears that the use of manual signing does not inhibit the development of speech in people with autism, even though the use may not always promote it.

The evidence for the effectiveness of visual strategies in enhancing speech development is less clear. Studies by Frost & Bondy (1994) and by Romski & Sevcik (1996), however, have supported the idea that, as in the case of manual signing, visual symbol use does not hinder and may, in fact, enhance the development of speech in children with autism.

Introducing visual strategies to young children with autism provides an immediate form of functional and effective communication that supports speech development, and lays the foundation for a functional alternative if children do not develop natural speech. Unlike manual signs, visual strategies are a functional alternative to natural speech development that are easily used and understood within the general community.

How do we develop and use visual supports?

In order for visual aids to effectively support communication interactions, help people organise their environments and facilitate the learning of functional skills, it is important to consider the following questions in order to ensure that the supports are being used most effectively and efficiently:

1. Who will be using the visual support?
   Consider the individual's functional skills when choosing the appropriate visual symbols to use.
2. Where will the visual support be used?
   Consider the learning environment when determining where the visual symbol should be placed and how it should be used. Consider the format of the visual support to ensure that it is easily accessible.

3. What will the visual support be used for?

Consider the possible functions when developing what is the appropriate content and format of the visual symbol to ensure that it remains user friendly.

4. How will the visual support be used?

Consider the diversity/content when deciding how the visual support may be generalised to different settings, situations and people and to ensure that the support is appropriate for real life situations.

Who will be using the visual support?

Any person with autism can use visual symbols, as well as people with other related disorders and people with no disabilities at all. In fact, we all use visual supports in our everyday lives to help us to remember things, to be better organised and to provide us with essential information. Sometimes visual symbols are the most efficient means of imparting general information to a wide range of people with different abilities.

The use of visual supports is not determined by a person's ability to talk. Visual supports may benefit both verbal and non-verbal individuals because their use is partly determined by a person's ability to take in information and to understand meaning. When using visual supports it is important to determine the most effective symbol to use for each individual in terms of the hierarchy of representation.

Figure 12.12 shows some examples of general information presented visually for maximum effect.

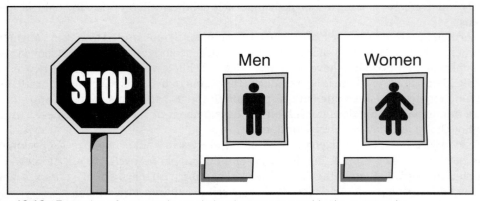

Figure 12.12 *Examples of commonly used visual supports used in the community*

When planning the development of an individualised program that incorporates extensive visual supports, it is essential to assess the person's cognitive skills before choosing what visual symbols to use. The person using them should easily understand the visual symbols; otherwise they will be of little benefit. The following steps are important:

1. Observe the individual in a number of different situations to determine what he/she likes and dislikes (it is important when introducing visual supports to start with something that is of interest to, and motivating for, the person).

2. Observe how the individual responds to certain everyday items such as objects, photographs, magazine pictures (this will give an indication of the person's ability to understand representations).

3. Determine what exactly you hope to achieve with the introduction of a particular visual support (this will influence the content of the visual support and how you present the information).

If a child loves to look at photo albums and picture books with realistic images, you may assume that such a child will recognise that a photograph of an object represents that object. Photographs will probably work well for this child.

If an individual is interested in transport and spends many hours looking at magazines, pamphlets and catalogues that contain drawings of items, then you may assume that they will recognise and understand some line drawings, as well as photographs, in their visual supports, as shown in Figure 12.13.

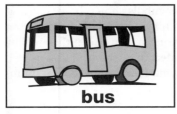 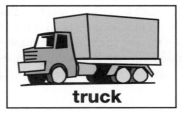 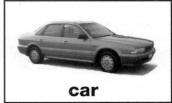

bus   **truck**   **car**

Figure 12.13 *Examples of line drawings and photographs of transport*

Real objects are the easiest symbols to understand and also the most concrete. Symbols become increasingly more abstract as you move through the hierarchy of representation. A variety of symbols may be used as long as the individual understands the meaning of each one. If a person is able to understand line drawings, it is still acceptable to use a combination of line drawings, remnants, and photographs in their visual supports. However, written words should not be included at this stage as they are further up the hierarchy or representation.

According to Hodgdon (1995), when we choose a visual symbol, we are making assumptions 'about the client's ability to see, interpret, attach meaning, and take action'. It is important to choose wisely to make sure that the symbols are appropriate. It does not matter if the symbols are easy and at a lower level than the person's current cognitive abilities suggest. Using easier symbols is perfectly suitable as long as the completed visual support meets the individual's needs. Symbols should not be considered inappropriate because they are too easy. Too easy is not an issue — too difficult to understand is the problem.

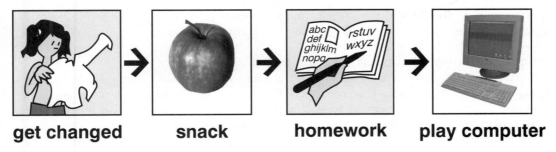

get changed   **snack**   **homework**   **play computer**

Figure 12.14 *Example of an after school visual sequence using a combination of photographs and line drawings.*

Figure 12.14 shows a visual sequence using various media.

Some visuals may be developed for group use, so the format and the type of symbols should take into account the skills of all possible users. Keeping in mind that too easy is not a problem; the visuals should be pitched to the least able students in the group.

Where will the visual support be used?

Visual symbols should be individually designed to meet the needs of the person using them. It is no use having visual choice boards for food if they are not placed in the kitchen, on the cupboard or fridge where the food is stored. A rules board for the classroom needs to be prominently displayed on the wall of the classroom where it can be seen by all of the children. A toileting sequence should be in the bathroom with a portable version available for different settings.

Some visual supports need to be portable so that they can be used in a number of different settings. However, it is not always practical to expect a person to carry all of their visual supports with them at all times. The environment itself should also be augmented with visual supports where possible and individuals taught to use a variety of different supports, some fixed and some portable.

Visual symbols are used to augment language, therefore the symbols should be visible and accessible to the user in order to be functional. Visual symbols may need to be developed in many different formats to suit the person using them and the situations in which they will be used. The format of a visual support refers to how it is presented (a portable wallet, a wall chart, a folder or a set of cards clipped together) as well as the layout (size, shape, colour, number and position of images).

The overall format of the visual support will be dependent upon who is using it, where it will be used and how it will be used. For example, a toileting sequence should be presented as a wall chart and placed in the bathroom, near the toilet and at an appropriate height for the user. A visual choice board for a child at preschool, however, is different and may consist of a series of photographs or line drawings that reflect favourite play activities. These may be clipped together on a ring clip making it portable, durable and readily accessible. It can then be used both indoors and outdoors at preschool and at home, and is easily transferable from one setting to another.

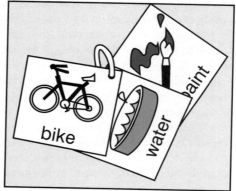

Where possible, visual supports such as wall charts, booklets and sequence boards should have detachable images so that changes can be made when necessary. The use of Velcro tape allows symbols to be removed and replaced easily without having to remake the entire visual support. This accommodates the need to change supports as the requirements of the person, the settings and the situations change.

Figure 12.15 *Example of a ring cluster of cards with play activities*

What will the visual support be used for?

When developing a visual support for a person, it is important to clarify what it will be used for to ensure that it achieves what it sets out to do. The purpose may be to provide information, to provide a way to request something, to teach a new skill, to support a previously learned skill, to provide rules, to pre-empt change or to manage problem behaviour.

The key to the successful use of visual supports is to make sure that they are relevant for the user and that the purpose behind their use is clear. All visual supports must be individualised for the user and should contain only information that is relevant to that person. The content of each visual support should clearly reflect its use in order to ensure that it can be used most efficiently. The content and layout of each visual support needs to be carefully considered so that it is user friendly and contains only information that is necessary for the person, place and time. Don't be tempted to add extra images that are not relevant for the current use. Extra images can always be added later as the person's needs change.

It is no use, for example, having a shopping list that is big and bulky. Formats of visual supports may vary from single photographs through to sequence boards, ring binders and wallets depending on their intended use.

In his day program, Thomas is being taught to do the grocery shopping. He has a shopp-ing list and is able to match items on the shelves with the pictures on his list. When he first started, Thomas was able to match two items but, with practice, he is now able to collect all eight items on his list. His list is portable so that he can carry it in his pocket.

Visual supports also need to be kept up to date for the person using them. If the information on the visual supports is out of date, then the supports themselves become irrelevant and useless for the user. One of the advantages of using products such as Velcro or Blu-Tack when originally making a visual support is that the images can be changed and added to as needed.

As far as possible, visual supports should be personalised for the user. If photographs are used to reflect actions or activities, then use photographs of the individual who will be using the visual support. If the visual support contains images of objects, these should also be elevant for the user. Often, having a photo of the person on a chart or choice board indicates ownership. This is illustrated in Figure 12.16.

Michael has a visual choice board on the wall, near the door that leads to the backyard. He has learned to point to what he wants to play with when he goes out-side. Michael loves to play out-side and the visual choice board has helped him to learn how to make choices. He has his photo-graph on the top of the board to remind him that the board belongs to Michael.

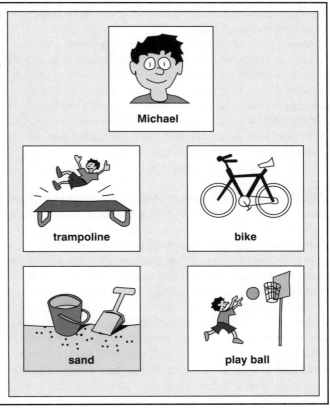

Figure 12.16 *Visual choice board*

How will the visual support be used?

It is important that visual supports are introduced and used in real life situations in order for them to be of benefit to the user. It is often difficult for people with autism to generalise skills learned in one situation to other situations. Just because a person has learnt and uses a skill in one situa-tion, it should never be assumed that they are then able to generalise that skill to other settings.

Visual symbols are most effective if they are portable and designed to be used in a number of different situations and with a number of different people. When first introducing visual symbols this may not always be possible, but emphasis is placed on moving toward more abstract, portable symbols. When first introduced to visual supports, individuals need to be taught how to use them initially in one situation. The visual supports should be introduced in a way that is positive and motivating so that the person sees the advantages and benefits for themselves and will be encouraged to use the supports again. The key to success with visual supports is to ensure that they are associated with positive, real life experiences.

As children become more familiar with particular visual supports, these can be extended to include additional examples and then introduced into different settings and with different people. This encourages children and adults to generalise their skills to different people, times and settings. All visual supports should be functional for the user.

If visual supports are well designed, functional and the user is taught how to use them in a number of different settings, then they should be appropriate in any situation. Visual supports are designed to augment communication, and to assist people with autism to understand what is happening around them. They may be used to teach new skills, explain changes to routines, provide information, and provide ways for the person to request or comment or to provide positive behaviour support.

Visual symbols should initially be associated with the thing that they represent by labelling; that is, attaching a label to the object or place it represents such as 'apple', 'milk', 'toilet'. Thus, a person learns to associate the symbol with a real object and learns to use the symbol to request. The rate at which new symbols may be introduced will vary from person to person but it is important to initially introduce symbols for objects that are motivating for the person with autism and to wait for clear signs of understanding before introducing additional symbols.

People with autism have difficulty learning how communication works and the importance of communication in their lives. To assist the person with autism to understand how communication works, it can be helpful to exchange a symbol for a desired object.

What materials are needed to make visual supports?

Visual supports can help children and adults with autism to communicate more effectively and to learn new skills. It can never be repeated enough that visual supports will only truly work well if they are personalised, functional, durable, accessible and easy to use. They should be introduced gradually and in a format that is appropriate for each person's level of understanding.

A list of basic materials you need to have in order to make simple visuals should include:

- cardboard — acts as a background for templates and as the basis for wall charts and visual sequences;
- felt — as an alternative to cardboard, may be used as a background for a template;
- Contact paper — used to cover cardboard or photos in order to protect them and strengthen them. Alternatively, visual supports may be laminated;
- adhesive Velcro — used to attach photos, remnants or symbols to cardboard, felt or other objects. Using Velcro allows you to change photos and remnants as needed. Velcro is available from craft and department stores;
- Blu-Tack — used as an alternative to Velcro;
- scissors — used to cut materials to the appropriate shape and size;
- glue and sticky tape — used to permanently attach photos or symbols to backing sheets of cardboard;
- ruler — used to measure and determine the size of visuals required;
- textas — used to outline pictures and photographs;
- coloured paper/cardboard — used to outline some images and to make arrows, ticks, crosses etc for use in some visuals;

- mini photo albums — great for portable choice boards, shopping lists and outing sequences;
- key rings and metal curtain rings — used to hold a number of individual cards together;
- fridge magnets — stuck to back of visual supports to attach them to metal surfaces;
- real objects including toys, foods, clothing, to be used as visual prompts to support language;
- remnants of relevant packaging — to be used to encourage a person to communicate;
- photos of relevant objects, actions and events; and
- line drawings such as 'Boardmaker' (this is also known as Picture Communication System (PCS) and is a computer graphics program commercially available) images of relevant objects, actions and events.

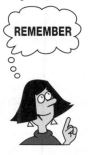

REMEMBER

- The hierarchy of visual supports — it is better to use visual supports that are easier for the individual to understand than to use visuals that are too abstract. The aim is to move towards more abstract images when ready.
- Visual supports are sometimes presented as a magic cure for autism or as a certain method of teaching children and adults to talk. A lot of their success is dependent on how they are developed and how they are used.

Why are visual supports so effective?

Visual supports assist people with autism to be more effective communicators because they present information in a concrete, tangible way for individuals who are visual learners. Research has shown that the visual skills of people with autism are superior to their auditory processing skills. Schuler and Baldwin (1981) suggested that the relatively strong visuo-spatial skills of individuals with autism would be most effectively used in conjunction with symbols such as real objects, photographs and line drawings. By the late 1980s, visual supports had been shown to be successful in a number of studies (Mirenda & Schuler (1989); Mirenda & Mathy-Laikko (1989)) and their use was becoming more widespread in everyday practice.

Most people with autism have auditory processing difficulties (part of the triad of impairments which form the basis of a diagnosis of autism). These difficulties have a significant impact on their ability to understand and use information that is presented verbally. As discussed previously, auditory processing difficulties include:

- hyper- or hypo-sensitivity to certain sound frequencies. This may be shown as a lack of response to certain sounds such as the human voice and/or an overreaction to certain sounds such as the sound of the vacuum cleaner;
- difficulty analysing auditory information and formulating appropriate responses. This may be seen in a child who repeats what has been said to him rather than responding appropriately to a particular request (immediate echolalia);
- problems focusing on relevant information while screening out irrelevant details. This may be seen in children who insist on having the television turned on even though they are not actually watching a particular program, who are very aware of any change in channel or volume but who, at the same time, do not respond when a parent calls them by name.

> Raoul is starting to use speech to communicate and he understands that speech works because it gets him what he wants. He does not always know what to say, especially when he is asked a question. When his mother asks him 'Raoul, do you want a biscuit or an apple?' he tends to repeat back 'biscuit or apple?' because he does not understand the verbal request. If his mother shows him the objects at the same time he is able to answer more appropriately.

Since the mid-1990s, most programs developed for children and adults with autism have included examples of visual strategies as an effective method of overcoming auditory processing difficulties, teaching new skills and supporting behaviour.

Visual supports provide information in a concrete non-transient format. This gives individuals a permanent reminder and reference as they attempt to take in information, process it, understand it and formulate appropriate responses. Visual supports may be used to facilitate comprehension and to support expression in children and adults who have difficulty with both receptive and expressive language (as indicated in the triad of impairments). It is commonly assumed that people comprehend more auditory information than they actually do.

We know that people with autism experience difficulty attending to, modulating, organising and understanding auditory input. With that knowledge, it is only common sense that dictates that these people require, and respond to, alternative methods of providing information. When we add to the equation the fact that many individuals are non-verbal or have disordered language but superior visual memory skills, it makes sense to focus on using visual supports to augment spoken language and to aid comprehension.

Visual supports facilitate learning and assist the teaching of skills, including many of the daily living skills children and adults require to function independently. For example, a visual sequence may be introduced to teach an adult to make a cup of tea, to follow a recipe or complete a work activity; to teach a child to clean their teeth, unpack a school bag or play with a doll. Visual sequences such as these are shown in Figures 12.17 and 12.18.

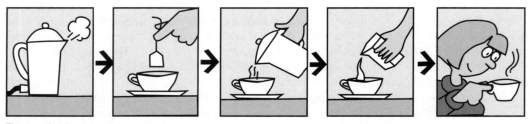

Figure 12.17 *A visual sequence showing an adult how to make a cup of tea*

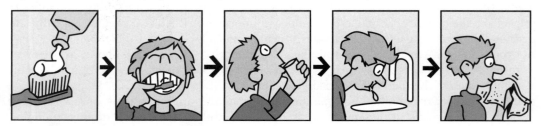

Figure 12.18 *A visual sequence showing a child how to brush teeth*

Visual sequences in the form of calendars, schedules, timetables and diaries help to clarify what is happening, when it will happen, what will happen next and any changes to the normal routine. Figure 12.19 illustrates a bedtime routine.

Visual supports assist people to cope with change (see Figure 12.20). Many children and adults with autism have difficulty coping with changes to normal routines and moving on from one activity, situation or setting to another (transition). They do not read their environment very well, have difficulty processing information presented verbally and have a preference for sameness. Visual supports are useful, as information is presented in a concrete way that allows a person to see exactly what is happening and what will happen next. (see information on planning for change in Chapter 16).

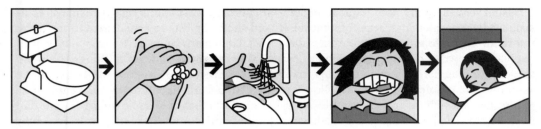

Figure 12.19 *A visual sequence to teach a child a bedtime routine*

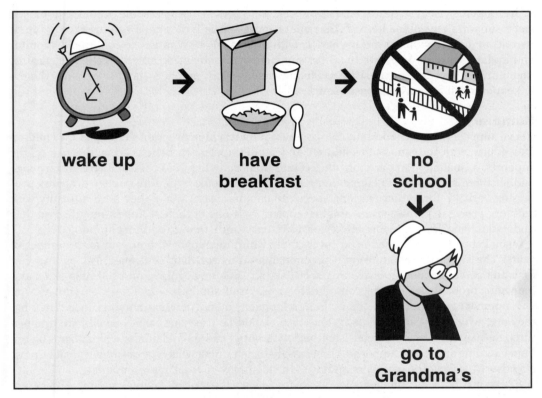

Figure 12.20 *A visual sequence to prepare children for a change in routine*

Visual supports are an effective means of decreasing problem behaviour and describing and prompting desired behaviour in children and adults with autism.

It has been discussed that children with autism have difficulty sustaining attention, shifting attention and difficulty focusing attention on what is important while blocking out extraneous stimuli. Common communication methods such as speech, manual signs and gestures are transient; they are present for a short period of time before they disappear. Children with autism have difficulty trying to take in the essence of a transient message in a noisy environment because of their problems establishing attention, maintaining attention and focusing attention while blocking out the irrelevant information. Usually a spoken or signed message is gone before the student is focused enough to receive it (Hodgdon 1995). A message presented visually allows the child ample time to establish attention and block out auditory distractions such as the sound of other voices or the sound of music from the radio.

Visual sequences are not unique to people with autism. Most adults rely on visual supports such as diaries, calendars, appointment books and shopping lists to assist them to remember information and to be organised in their daily lives. How many of us have a calendar near the telephone to write in important appointments? How many of us keep a 'things to do' list, take a shopping list with us to the supermarket, rely of written instructions to tell us how to assemble and use new equipment, follow a recipe and look at a menu to decide what to order in a restaurant? These are all examples of visual supports that are used regularly in our daily lives. These visual tools are used widely because they work for us. They help us to remember information and to organise our thoughts. People with autism use visual supports for many of the same reasons.

Introducing visual supports varies from person to person, because some people require only basic supports and other individuals require more specially designed resources. It is up to parents and professionals working closely with individuals with autism to continually monitor and update supports to create the most supportive and nurturing environment for learning. The ultimate goal is to be sensitive to the individual's skills and needs and to provide whatever supports will produce the best results.

Summary

Visual supports are an important component of any teaching program developed for children and adults with autism. Both children and adults appear to benefit from the use of the supports. Visual supports are introduced into their daily lives in order to augment language and let them know what is happening around them. People with autism have difficulty processing verbal information or using speech to communicate. While they have difficulty with auditory processing, their visual abilities appear to be one of their relative strengths and they understand and respond more effectively to visual stimuli than to auditory stimuli.

Visual supports have been used successfully with individuals with autism for a number of years. The list of professionals and parents advocating for their continued use, as a way of assisting communication, developing social skills, teaching cognitive and self-help skills and managing problem behaviours, continues to grow. Visual supports work for people with autism.

A number of questions arise about the development and use of visual supports, including what they are, why they should be used, how they should be used and what benefits are attained through their continued and consistent use with both children and adults with autism. Before implementing any visual supports, it is necessary to determine what type of supports will be most effective. This includes an understanding of the hierarchy of visual representation.

There are both advantages and disadvantages to the use of manual signing and visual supports in autism. Parents and teachers should consider these before choosing a communication system to augment speech. Whatever system is chosen, it should be emphasised that the focus remains on using speech, especially with children, in the expectation that they will eventually learn to talk. However by introducing visual supports, parents are also establishing the basis of a functional communication system for those children and adults who are not comfortable using speech to communicate. When setting up visuals, one has to consider how, when, why and where to use visuals and what materials are needed to develop visual supports. Visual supports have proven to be very effective when properly developed and introduced with individuals with autism.

13

Understanding Emotions and Feelings

The basic emotional needs of all children include forming attachments and experiencing consistency, affection, respect, empathy, comfort, compromise, safety, success, and joy. A child's emotional well-being must always be considered during intervention.

Quill 2000

Before it is possible to meet the emotional needs of children and adults with autism, it is important to understand their uniqueness. This is not an easy task because they tend to give out conflicting signals that make it difficult to interpret their thoughts and feelings.

The nature of the disability of autism, especially limited social interaction skills, may preclude individuals from establishing meaningful social relationships. This is so frustrating for people who desperately want to form friendships but don't know how to do so. For most children, basic social skills such as turn-taking and initiating conversation are easily acquired but for children with autism the process is much more difficult. Among the social skills deficits commonly associated with people are difficulties with reciprocity, initiating interactions, maintaining eye contact, sharing enjoyment, inferring the interests of others and an inability to read or understand emotion in themselves or in others (empathy).

Most individuals with autism are visual learners and concrete thinkers. Abstract concepts such as empathy or reciprocating emotions are difficult for them to process, and so they often experience problems interpreting other people's emotions, facial expressions and body language. In addition, children and adults with autism frequently have difficulty identifying their own feelings, dealing with them, controlling them and sharing them with others. Their emotional responses may be inappropriate for the particular situation and, as a result, other people may misinterpret their behaviour.

These problems may lead to feelings of anxiety such as increased heart rate, sweaty palms, noticeable shaking, difficulty concentrating and a tendency to avoid social situations altogether.

Most people with autism, especially high-functioning autism, have difficulty identifying, expressing and controlling their own emotions as well as reading and interpreting other people's emotions. Some children and adults appear to display few emotions, having a very flat affect and remaining very passive and disinterested in what happens around them. In contrast, other individuals may appear to over-react in many situations, either laughing hysterically when they are happy or becoming furious when the situation is merely annoying.

Many individuals feel more comfortable around logical thought and concrete facts and figures than they do around emotional issues. Among the problems associated with emotions are the lack of rules that assist in defining emotions and the range of nuances, subtleties and shades that are present within particular feelings and emotions. Emotions are not black and white, but rather contain all the different shades of grey. These shades of grey make it very difficult for the individual with autism not only to express their own feelings but also to understand the range of emotions present in other people.

> Daniel enjoys watching the other children in his class play games at lunchtime. He would quite like to join in with them but he does not seem to understand why they get so excited and make so much noise yelling and shouting and running around like crazy.
>
> He tends to stand on the sidelines watching, smiling and trying to imitate their actions but refusing to play.

While recognising and understanding the thoughts, feelings and emotions of self and others is a fundamental weakness among individuals with autism it is something that is so important for successful social interactions. Non-verbal feedback from others, for example, enables us to modify our behaviour but a failure to recognise these non-verbal cues leads to an inability to modify behaviour to meet the emotional and cognitive needs of other people.

Researchers believe that individuals with autism have not developed a theory of mind; they are unable, therefore, to infer mental states of others. Baron-Cohen (1985), in particular, has suggested that they are 'mind-blind' and therefore are unable to engage in social interactions with others. This leads to significant problems with social relationships, communication and interaction because they are unable to understand that other people have different thoughts and feelings to themselves. They are unable to predict or anticipate what people may say or do in different situations. In addition, they may have difficulty understanding that their peers, classmates, family members and other people they meet will actually have thoughts and emotions, and they may therefore appear to be self-centred, eccentric or uncaring (Edelson 1995).

According to Berk (2002), 'Children with autism have great difficulty with false-belief tasks and are frequently unable to attribute mental states to themselves or to others. Words such as believe, think, know, feel, and pretend are rarely part of their vocabularies.'

How do people with autism acquire basic social skills?
Despite many difficulties, children and adults can acquire social skills over a period of time, given appropriate intervention. Attempting to teach people with autism about emotions using conventional strategies, such as trying to get them to understand another person's point of view, is seldom effective, and a more concrete approach is often called for.

Carol Gray has developed a method to teach individuals with autism to understand and acknowledge the thoughts and feelings of others through 'social stories'. These short stories describe scenarios that enable individuals to improve their understanding of themselves and others. These stories prompt both children and adults to ask questions about other people and attempt to recognise that different individuals think in different ways. There are four types of sentences used in social stories:
- descriptive;
- directive;
- perspective; and
- affirmative.

Each sentence has a specific purpose.

Descriptive sentences indicate what the person does in a particular situation and why they do it. Social stories often start with a descriptive sentence because they set the scene. Descriptive sentences are factual and free from assumptions. For example: 'My name is Sue. I catch a bus to work every day.'

Directive sentences are individual statements of desired responses. They provide an outline of expected responses to a particular situation and provide the individual with specific information about what they should do in a situation to achieve their desired outcome. Directive sentences should always contain positive statements. For example: 'I always give the driver the correct money for my fare. I will stand at the back of the bus if there are no empty seats. I will stand quietly and not push other people on the bus.'

Perspective sentences present other's reactions to a situation so that the individual can learn how others perceive various events. The sentences in the following social story are examples of perspective sentences.

When the bell rings for recess to end, the teacher is happy to see all of the children line up quietly and walk to their classroom. Many of the children are excited because the teacher is going to read the class a story. The teacher enjoys seeing the children so happy and listening to the story. The teacher likes it when the children are quiet in class.

Affirmative sentences enhance the meaning of the other sentences and share a commonly held opinion. For example 'Children should line up and not push so that no one gets hurt. Everyone should go to their correct class line as soon as the bell rings.'

Social stories should be literally accurate, use concrete, simple text and general terms. The text should be supported by visual supports such as photographs, symbols, maps or drawings.

Picture cards can be used to determine the child's understanding of the feelings of others. The pictures may portray characters participating in a variety of social situations while emoting various feelings. The child may be asked to discuss how the characters are feeling based on clues such as facial expression, posture and what is happening in the picture. The child is encouraged to make inferences based on the context and cues in the picture. Other possible strategies include the use of video footage and thought bubbles to teach the concept that it is often possible to understand the thoughts and feelings of others by listening to what they are saying See Figure 13.1.

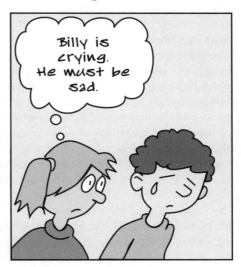

Figure 13.1 *Use of thought bubbles in understanding feelings of others*

What is video modelling

Modelling may be defined as the process in which an individual, referred to as a 'model', demonstrates a behaviour that can be imitated by another person. According to Corbett (2003), video modelling facilitates observational learning by:

- selectively focusing a child's behaviour on a relevant stimuli (attention);
- maintaining learned material through repetition (retention);
- reproducing observed behaviour through rehearsal and practice (production); and
- rewarding all attempts and progress (motivation).

Video modelling has been considered an easy and effective means of getting through to individuals with autism and teaching skills such as taking turns, pointing to objects, requesting, sharing and self-help skills such as dressing, and washing. Videotaping and then playing back certain behaviours encourages individuals to memorise, imitate and generalise these behaviours.

Using video modelling to teach children and adults with autism may speed up the rate of learning and also provide a means of motivating them when traditional teaching methods have been unsuccessful. The approach seems to work particularly well for those individuals who love to watch videos and television.

Why use video modelling?

Effective modelling in child development is the major means of conveying information in the process of social referencing (Bandura 1993).

Over the past decade, the effectiveness of video modelling as one component of intervention packages designed to promote self-care, vocational and play skills in individuals with autism has been examined. Video modelling has been identified as an efficient teaching procedure for individuals with autism for skills such as perspective taking, play, and social language (Le Blanc et al 2003).

Autism is a neurodevelopmental disorder. People with autism exhibit difficulty with organisation, conceptualisation, processing, planning and integrating information. Behaviours therefore often need to be taught in systematic step-by-step formats. Even children who do not readily imitate models will often reproduce verbalisations and actions from television and videos. The message to parents therefore is not to hide the television and videos but rather to change the programming and content. According to Charlop-Christy, Le & Freeman (2000), video modelling has yielded better results than live modelling in some individuals with autism.

What is video self-modelling?

Video self-modelling is based on the principles of social learning. According to Bandura (1969), the age, sex and similarity of a model to the observer are important factors in modelling. It follows therefore that using an image of one's self as a model would be a most effective means of changing behaviour. Buggey (1995, p 39) defined video self-modelling as 'a procedure by which children are allowed to view themselves at a slightly higher level than their normal ability through the creative use of videotaping and editing procedures'. During the process, a behaviour that is targeted for change is identified and an alternative, appropriate behaviour is determined. The child is then videotaped in either a role-playing situation or a natural setting, and the tape edited to show the desired behaviours.

Why use video self-modelling?

Video self-modelling is effective with individuals with autism because it does not require social interaction, it is based on the concept of visual learning, it is predictable as well as being easy to control. According to Charlop-Christie, Le & Freeman (2000), video self-modelling is also cheaper and less time consuming than other forms of video modelling.

Video self-modelling has been used successfully to treat a number of disorders and problem behaviours. Buggey et al (1999) found that the use of video self-modelling increased the level of appropriate responding in a group of children with autism and Bellini found it helped individuals to recognise thoughts and feelings in social situations and therefore reduced their anxiety and depression.

The majority of research using video self-modelling indicates that this procedure is effective in eliciting positive behavioural changes. According to Buggey (1995, p 41), 'children's confidence and self-rated ability on a task tends to increase as a function of viewing their own success'.

The development of an appropriate emotional state relies on an accurate perception and comprehension of visual stimuli, such as facial expression (Heilman & Valenstein 1993). It is certainly possible that the emotional development of individuals with autism may benefit from the use of video modelling, and video self-modelling, to teach them to interpret emotions in others. Research is in the early stages of testing whether video modelling can improve the perception and expression of emotion in children with autism. Visual images, however, are already used extensively to teach an understanding of different emotions.

What impact does autism have on an individual's emotions?

It is important to understand that how individuals respond to different emotions and feelings is related to their previous experiences. Do not make assumptions about how a person may be feeling in a particular situation. Most feelings are subjective, especially for individuals with autism, and their feelings of happiness, sadness and anger may differ from the feelings of other people. A child with autism may feel happy at being alone in the playground at school, a child may feel sad at a birthday party because there are too many people and too much noise or a young adult may feel angry when someone wants to share the same seat on the bus to work.

Many people with autism tend to interpret things literally. The person with autism will interpret 'I feel sick' as someone being physically ill or 'I feel cold' as someone turning blue and icy cold to touch. Try to select teaching resources that are literal, concrete and visual and avoid any resources that rely on an expectation of abstract reasoning abilities.

Most children and adults with autism have no basic understanding of empathy. Empathy is not an emotion that can be taught to people but individuals can learn to recognise different emotions in people by looking for certain physical signs (see Figure 13.2).

How may visual supports be used to understand emotions?

When teaching individuals with autism about emotions, it is important to describe each feeling pictorially, using pictures with clear outlines, minimal detail and colour and to keep explanations about emotions as simple and as concrete as possible. Relate the emotion to what can be seen, such as facial expression or body language. For example, smile means happy, frown means anger, mouth downwards means sad or hands on hips means anger and head lowered, tear in eye means sad (see Figure 13.3).

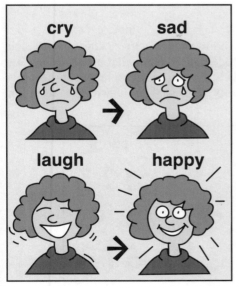

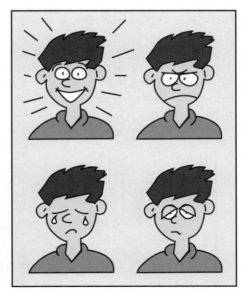

Figure 13.2 *Example of a visual strategy to help recognise feelings*

Figure 13.3 *Examples of visuals to describe feelings such as happy, angry, sad and tired*

For young children, it is advisable to keep to the basic emotions such as sad, happy, angry, sick, scared and tired, rather than to try to explore emotions that the child may not understand. It is also advisable to describe the basic emotions in concrete terms and give examples of situations that occur where a child may feel a particular emotion. Children may not realise that they are experiencing an emotion because no one has told them that what is happening is an emotional response to a particular event.

Joseph started to cry and throw himself on the floor because the wheel broke off his toy train and his mother was not able to fix it for him. Joseph was feeling angry because he couldn't push his train along the tracks any more. His mum said: 'You are crying and yelling because you are angry. You are angry because your train is broken.'

Use visual sequences to explain how to manage particular feelings. If a person is feeling tired, he should go to bed. If a person is feeling sad she should try to do something that will make her feel better (such as watching a favourite video, having a warm bath, visiting the local park or listening to favourite music). If a person is feeling sick he should tell someone or see a doctor. This type of strategy is illustrated in Figure 13.4.

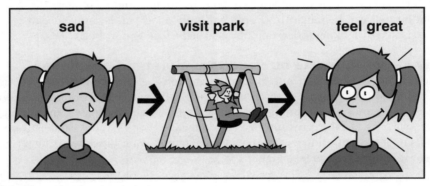

Figure 13.4 *Example of a visual strategy*

Assist individuals to recognise different emotions and to deal with these effectively. Teach alternative behaviours through visual cue cards and modelling to ensure that people know how to respond appropriately. For example, if a person is angry, he could be taught to keep his hands by his side, take a big breath and then count to 10. The visual strategy for this situation is shown in Figure 13.5.

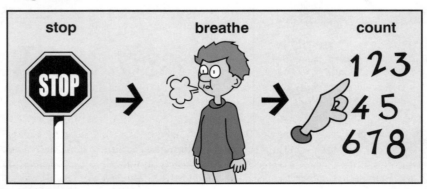

Figure 13.5 *Example of a visual strategy*

Children and adults may be encouraged to describe their feelings in different situations or for different people. Provide visual prompts to augment language, such as providing cue cards to prompt appropriate questions about a range of different emotions (see Figure 13.6).

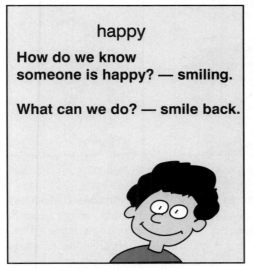
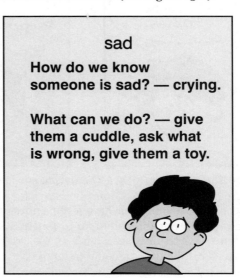

Figure 13.6 *Example of a visual strategy*

Sometimes facial expressions and body language need to be exaggerated and vocal tone altered when interacting directly with individuals to assist them to interpret different emotions. Introduce opportunities throughout the day to discuss feelings and emotions in everyday situations. Model appropriate social phrases and responses if a person seems unsure about how to react in a particular situation. For example, parents may need to model for their child how to take a deep breath and sit quietly when he feels anxious or stressed by a particular situation. They can also model phrases such as 'help please' or 'more' to aviod distress when their child requires assistance to complete an activity.

Help children and adults to understand their own emotions and feelings by vocalising what they may be feeling. For example, 'You're crying because you are sad.' Try to encourage them to share information about what they think has made them sad.

Some people with autism have a flat affect and may not show their feelings through their facial expressions. Their faces and body language may not always indicate their true feelings. When working or socialising with a person with autism, it is necessary to watch for other indicators of how they may be feeling. For example, if a person is feeling stressed and anxious, the signs may include an increase in repetitive/ritualistic behaviours, sensory issues or withdrawal.

Always acknowledge any attempts to respond to other people's emotions or to recognise and understand their own feelings. If using visual supports to teach new emotions or to acknowledge current emotions in individuals, there are a couple of widely recognised symbols to illustrate emotions and feelings. These are a speech bubble, thought bubble and feeling bubble.

Visual supports can therefore assist individuals to understand emotions through the use of speech, thought and feeling bubbles (see Figure 13.7). The bubbles are used in social stories and other strategies to indicate whether the information they contain is actually speech, or to describe the individual's thoughts or feelings. The speech bubble is a visual indication of speech while the cloud shape is used to indicate the person's thoughts and the heart shape indicates their feelings.

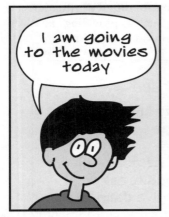
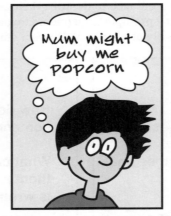
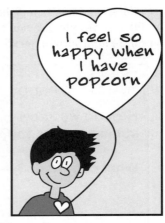

Figure 13.7 *Examples of speech, thought and feeling bubbles to explain emotions*

It is important to teach children and adults to cope with any emotions that they find overwhelming and difficult to control such as anger, fear and anxiety. Introducing cue cards for pleasurable activities (see Figure 13.8), writing social stories or repeating coping sentences such as 'I can do this' or 'count to ten if you feel angry' will often help individuals to acknowledge their feelings and regain control over their emotions in stressful situations.

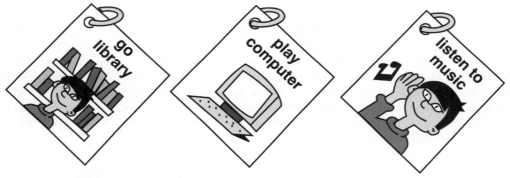

Figure 13.8 *Examples of visual cue cards*

It is also important to seek advice and assistance from experienced professionals, such as psychologists and occupational therapists about individual intervention strategies and programs. At times, medical advice and intervention may also be necessary when dealing with extreme anxiety or stress.

What are anxiety disorders?

Most people experience feelings of anxiety before an important event such as a big exam, business presentation, or first date. Anxiety disorders, however, are illnesses that fill people's lives with overwhelming anxiety and fear that are chronic, unremitting, and can grow progressively worse. Tormented by panic attacks, obsessive thoughts, flashbacks of traumatic events, nightmares or countless frightening physical symptoms, some people with anxiety disorders even become housebound.

(National Institute of Mental Health – NIMH, p 1)

Anxiety is a state or emotion that is characterised by negative affect, somatic symptoms such as rapid heart rate and increased tension and/or a feeling of fear or apprehension about some future event. Anxiety disorders, as a group, are the most common mental illness in the United States of America with more than 19 million adults affected by these debilitating illnesses each year. Anxiety disorders also affect children and adolescents. Approximately one in every ten young people may have an anxiety disorder. About half the children and adolescents with anxiety disorders also have another mental or behavioural disorder such as depression or autism.

If not treated early, anxiety disorders can lead to major problems among individuals, including impaired relations with peers, low self-esteem, drug and alcohol use, inability to work or function in the general community and anxiety disorders in adulthood.

According to Tonge & Einfeld (1999), there are high prevalence rates of anxiety disorders and anxiety problems among individuals with autism and significantly higher prevalence rates of anxiety problems in the autism population than the regular population. This growing awareness of anxiety problems has not yet been matched by a corresponding growth in scientific research about assessment or treatment of these disorders in children and adults with autism.

Why are anxiety problems associated with autism?

Because the deficits of autism are so pervasive and affect all parts of a person's life, many individuals with autism are under a great deal of stress as they attempt to make sense of the world they live in. They are under constant pressure in all aspects of life as they struggle to understand the most elementary social and communication concepts, to cope with problems involving planning and organising, to process and understand information from the senses and to deal with major difficulties involving emotions and abstract concepts. It is no wonder that many children and adults with autism are chronically stressed and that they develop problem behaviours in response to their constant stress and anxiety.

Many individuals with autism are prone to high levels of anxiety. Sometimes anxiety may be attributed to biological factors, at other times anxiety may be due to the overwhelming and unpredictable nature of the environment people live in. Because of the cognitive deficits of autism, people may have difficulties understanding what is expected of them in different situations and what is happening around them. Anxiety is an understandable reaction to this constant uncertainty.

Many children with autism become anxious and are harsh judges of their own performance. Challenging behaviour, repetitive actions, ritualistic behaviours and aggressive outbursts may arise because of the anxieties they face during a normal school day. Anxiety in children and adults with autism, unless treated, can become extreme, with prolonged periods of anxiety leading to secondary conditions such as:

- phobias;
- obsessive-compulsive disorder;
- panic disorder;
- post-traumatic stress disorder; or
- generalised anxiety disorder.

Phobias

Phobias are unrealistic and excessive fears of some situation or object. The two major types of phobias are social phobia and specific phobia. Children and adults with social phobia experience an overwhelming and disabling fear of being criticised or judged harshly by others, of being scrutinised, embarrassed or humiliated. This can lead to the avoidance of many potentially pleasurable and meaningful activities. Specific phobias centre on animals, storms, water, heights or particular situations, for example. People experience extreme, disabling and irrational fear of something that poses little or no actual danger and leads to avoidance of objects or situations that cause people to restrict their activities unnecessarily.

Obsessive-compulsive disorder
Obsessive-compulsive disorder is a pattern of repetitive, unwanted thoughts and compulsive behaviours that seem impossible to control or to stop. The behaviours may include repeated hand washing, counting, or arranging and rearranging objects.

Panic disorder
Panic disorder results in repeated episodes of intense fear that strike often and without warning. They are usually accompanied by pounding heartbeat, sweating, dizziness, nausea, a feeling of unreality and fear of dying. People will tend to avoid situations that may bring on a panic attack.

Post-traumatic stress disorder
Post-traumatic stress disorder shows in persistent symptoms that occur after experiencing or witnessing a traumatic event such as rape or other criminal assault, war, abuse crashes or other disasters. Common responses include nightmares, flashbacks, numbing of emotions, depression, anger and troublesome thoughts.

Generalised anxiety disorder
Generalised anxiety disorder manifests as constant, exaggerated worrisome thoughts and tension about everyday routine life events and activities lasting at least six months. People usually anticipate the worst even with little reason to expect it. The anxiety is usually accompanied by physical symptoms such as fatigue, trembling, muscle tension, headache and nausea.

Among children and adults with autism, anxiety may be associated with a number of factors including the need to socialise with peers and others, the inability to express emotions and understand the emotions of other people, the changes that occur daily as part of real life situations, the lack of understanding of the feelings and needs of other people and unexpected and uncontrollable events that may have disastrous consequences.

When 'stress affects a child with a neurological disorder, the child is less able to access the thinking area of the brain. Therefore the child does not act in ways others perceive to be logical or rational' (Myles & Southwick 1999, p 6). Individuals with autism, even if they have been taught how to handle a stressful situation, may not be able to recall their coping strategy when anxious or under stress. The problem does not lie in an inability to learn, it tends to lie in the way that information is presented. People with autism have difficulty tuning into the thinking part of their brain under duress, so it is important to provide functional ways to help them to recall their coping mechanisms to bring their anxiety under control. Visual strategies and supports offer the most effective means of teaching coping skills and providing visual reminders of what to do in particular situations.

How is anxiety managed in people with autism?
People with autism manage their anxiety in many different ways, sometimes successfully but in unusual and inappropriate ways. People with autism seek predictability and familiarity in their surroundings. Sticking to a fixed routine is the most effective way for them to avoid feeling anxious.

Individuals may attempt to manage their anxiety by withdrawing into their own world among their special interests and becoming preoccupied with their obsessions. The more anxious a person becomes, the more preoccupied and intense the focus on their special interest. Other individuals with autism may become more physically active, increasing their pacing, rocking, flapping or spinning or appear unable to control emotional responses such as crying, outbursts, rages or physical withdrawal. The most common reaction to increased anxiety is to develop routines or rituals. These actions operate as a means of reducing anxiety.

Strategies for recognising and managing these anxieties will differ for each person but the following suggestions may be included to help individuals cope with and avoid extreme levels of anxiety:

- Establish predictable routines to ensure consistency and present these visually with contingencies for change.
- Introduce visual supports to assist individuals to recognise and manage their anxiety by providing information in a concrete and readable format. Refer to the hierarchy of visual representation to determine levels of visual understanding before developing visual strategies. For example, does a person understand visual material presented via remnants, photographs or line drawings?
- Encourage relaxation and provide activities within the person's abilities to ensure achievement. Provide positive feedback for work completed.
- Determine a person's comprehension level, as this may be lower than their actual reading age, to make sure that understanding occurs.
- Be aware that during times of anxiety or stress, levels of visual understanding may decrease. Be prepared to use more concrete forms of visual representation such as photographs, even though a person may normally comprehend information presented through line drawings.
- Introduce physical activities at different times during the day to help individuals remain calm.
- Teach social skills and acknowledge the difficulties individuals have socialising.
- Limit unstructured break times. These periods may be stressful for people with autism because they do not know what to do and find unstructured socialising a problem. This can also present problems for staff in mainstream settings where unstructured times are part of daily routine. During these periods it is still possible to maintain some structure by providing individual visual sequences or choice boards of activities for those children who need them without compromising the free choice of the other children. It is also necessary to 'build in' down-time within any structured program for individuals with autism where expectations are lowered and they are allowed freedom to engage in favoured activities without any demands placed upon them.
- At certain times during the day, provide a quiet area of solitude. For example, individuals may be allowed to go to a pre-arranged, alternate place for a few minutes until calm when they indicate that they are stressed.
- Reduce the amount of time a person is expected to engage in a particular activity to minimise stress and anxiety. Schedule breaks within the regular daily and weekly timetable to allow the person to relax and regroup for the next series of activities.
- Develop a secret sign for help if a person is too embarrassed to indicate they are becoming anxious or to ask for help.
- Work closely with the individual's parents. Someone who is exhibiting a high level of anxiety outside home is also probably having similar issues at home. Monitoring anxiety levels across different settings provides information about current and potential stressors.
- For some individuals, the symptoms of stress/anxiety may be more evident at home outside school or work hours. Some people try so hard to conform and 'do the right thing' at school or work that they end up overloaded and take out their distress at home. It is therefore essential to maintain that collaborative approach between home and school/work to ensure that both parties are aware of any marked changes in behaviour.

- Challenging behaviours may serve as indicators of anxiety, stress or sensory overload. There is a need to look closely at challenging behaviours to determine possible causes.
- See each person as an individual. Each person will have unique needs that are different from the other people in the group. Allow for individual schedules, preferences and needs.
- Signs of anxiety or stress may be subtle and not always evident.

Commonly observed anxiety indicators include:
- picking at parts of the skin or pulling at the mouth;
- agitation or confusion during transition times;
- change in vocal tone, such as whispering, adopting an unusual voice, garbled speech, shouting or dictatorial tone of voice;
- wringing hands not obviously for pleasure or excitement;
- increase in obsessions, rituals or repetitive behaviours;
- increase in sensory sensitivities including auditory, tactile or visual senses;
- changes in regular toileting, eating and sleeping behaviours;
- increased pacing or other repetitive physical movements or actions;
- increase in fears or phobias;
- adopting another persona, such as becoming an animal;
- overreaction when spoken to or touched by peers;
- increased levels of withdrawal or detachment;
- catastrophic reaction to new tasks;
- refusal to go to school or leave the house;
- complaints of vague aches, pains of no apparent cause; and
- seeking deep pressure or vestibular movement more than normal.
  (Adapted from Brennan, Dodd & Fryer (2002) *Transition to School Manual*)

What treatment options are available?

There are a number of recognised intervention strategies available to treat anxiety problems. The interventions may be used alone or combined, depending on individual needs.

A number of medications, originally approved for treating depression, have been found to be effective for anxiety disorders as well. Some of the most recent antidepressants are called selective serotonin reuptake inhibitors (SSRIs). Other anti-anxiety medications include groups of drugs called benzodiazepines and beta-blockers.

Two clinically proven effective forms of psychotherapy used to treat anxiety disorders are behavioural therapy and cognitive-behavioural therapy. Behavioural therapy focuses on changing specific actions and uses a number of different techniques such as diaphragmatic breathing or gradual exposure to the actual fear of phobia. Cognitive-behaviour therapy uses similar approaches but also teaches individuals to understand and change their thinking patterns to help them to react differently to anxiety invoking situations.

Relaxation techniques are also commonly employed to decrease a person's anxiety in stressful situations. Techniques include deep breathing and progressive muscular relaxation. The deep breathing technique helps people regain control. When the individual focuses on breathing slowly and rhythmically, the body gradually begins to relax. The progressive muscular relaxation technique involves tensing and relaxing specific muscle groups. When the tense muscles become relaxed, one naturally feels less anxious.

The individual can be taught to employ this technique when anxious before or during a tense situation.

It is becoming more and more widely acknowledged that emotional issues are a major concern for individuals with autism, especially individuals with Asperger's syndrome, who are trying to live and function in society with minimal support. Individuals with autism are not good at reading emotion in other people, nor are they very good and recognising, understanding and expressing their own feelings. Many individuals with autism become overly anxious and stressed because of the difficulties they have trying to understand themselves and others.

Summary

The chapter has looked at the emotional needs of children and adults with autism. The communication and social skills deficits common to autism preclude people from establishing meaningful social and emotional relationships because of their inability to recognise and understand the thoughts, feelings and emotions of others.

Strategies have been suggested to assist individuals to develop effective social skills and to teach them to become more aware of the importance of emotional issues in starting and maintaining relationships.

Because of the unique characteristics associated with autism, many individuals develop anxiety disorders. Anxiety is a common problem among all people with one in every ten individuals suffering from some form of anxiety disorder. At least half of the children and adolescents with severe anxiety disorders have some form of mental or behavioural disorder such as depression or autism.

Discussions about causes of anxiety disorders and management strategies for people with autism have also been included.

Inappropriate, difficult behaviour is frequent in children with autistic disorders. The causes include confusion and fear of unfamiliar situations; interference with repetitive routines; failure to understand social rules; inappropriate attempts to control events; oversensitivity to sensory input from loud sounds, bright lights, crowds of people; pursuit of preferred activities without any ability to consider the consequences.

Wing 1996, p 56

Challenging behaviours threaten the safety and general wellbeing of individuals and prevent them from participating in everyday community activities. Challenging behaviours are usually measured in terms of the frequency of occurrence, the duration of the outburst and the intensity of the behaviour itself. Children and adults who engage in challenging behaviour may end up being excluded from school, work and local community events. They may also miss valuable opportunities to learn new skills or to become involved in new experiences. A number of factors cause behaviour problems for children and adults with autism including:

- poor comprehension and difficulties communicating verbally and non-verbally;
- high levels of stress and anxiety that may partly be due to overwhelming fears and phobias;
- sensory distortions;
- dependence on routine and structure as well as a need for sameness and resistance to change;
- obsessive and compulsive behaviour;
- lack of empathy for others; and
- inability to grasp overall concepts.

What approaches have traditionally been used to manage behaviours?

Most traditional approaches to dealing with challenging behaviour emphasise reactive strategies rather than developing a proactive approach. For example, most traditional methodologies involve some form of punishment (a reactive strategy that follows after a particular behaviour has occurred). Punishment may take the form of aversive stimuli or the removal of a desired object or activity. In traditional approaches, the majority of effort is focused on consequences, what happens after the behaviour. Little effort is made to look at what happens before the behaviour, the antecedents that serve as the triggers to the behaviour.

Pete is a young adult with many challenging behaviours. He becomes aggressive and kicks or hits anyone near him whenever he is not allowed to watch his favourite videos. As soon as Pete hurts someone he is forced to go to his bedroom and is not allowed to watch anymore TV that day. No one has bothered to teach Pete a more appropriate way of requesting his videos.

Children and adults with autism do not always respond positively to traditional behaviour management techniques. In current trends, the focus has shifted away from eliminating or suppressing challenging behaviours to looking closely at the possible cause or function the behaviour serves and teaching people more appropriate and effective alternative responses.

Why do challenging behaviours occur?

The severe communication and social interaction difficulties associated with autism result in individuals feeling confused, frustrated and anxious. People with autism have disordered communication that includes both receptive and expressive language as well as problems relating socially.

Individuals with disordered expressive language communicate in the most effective manner that works for them. This often includes some form of challenging behaviour. This is effective because it achieves a response. Some people with autism have no effective means of communicating apart from challenging behaviour. Other individuals may have more appropriate means of communicating (either verbally, through signs or gestures or visually) but still find that certain challenging behaviour usually generates an immediate reaction and, therefore, achieves better results.

Disordered receptive communication leads to confusion and anxiety when individuals are unable to understand what other people are talking about. When they are unable to understand what is happening around them or what is about to happen, the confusion and anxiety may trigger challenging behaviour.

Behaviour problems are more easily solved when they are viewed as logical and predictable responses to particular situations. Once the meaning behind a behaviour is understood, solutions or modifications to the environment can be put into place. According to Janzen (1996, pp 47–9), an understanding of behaviour involves a knowledge that:

Behaviour is communication: it is a logical response to a particular situation and challenging behaviour is an effort to regulate conditions that do not match a person's needs.

Behaviour is a logical response to the environment in which the behaviour was first learned. Over time, however, the behaviour is generalized to other situations that are not appropriate and the purpose behind the original behaviour may be lost.

Behaviour is an attempt by the person to keep the brain stimulated and in equilibrium. Self-stimulation and repetitive behaviours are examples.

Behaviour is an outward expression of an inward state. Fears and phobias, illness, anxiety and fatigue all have a significant effect on a person's tolerance and control and ability to cope in different situations.

It is only recently that people have begun to understand and acknowledge the relationship that exists between the severe behaviour problems of autism and the inability of these children and adults to communicate and relate to others.

People with autism:
- have limited understanding of the meaning of words — they use words literally and concretely;
- are frequently 'tuned out' and miss most of the information that other children pick up through incidental learning;
- have difficulty remembering the correct order or sequence of events — this leads to a lack of understanding of cause/effect relationships;
- don't know how to communicate their wants, needs and feelings;
- have limited communication skills so are unable to communicate in an appropriate manner;
- learn routines without understanding the concept behind, or the reasons for, the routine; and
- have difficulty relating to other children or adults and often do not know how to initiate any form of interaction.

Individuals with autism display inappropriate and embarrassing behaviour because they have difficulty adapting to and interpreting the different environments and people that they come into contact with. They often find it difficult to learn new skills. There are times when an individual may be under particular stress or when physical and emotional changes occur that can trigger problem behaviour. A number of adults and children with autism also have other difficulties such as learning difficulties, hearing and visual impairments or attention problems and these conditions themselves can lead to problem behaviour.

Problem behaviour is often an attempt to cope with the environment and the frustrations that are encountered daily. We all try to arrange our world to avoid confusing and unpleasant situations. People with autism, who meet more of these situations than anyone else, try to organise their world to remain stable and unchanging. They have limited expressive and receptive language and are often unable to communicate their feelings and desires. Management strategies for both children and adults with autism are based on a clear identification of any problem behaviour and when it occurs. Is it an inappropriate behaviour? Is it a learning related problem? In order to understand people with autism, it is essential to listen to the language of their behaviour.

How prevalent is problem behaviour in children with autism?

A synopsis of published research on behavioural interventions for young children with autism by Horner et al (2002) found that problem behaviours are a common concern for young children with developmental disabilities, including autism. Between 13 and 30 per cent of young children engage in problem behaviours that require intervention and young children with limited communication skills and poor social relating skills are particularly at risk of developing problem behaviours.

Challenging behaviours such as physical aggression, self-injury, pica, destruction of property, defiance, and tantrums are major barriers to effective education and social development and young children who engage in problem behaviours are at increased risk of becoming isolated and excluded from educational settings, social relationships, typical home environments, and community activities (Sprague & Rian 1993).

It has been found that once problem behaviours become established as part of a child's behavioural repertoire, the problem behaviours don't tend to go away or decrease without some form of structured intervention. Therefore not intervening, or waiting for children to outgrow their problem behaviours is not an effective method of dealing with them (Oliver, Murphy & Corbett 1987; Rojahn 1994).

What is meant by positive behaviour support approaches?

Positive behaviour support approaches emphasise proactive strategies that focus on preventing challenging behaviour from occurring. The focus is upon looking at the antecedents, or what was happening before the behaviour, in an attempt to obtain information about what caused the behaviour and then develop strategies to prevent it from happening again.

Positive behaviour approaches emphasise the fact that most challenging behaviour is learned rather than inherent. It is no longer acceptable to justify a particular behaviour by stating that the person 'has always been like this and is just like his uncle/father/etc'.

It has also been recognised that challenging behaviour is communicative — the behaviour serves a purpose for the individual and sends a clear message to others. The cause of problem behaviour is frequently related to either receptive language difficulties and/or difficulties with expression. The remedy seems to lie in improving communication skills through the use of visual strategies to support communication.

It has also become clear that challenging behaviour may be due to environmental factors, especially among children and adults with pronounced sensory impairments.

A positive behaviour approach is, therefore, concerned with more than decreasing a particular behaviour. The approach aims to promote every individual's overall success. Positive behaviour approaches teach the skills that are required to function in the general community and decrease stress and anxiety levels. This approach, for both children and adults with autism, focuses on developing communication-based strategies that are pitched at each person's level of understanding. There is a direct correlation between the existence of challenging behaviour and a person's lack of understanding and awareness of the social rules that govern their world and their inability to use socially acceptable means to influence the behaviour of others.

A positive behaviour approach is concerned with the factors that influence the behaviour of people with autism and establishing a multi-element procedure to address the problems, provide alternative responses and teach new skills. Current research supports this approach as an effective means of reducing the intensity and frequency of challenging behaviour while increasing the individual's skills and independence. 'We must go beyond the use of single interventions and develop comprehensive, multicomponent plans of support that are responsive to the unique demands of each person and setting and are guided continually by functional assessment data' (Lucyshyn et al 1995).

What is a multi-element approach to behaviour problems?

A multi-element approach involves looking beyond the behaviour itself in order to understand the background of the problem and to identify possible skill deficits. Once probable causes have been identified, the next step is to develop appropriate strategies that take into account the learning strengths and interests of the individual and also the particular learning styles common in autism. Positive interventions address all possible aspects of the particular situation and the challenging behaviour through multi-element programming.

A multi-element approach incorporates the following processes:

- providing environmental supports that take into account the necessary physical, social and program changes to prevent anxiety and support an optimal learning environment to suit the needs of the person with autism;
- teaching new concepts, skills and rules to develop independence and competence in a variety of different situations. The emphasis is on teaching the skills necessary for overall success and building confidence rather than merely reducing challenging behaviour. This includes teaching alternative, more functional ways of communicating needs and wants;
- organising and structuring the environment to take into account any sensory processing problems and provide consistency and ongoing support;
- providing positive reinforcement to encourage desired behaviours and ignore problem behaviours. This contradicts the traditional approach of focusing on the problem behaviours

by applying consequences in the form of punishment and ignoring desired responses;

■ continually evaluating the problem situations and modifying programs to address changing needs; and

■ establishing a crisis management plan as part of the multi-element approach to provide a consistent and immediate procedure that will protect the person and others if necessary. This is based on providing an immediate consequence when severe challenging behaviour occurs and is a reactive strategy.

What does a functional assessment of behaviour involve?

As part of a positive approach to behaviour, it is necessary to collect information about the behaviour and also about the situation in which the behaviour occurs. This information will assist understanding of why the behaviour is happening and also determine what strategies should be developed to help prevent the behaviour from occurring again.

A functional assessment looks at the relationship between the challenging behaviour and the environment. The assessment identifies the variables that reliably predict and maintain problem behaviour. Functional assessments are useful when other behaviour support programs have proved ineffective, when behaviour appears to be increasing or is not decreasing over a period of time, or in complex situations where ongoing behaviour support seems to be necessary.

The logic for functional assessment comes from research findings that operant behaviour is affected by the consequences that the behaviour has on the environment; the antecedent events that signal a link between occurrence of a behaviour and a consequent event; and setting events that alter the value of available consequences. A functional assessment therefore looks at a number of factors that may influence a particular challenging behaviour including:

■ the individual — including likes and dislikes, interests and obsessions, fears, sensory sensitivities, learning style, strengths and weaknesses;

■ the challenging behaviour — including what it looks like, how often it occurs, when it occurs, how long it lasts and how intense it is. The behaviour should be described in observable, measurable terms;

■ the setting events — including anything that influences the behaviour such as biological factors in the individual (pain, hunger, tiredness), the physical environment or social factors;

■ the antecedents — including anything that occurs before the challenging behaviour that triggers it or predicts its occurrence;

■ the consequences — including any event that follows the challenging behaviour and affects whether it will increase or decrease over time.

Once these factors have been studied and information has been collected, it should be possible to generate hypotheses about the function of the behaviour.

What critical questions need to be addressed?

When a functional assessment has been completed and hypotheses generated, the next step is to develop intervention strategies.

A number of critical questions should be considered when developing appropriate intervention strategies to manage challenging behaviour. Questions should be asked about the needs of the client, the learning environment, the influence of other people involved, the use of visual supports and the methods used to teach any changes to regular routines. Questions may include the following:

■ Do the intervention strategies reflect the interests, abilities and needs of the individual?

■ Is there recognition of the individual's areas of interest, obsessions and communicative and social limitations?

■ Are strategies presented in a way that accommodates the individual's particular learning style? For example, are visual strategies introduced to augment language and provide rules and routines?

■ Is the learning environment structured and predictable and are routines established and consistently followed?

■ Are there procedures in place to assist the individual with transitions and changes to routines or to the environment?

Challenging behaviour itself is not a characteristic of autism. It is a common reaction to the difficulties people with autism face in a confusing world where they cannot communicate their frustrations and anxieties or control the actions of other people. Challenging behaviour tends to decrease as individuals develop better communication skills, a better understanding of other people and ways of reading their environment or predicting changes to normal routines.

In addition to developing a functional means of communicating, individuals must learn to function in different settings and to generalise skills to become more independent. They have to learn social interaction skills such as sharing, turn-taking, listening and waiting so that they can interact with their peers, family and the general community. Young children with autism require help to learn the skills that other children pick up incidentally as they mature. They also need help to manage difficult behaviour. Encouraging both children and adults with autism to be more independent requires a consistent, planned approach that incorporates an assessment of their current skills, teaching of new skills and management of problem behaviour.

Once problem behaviour is identified, it should be possible to determine probable causes. The cause, or causes, will often relate to the deficits of autism: a sense of frustration due to poor social interaction and communication skills and an inability to understand what is expected of the person in particular situations.

What basic principles apply to behaviour support programs?

Some of the basic principles that apply when dealing with children and adults with autism are:

■ determine the message;
■ importance of consistency;
■ encourage participation;
■ provide clear messages;
■ use visual supports;
■ provide positive reinforcement;
■ plan for success; and
■ choose priorities.

Determine the message

It is important to recognise that people behave in certain ways for different reasons, and they learn to modify behaviour according to the results of it — how others receive it and what they obtain from it. Sometimes the reason for an inappropriate behaviour is quite obvious; at other times the reason may appear quite obscure.

When working with individuals with autism, try to identify all of the problem behaviours. This information may help to determine the message behind the behaviour. It may seem to be a priority to target overt behaviours such as a child's screaming, or tantrum behaviour in the shopping centre, while other everyday problems, such as crying when the video won't start, or head-banging when food is not presented quickly enough, are overlooked or not given priority. The different behaviours, however, may have the same underlying cause. In the examples above, the common element may be the child's inability to wait. By identifying all of the problem behaviours it becomes easier to see a pattern that helps identify the common elements. It then becomes possible to work on the behaviour in the least difficult setting — at home rather than in the shopping centre — and then gradually generalise the skill to other settings. A visual strategy may be introduced to assist children to understand the idea of waiting and one such strategy is shown in Figure 14.1.

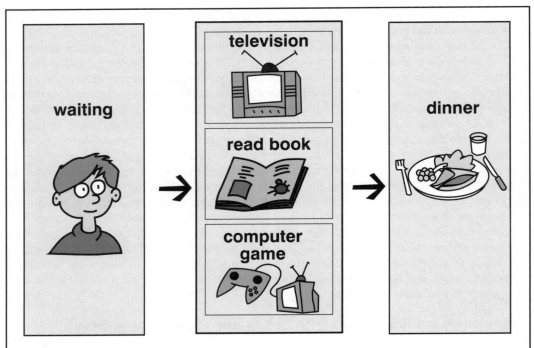

Figure 14.1 *Visual strategy*
Jack has difficulty waiting for his dinner so his mother made him a visual sequence that pro-vided him with a favourite activity to complete while he waited for his meal. She offered him a choice of activities so that he was not only learning to wait but he was also learning to make choices. Jack knows that as soon as he finishes his chosen activity his dinner will be ready. This has helped Jack learn to wait.

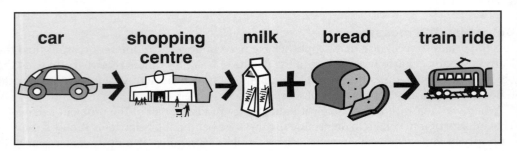

Figure 14.2 *Visual sequence to explain an outing*
When Jack goes to the supermarket with his mother, she shows him a visual sequence to explain where they are going and what they need to buy. She also includes a reward for Jack for good behaviour as an incentive to remain calm and to teach him to wait. Jack's waiting skills have improved since he started using his visual sequence cards.

Additional visual supports that may be introduced to assist a person to wait include cooking timers, counting to a number and a clock face (see Figure 14.3).

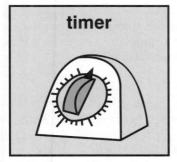
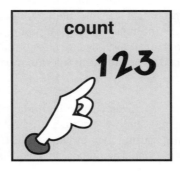
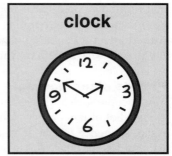

Figure 14.3 *Visual supports*

Initially children and adults should only be expected to wait for very short periods. The waiting time can be increased as people are able to cope for longer periods, as they learn skills and as they develop interests to occupy them while waiting.

Importance of consistency

Consistency in giving clear messages is essential when working with children and adults with autism because of their inability to read their environment accurately. This consistency needs to cover all people, programs and places.

The success of particular intervention strategies depends on the consistency of approach. Without the consistency of regular management, strategies are less effective. Consistent messages are often best given in a visual format that individuals can process easily and that remain constant for future reference.

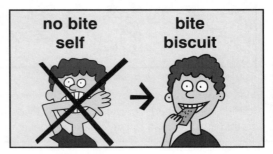

Figure 14.4 *Visual sequence*
James has a visual sequence card that reminds him not to bite himself. It is OK to bite biscuits or his piece of rubber 'chewy'.

Encourage participation

Encourage participation in family, school, work and community routines. Individuals with autism should be allowed to withdraw sometimes when their sensory overload suggests that they need space or time alone.

Children and adults with autism generally prefer to function in isolation. Even when they may want to be with others, their ability to interact is limited, and they may react in a negative way to the approaches of others. Parents and professionals must learn to 'read' the signals they put out — sometimes the non-verbal messages should be respected and complied with, while at other times the 'warning-off' signals should be ignored. Continue through any resistance, but take it slowly. It is important to determine the best approach — the indirect versus the direct approach. With a young child, for example, is it better to engage in parallel play or the more direct 'hello, what's your name?'.

In order to develop social interactive skills, each person with autism must learn to tolerate the intrusion of others. They need to learn the importance of social interaction and how this may be achieved. They should be supported and praised as much as possible for tolerating intrusion from others.

Intrusion can take many different forms. These forms may include tolerating another person within personal space, body contact such as holding a child's hand or giving a person a hug, approaching and attempting to interact verbally, stopping an inappropriate behaviour, or extending a particular behaviour. Intrusion occurs at one time or another in everyone's lives, but people with autism may need to be taught to tolerate intrusion from others.

Provide clear messages

Most people with autism prefer to be given clear rules and messages that assist them to understand what others expect of them. Usually these rules are best stated in a visual form. A simple visual sequence for the morning routine may assist a child to get ready for school/preschool without fuss or distress. The same visual sequence can easily be adapted for a young adult who may be attending a supported work placement or an older adult who lives at home.

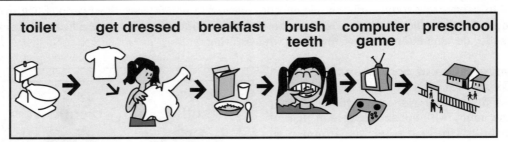

Figure 14.5 *Visual sequence*

Mary is more organised in the mornings since her mother started using a visual sequence to help her get ready for preschool. She loves her computer game so is eager to get ready so that she has time to play before school.

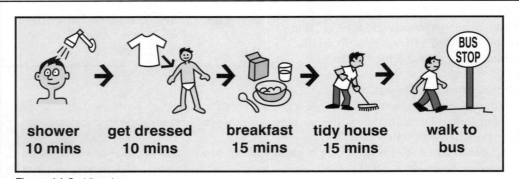

Figure 14.6 *Visual sequence*

George was always late for work and was likely to lose his job until he started to use a visual sequence to help him to be more organised in the mornings. Because he loves numbers, George also gave himself time limits to complete each step of his morning routine.

Clear rules assist individuals to overcome confusion in different situations. They may test the limits of these rules until they are firmly established. That is why it is important to develop a consistent approach.

Use visual supports

Some people with autism will respond to teaching programs presented verbally, but the vast majority of children and adults will respond more appropriately to programs and information presented visually. Different thinking and learning styles should be accommodated to ensure that a high level of understanding occurs. If in doubt, augment language with visual strategies to assist individuals to process the relevant information.

Provide positive reinforcement

Rewards should be individual and highly motivating. The best rewards may not always be what we would consider motivating. Obsessions, if controlled, may be used as rewards.

The list of possible reinforcements should include both tangible and non-tangible/social rewards. Often non-tangible or social rewards such as praise, attention, or a hug may not succeed if used on their own. To begin with, children and adults may respond more consistently if a non-tangible reward is paired with something more tangible such as food or a special toy. Social rewards are often ineffective when used alone. Individuals with autism do not usually behave to please other people, and may in fact prefer when other people withdraw social attention rather than give it. Social attention may be seen as something to avoid rather than reinforcement for desired behaviour, and an incompatible inappropriate behaviour may actually increase. When pairing a social reward with something more tangible, the aim is to gradually decrease the person's dependency on the tangible reward so that the social rewards and/or the activity alone become reinforcing.

Whenever rewards are introduced to reinforce appropriate behaviour, the rewards must be given consistently, and given as soon as the desired behaviour occurs.

Plan for success

Success is highly motivating, and encourages people to try harder. Highlighting failure is discouraging, and makes a person less likely to try again.

Children and adults with autism are as motivated by success as others. It is therefore important to control situations so that the individual succeeds and is reinforced for achieving. Plan for success by making sure that all of the conditions are right for the desired behaviour to occur. Behaviour should be managed, even to the point of manipulating the environment or situation to ensure a successful outcome. It is important to understand each person's limits and, if necessary, compromise a little to ensure their success. It may be necessary to reduce the demand a little: 'One more, and then finished' when asking a child to complete

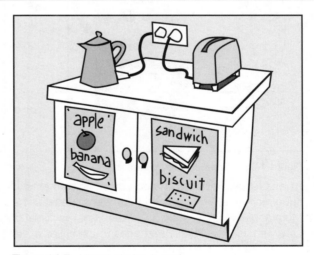

Figure 14.7 *Visual choice board*

Anthony has learned to make a choice between objects and is now starting to use photographs and line drawings. This choice board of Anthony's favourite food is on the cupboard in the kitchen at home. The pictures are attached with Velcro so that they can be changed if the item is not available. This allows Anthony to be more independent and avoids the frustration when he cannot communicate what he wants.

an activity with multiple parts. Avoid threats, especially if unable or unwilling to carry them through. If a reward is given when a desired behaviour occurs, the behaviour is reinforced and is likely to be repeated more frequently in the future.

In addition to reinforcing appropriate and acceptable behaviours, emphasis should be placed on teaching new skills to enable children and adults to communicate, socialise and manage better in a number of different settings.

Use positive rather than negative statements with both children and adults with autism and avoid situations of no win confrontation where no one can back down.

Avoid physical confrontation with young children such as smacking or shaking, or the threat of these. Physical confrontation may teach children to be aggressive and, as some children with autism have a high tolerance of pain, an unacceptable level of force may be required before it makes an impact on a child.

Always provide people with choices if they can make choices between objects, either verbally or non-verbally. Making choices provides some control over decisions and, hopefully, more willingness to comply. The choice should be between two objects or activities. Neither children nor adults should be given the choice to do something that must be completed — offer this choice and the answer may be no. Visual strategies, such as choice boards, may be introduced to assist people to make choices.

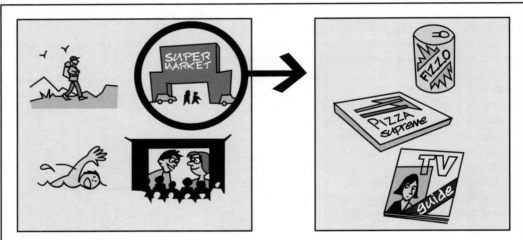

Figure 14.8 *Visual choice boards*

At weekends, David likes to go out with his parents. He loves to go to the park, to the supermarket, swimming or to the movies. Because he is non-verbal, David cannot tell his Mum and Dad where he would like to go. His visual choice boards help him to communicate with others. When David goes to the supermarket he uses a visual shopping list to choose his favourite items.

Choose priorities

The problems for people with autism often extend over many different areas of their lives. It is not possible to address all of these issues concurrently so it is necessary to prioritise:

- any behaviour that risks physical survival (such as pica, self-abuse, running away);
- any behaviour that impinges on the rest of the family (such as aggression against family members, poor sleeping habits);

- any behaviour that affects school/work placement (such as throwing objects, refusal to follow routines, loud screaming); and
- any behaviour that makes it difficult to take the person into the general community (such as obsessions and rituals, fear of dogs or using public toilets).

What is positive behaviour support?

Positive behavioural support provides the means to change or control inappropriate behaviours by providing a consistent, firm, and positive approach; introducing visual supports to facilitate understanding and teaching new skills and more appropriate ways of behaving in different situations.

Behavioural support should be applied firmly and consistently over time and care taken not to inadvertently reward inappropriate behaviour. It is not necessary to be loud, forceful or overbearing to convey a message of firmness. It is important to clarify all the elements of the problem — the 'why' as well as the 'what'.

When an inappropriate behaviour occurs, it is important to look not only at the behaviour itself but also at why it is occurring (that is, what does a person achieve from a particular behaviour?). This is known as an ABC approach to behaviour management where:

- A = antecedent conditions (what were the circumstances before the behaviour occurred?);
- B = behaviour (describe the behaviour); and
- C = consequences (what happened after the behaviour occurred).

Based on this information, new skills may be taught to provide alternative responses to a particular situation. Visual strategies may be introduced to clarify rules, teach alternative responses and provide clear messages to individuals who have difficulty processing verbal information.

Immediate behavioural intervention may be necessary, but it is generally not the only form of intervention required, and may not be motivation enough to eliminate a particular behaviour completely.

Consider the antecedent of the behaviour — what happened to cause the behaviour to occur. It may be possible to prevent the behaviour from occurring again by controlling or limiting the antecedent. If a particular problem behaviour occurs when a person's routine is changed, the behaviour may be eliminated by providing an early warning about the change to routine and providing a clear message about what will be happening instead. This may be achieved visually if the person has limited understanding of language.

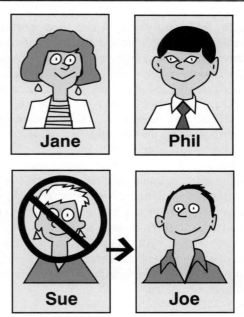

Figure 14.9 *Visual strategy*

Jonathon has a great relationship with his teachers at his day program. He enjoys attending and his behaviour has improved since he settled in and learned the routines. Jonathon does not cope well to changes in his life and staff members are worried because his favourite teacher is going on holidays for a week. A visual strategy was developed for Jonathon to help him to understand the change in his routine when his teacher is away.

It may be necessary to teach some coping strategies to assist an individual to handle certain situations by replacing inappropriate reactions with more appropriate responses in a particular setting. This strategy may include teaching some form of communication ('Go away.'), self-control (relaxation exercises), or avoidance (walking away from the situation).

It may also be possible to teach specific skills for specific situations so that coping strategies are not required. Teaching a child how to approach another child and to take turns with a particular toy may eliminate a number of inappropriate behaviours caused by frustration. Teaching a non-verbal adult to point to a line drawing to request a particular food item encourages an appropriate requesting response that is more effective and acceptable than hitting or yelling.

It is important to consider why problem behaviour occurs in order to determine how best to deal with it. Most problem behaviour occurs because of limited communication, a sense of frustration, self-protection, pain or to obtain attention.

Children and adults with autism have difficulty processing verbal information and may require a visual prompt or cue to support a verbal request. An effective way of learning is through experience. Most individuals with autism are visual learners. They can process information presented visually as long as it is presented at an appropriate functional level and they are allowed enough time to process the information. For some individuals, it may take from 5 to 30 seconds, or even longer, for information to be processed.

Where possible, language should be augmented with visual cues and prompts in particular situations and routines. Both children and adults with autism learn what is expected of them in certain places and through procedures that are familiar to them. Verbal language, though not always understood, will often appear to be understood when used in particular contexts. People with autism, however, have difficulty generalising any skills to new and unfamiliar situations and so should be given opportunities to practise new skills in many different settings.

Although challenging behaviours caused by a person's inability to cope must be considered and intervened upon, it is most important to teach alternative and more acceptable behaviour for a range of different situations.

Many people with autism lack skills in the areas of communication, socialisation, and play and they should be taught these skills as part of any intervention strategy. It is also important to be aware of possible sensory impairments as these also affect how a person responds in different situations.

What are the accepted procedures to manage behaviour?

A simple procedure to follow in managing challenging behaviour is to:

1. Determine the communicative intent of the behaviour — observe and record the events that lead up to and follow a specific behaviour.
2. Focus on the message or intent of the behaviour and do not give feedback on any inappropriate behaviour.
3. Provide enough information in a simple form so that a person can understand what is expected of them.
4. Teach a more effective and understandable way of communicating a message — encourage alternative, more appropriate and socially acceptable responses. The use of visual communication systems is often the most effective means of communication for both children and adults with autism.
5. Teach social play with peers using a range of different materials and equipment.
6. Show individuals how to initiate and how to respond in different situations. As most people with autism are visual learners, it is important to show them how to initiate and respond in different situations. Modelling is an effective teaching method to use.

7. Organise environments or situations to avoid confusion. Environments can be modified to make more sense to anyone having difficulty relating to the world around them.
8. Look carefully at the outcomes that are maintaining the problem behaviour — alter the consequences that have been rewarding and maintaining particular behaviour.
9. Individualise expectations — set priorities and aim for success by choosing to work on only one or two problems at a time.

What strategies are recommended?

There are a number of strategies that can be easily implemented to assist individuals to cope and feel comfortable in different situations to avoid problem or inappropriate behaviour. The important thing to remember is to ensure that individuals understand what will happen and what is expected of them in different situations.

Provide information

People with autism have a severe communication disorder, but they still learn. Since they tend to learn information exactly as taught, it is essential to provide clear and accurate models of language meaning and use. Introduce a number of visual supports to assist in different situations. In addition:

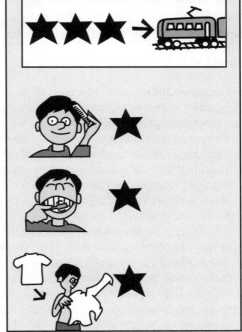

- obtain the person's attention;
- speak clearly: and clarify meaning through the use of visual supports such as facial expression, gesture and pictures;
- speak positively — tell the person what to do rather than what not to do;
- speak literally — keep language simple and functional; for example, 'put the toy in the box' or 'toy', point, 'box' rather than 'put it away';
- teach the meaning of rules and directions in natural contexts — state the request or rule both verbally and non-verbally (visually) to ensure understanding, and physically assist people to complete a task while repeating the words in different functional contexts;
- ask questions only when a choice is available, otherwise don't offer different options;

Figure 14.10 *Example of a visual reward chart to help with the morning routines*

- comment on what people are doing and praise appropriate responses;
- teach people to understand contingencies — these are contracts that allow people to organise themselves and to predict and prepare for what happens next. These should be presented visually to assist understanding;
- teach people to follow written or picture schedules or lists — visual timetables give a very clear message of what to expect at different times during the day (see Figure 14.11).

Help people to communicate information

Both children and adults with autism have a severe deficit that affects their ability to communicate their wants, needs and feelings. It is essential to provide them with a means of communicating with the people they come in contact with.

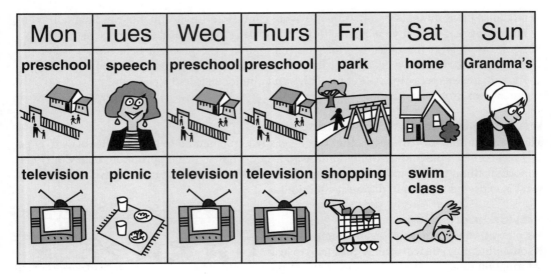

Mon	Tues	Wed	Thurs	Fri	Sat	Sun
preschool	speech	preschool	preschool	park	home	Grandma's
television	picnic	television	television	shopping	swim class	

Figure 14.11 *Example of a visual timetable to assist a child understand his weekly routine*

- Recognise the signals — be alert to any non-verbal signs of boredom, tiredness, hunger or frustration and teach the means to express feelings either verbally or nonverbally;
- Acknowledge individual's messages — if you cannot understand the message, acknowledge their attempt to communicate and then try to direct them to something else. It is most important to respond to any attempts by a person to communicate in order to encourage further attempts.
- Teach ways of obtaining attention — model appropriate ways to obtain attention by vocalising, touching, pointing etc.
- Have children or adults participate in some way before they obtain what they want, even if physical assistance is necessary. This may include pointing to objects or pictures or vocalising — at this stage do not insist that they say the words, it is more important for them to learn to communicate than to repeat words.
- Teach signals to indicate rejection or finished — this allows each person to have some control over their environment. The use of a 'finish box' is an excellent example of a visual support that signals the completion of a task or activity. A 'finish box' may be an empty tissue box or shoebox with a slot cut in the top in which to post photographs or pictures. A finish box is more appropriate for children than adults, who may be taught a sign or gesture for the word 'finish'.

Individualise expectations

Every person with autism is different and what works with one person may not necessarily work with another. It is essential to look not only at the challenging behaviour but also at the individual:

- Set priorities, adjust the environment and each individual's schedule — aim to prevent or avoid as many problems as possible in order to focus consistently on one or two.
- Start small and gradually expand expectations when successful — children and adults with autism should be expected to follow the same rules as others after learning what the rules mean. Expectations should be kept realistic during the teaching period. It is important to remember that people with autism often learn differently so it may be necessary to modify teaching approaches to accommodate individual learning styles.
- Use natural consequences in order to help people to learn cause/effect relationships and to be responsible for their own actions.

■ Keep records — a descriptive anecdotal record of behaviour and significant events may help to determine any pattern to the behaviour.

Additional strategies

Repetitive/stereotypic behaviours, tantrums and occasional aggressive behaviour will occur in spite of diligence and careful programming. In the event of challenging behaviour occurring, the primary goal is to prevent serious injury to any individual and to defuse the situation:

■ stay calm and relaxed, speak and move softly and soothingly;
■ do not attend to or talk about the behaviour itself — avoid nagging and scolding;
■ teach children and adults with autism to respond to signals such as 'stop', 'quiet', 'hands down'. These may be presented verbally or in a visual format;
■ treat all behaviour as an attempt to communicate;
■ allow the person time to process information;
■ structure the environment and provide familiar routines;
■ allow regular breaks or down time — a chance to relax and calm down in a quiet, undemanding area;
■ keep a record to check if a particular behaviour is getting worse. It is beneficial to record what is happening when a particular behaviour occurs and what happens immediately after;
■ use this information to develop additional skills and also to modify your approach; and
■ also make any necessary environmental changes to assist the individual to cope more easily.

Positive behaviour support may best be seen as an overall approach that encompasses teaching, modifying the general environment and developing an understanding of the individual's needs and limitations.

At all times when working with children and adults with autism, the emphasis should be on teaching new skills in a positive way. Emphasis should also be placed on understanding each person as an individual with different learning styles and different interests.

How do you manage obsessions?

If appropriate, work with the obsession, not against it. Use it as a teaching tool or as a reinforcer:

■ provide alternative appropriate ways of gaining the same kind of pleasure;
■ reduce opportunities to engage in the obsessive behaviour;
■ confine obsession to a particular place or time of day, *but make it contingent on something else*; and
■ do not exert all your energy attempting to extinguish an obsession (unless highly inappropriate) — it will often be replaced with another.

How important is use of reinforcement in behaviour support programs?

Research has shown that the strength of behaviour is influenced by the consequences that immediately follow it (that is, the event that occurs as a result of the behaviour). The type of consequence, either positive or negative, and the timing (how close the reaction is to the action) has an impact on whether the behaviour is more or less likely to occur in the future and whether it might be modified. If behaviour is followed by a pleasant consequence, the particular behaviour is more likely to occur in the future. In other words, to reinforce is to strengthen or to increase behaviour. If behaviour is followed by an unpleasant consequence (punishment), that behaviour is less likely to occur again. By applying pleasant consequences to desirable behaviour, such as a hug and smile if a child helps to pack away their toys or a doughnut for helping to complete the grocery shopping, the likelihood that the behaviour will occur more often in the future is increased. The use of punishment as a way of decreasing behaviour is highly questionable, particularly in children with autism, where problem behaviour is usually due to confusion, lack of skills or frustration.

Reinforcement occurs immediately after a particular behaviour, thus encouraging the behaviour to occur again. In short, reinforcement strengthens behaviour. There are two different types of reinforcement — positive and negative.

Positive reinforcement is a reward (something a child likes) given for good work or appropriate behaviour, the good feeling a child has on completing a task successfully, payment for work completed — all are examples of positive reinforcement.

Negative reinforcement is a behaviour occurring to avoid or stop something unpleasant from happening. This may be negatively reinforced if the child successfully avoids the situation in future. If a child avoids going shopping by screaming, the behaviour has been negatively reinforced and the behaviour is likely to occur again when the child wishes to avoid an unpleasant situation.

Problem behaviours are sometimes accidentally reinforced. People's natural response to inappropriate behaviours occasionally makes things worse and strengthens the particular behaviour that they are trying to eliminate. If a child expresses displeasure at a certain activity by having a tantrum and throwing toys, and the adult responds by stopping the disliked activity, the tantrum will be reinforced and be likely to occur in other situations in the future.

Chloe is obsessed with TV and videos. She insists on having the TV on all day and screams and bangs her head if it is turned off. Her Mum tries to turn the TV off at mealtimes but Chloe gets so upset and angry that, whenever Chloe screams, her Mum lets her turn the TV back on. Chloe has learned that if she screams she will get whatever she wants.

How effective is time-out?

Inappropriate use of some behaviour management techniques can also strengthen problem behaviour. Time-out is only effective when it is time away from something positive. Research has shown that time-out can strengthen problem behaviour if it represents time away from a disliked situation or if the child simply enjoys quiet time away from an over-stimulating situation.

Whenever Michael was aggressive towards any of the other children at school he was given time-out. Michael had to go and sit on a chair outside the classroom for 10 minutes. Michael did not enjoy loud noises and often found the classroom too noisy. He realised that if he hit one of the other students he was given time-out in a quiet area.

When should reinforcement be used?

Reinforcement strengthens behaviour. Reinforcement should always be given immediately after behaviour occurs, to increase the likelihood that the behaviour will occur again. It is important to determine what is reinforcing to an individual when working to encourage a particular behaviour. What is reinforcing for one person may not be reinforcing for another. This simply means giving someone something that he or she likes, after behaviour occurs, in order to strengthen that behaviour. People receive reinforcers hundreds of times every day. When they are rewarded for certain behaviours they will continue to repeat them. If a person is praised for helping around the home, that person will be more likely to continue to do so in the future.

Individuals with autism do not naturally like the same rewards enjoyed by others. Social rewards such as smiles, hugs, being told 'good boy' or 'clever girl' are not necessarily rewarding or reinforcing for children or adults with autism. They may be motivated by different reinforcers, these may be very specific and powerful for a particular person and may include things such as watching favourite videos, spinning a top, jumping on a trampoline or playing with a piece of string.

Children are reinforced hundreds of times everyday. Smiling and praising a child for helping to put toys away, finish their dinner, and clean their teeth will ensure that these desirable behaviours are likely to occur again. However, it is only reinforcing for a child if it is 'positive' for that child. Perhaps the best example of a reinforcer is the attention that is paid to children when they are being good. Reinforcement is a powerful method of increasing desirable behaviours in the future. It is important to understand how reinforcement works, the different types of reinforcement and when to use reinforcement to maximise a teaching situation.

Reinforcement does not always work immediately, but can influence future behaviour. Parents and teachers need to be consistent in any attempts to reinforce an individual and to maintain that consistency over a period of time. This will allow the reinforcement program time to work.

Although challenging behaviour should be dealt with immediately it occurs, it is also necessary to teach appropriate and alternative skills for communicating, socialising and behaving. Self-stimulating behaviours such as spinning, rocking and pacing, for example, often decrease as individual's social and communication skills improve. It is preferable to allow self-stimulatory behaviour to decrease naturally over time as the person's need for such behaviour also decreases. Trying to eliminate self-stimulatory behaviours in children and adults who need to spin or rock in order to calm themselves or reduce anxiety, is not recommended. The frustration and aggression of children and adults also tends to decrease as they learn to communicate and interact more effectively.

> Matthew always lined up his toys and turned his cars over to watch the wheels spin. He used to line up everything because he did not know what else to do with objects and he needed stimulation. As his play skills improved, Matthew spent less time spinning and lining things up and more time playing appropriately.

What types of reinforcement are appropriate?

A reinforcer is something that a person feels good about. It may not always be something that would be conventionally motivating. Reinforcers may be food or favourite outings such as muesli bars, pasta, sultanas, or juice or a trip to the park, railway museum or beach. Reinforcers may also be activities such as helping to mow the lawn, banging two sticks together, watching a favourite video, tearing paper or opening and closing all of the cupboard doors. Reinforcers may include hugs and kisses, smiles, attention, praise, and touching, or watching TV, playing a game, jumping on a trampoline or going for a walk together.

As a person is rewarded for appropriate behaviour it is important to also acknowledge why they are being reinforced. For example, 'Good boy, you came when I called you' or 'Well done, you have cleaned up all of the mess.'

How often should reinforcement be used?

When initially attempting to increase a desired behaviour, it is important to reinforce the person every time the behaviour occurs. This is called *continuous reinforcement*. If the reinforcement chosen is sufficiently rewarding, then the behaviour will be strengthened.

Once the desired behaviour begins to occur regularly, it may only require occasional reinforcement. This is called *intermittent reinforcement*. During intermittent reinforcement, the rewards are faded so that the reinforcement is offered sometimes rather than every time the desired behaviour occurs. The desired behaviour should continue to be intermittently reinforced otherwise it may decrease or stop altogether.

> When Kate was learning to do puzzles, her Mum used to give her a reward every time she put one piece in the puzzle. Eventually, she only needed to give a reward when Kate completed the puzzle. Now, Kate is happy with a hug from her Mum every two or three times she completes a puzzle. Kate is reinforced by the satisfaction she gets from completing the puzzles without help.

How do you reinforce behaviours?

Behaviour may be reinforced in a number of different ways, depending on the behaviour and the situation in which it occurs. For example:

- catch people being good — observe them so that you know when to reward appropriate behaviour;
- decide on some appropriate reinforcers for the particular person — remember that people with autism often like rewards that are outside the traditional reinforcers used by most people;
- specify what behaviour is being reinforced;
- use your reinforcers contingently, immediately and consistently; and
- use visual supports to assist individuals to understand the reinforcement process.

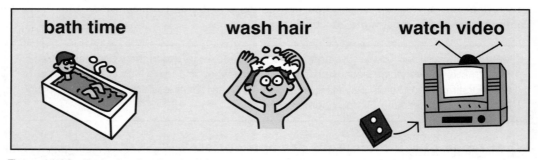

Figure 14.12 *Example of a visual reinforcement strategy to encourage children to wash hair*

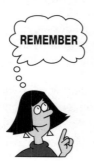

REMEMBER

- Remember that all behaviour is communication.
- Treat challenging behaviour as a means of expression.
- Consider echolalia an attempt at conversation.
- Support verbal information with visual cues, as much as possible.
- *Structure* the environment; provide familiar routines.
- Give information one step at a time.
- Allow time for processing (usually between 5 to 30 seconds, or even longer).
- Tell what to do, not *what not to do*.
- Keep language short and simple.
- Introduce the idea of language as a means of communication by commenting simply on what is happening rather than giving a lot of verbal directions.
- Avoid abstract concepts and multiple-meaning words.
- Be aware of potential sensory problems.

- Build communication skills — teach alternative, more appropriate ways of expressing the same thing such as visual aids and signing.
- Teach new skills to help individuals cope with any problems; for example, improve play skills and teach how to share.
- Teach specific social skills and conversation skills.
- Avoid certain situations that can lead to problems.
- Desensitise individuals to things that cause fear.
- Use strategies specifically designed for managing people with autism; for example social stories, visual systems, schedule boxes, teaching rules to be followed, and providing structure.
- Also employ other general strategies such as redirection, ignoring, positive reinforcement, and contracts. A contract, or formal/informal agreement, may be developed with the individual to outline what behaviours are acceptable in particular situations. An individual contract may be accompanied by some form of reward or reinforcement as an incentive to follow the rules of agreement. A contract may be either a verbal or written agreement and should, if possible, also be presented visually.

Learn to use children's obsessions as a tool for managing other problem behaviours.

Dealing with challenging behaviours requires a two-step procedure of functional assessment and positive behavioural support. These approaches are based on two premises:

1. that behaviour problems often reflect learned ways of responding to difficult situations; and
2. that systemic ways of responding to these behaviours have proven ineffective.

The first step in designing a comprehensive management program for behaviour problems is to identify why the person is engaging in these behaviours. The second step involves using information from functional assessments, along with a consideration of the individual's current strengths and needs as well as future goals to design a comprehensive positive behavioural support plan.

Summary

Challenging behaviours may be described as those behaviours that occur with such intensity, frequency and duration that they interfere with the person's ability to maximise their potential. In order to understand challenging behaviour and why it occurs among children and adults with autism, it is necessary to firstly understand the nature of the disability and its impact on the ability of individuals to function in everyday situations.

Available research indicates that young children with autism are at significant risk of developing problem behaviours and without structured intervention the behaviours are likely to worsen rather than improve. The impact of problem behaviours on educational, social, and community opportunities is both dramatic and detrimental.

Individuals with autism are focused on detail, rather than organising information to form the whole picture. Ritual and routine are relied upon to make sense of an overly complex environment. Obsessive behaviours can result and their impact on behaviour is substantial, as individuals focus exclusively on their own needs and interests and take little note of what is happening around them.

Once we have an understanding of the nature of autism, it is important to conduct a functional assessment to establish why the difficult behaviour is occurring. This includes looking closely at the individual, the behaviour itself, what it achieves for the individual (consequences), what causes the behaviour (antecedents). as well as looking at the environment (setting events).

Frequently, specific behaviours occur because they are the only functional means the person has to make a request, escape from a confusing or stressful situation, obtain attention or demonstrate boredom or frustration. If the primary function of the behaviour is to communicate a need, a want or a dislike, it is important to look beyond the behaviour to the message it conveys and teach the person alternative, more appropriate means of having their needs understood and acted upon. This usually requires the teaching of new skills and/or alternative behaviours.

The use of visual supports is widely recommended as part of any positive behaviour support programs. Other positive behaviour support strategies include:

- preparing the person in advance for change;
- using concrete, precise speech;
- gradually desensitising individuals to sensory stimuli;
- organising play and work to take into account the person's difficulty sequencing and seeing the whole picture;
- allowing controlled access to obsessions; and
- understanding the person's limited comprehension abilities.

15

Play

Play is a natural activity that fosters the development of cognitive skills, positive social and emotional behaviours, verbal and non-verbal communication and motor proficiency. Play based intervention, therefore, is an effective approach to use with children who have disabilities.

Clifton & Dodd 1998, p 1

Play is a diverse and complex behaviour that is a central part of the normal development of children. For most children, play is an intrinsic activity that is done for its own sake, rather than as a means of achieving any specific end. Play itself is difficult to define. Even dictionaries vary in the definitions they offer. Most, however, seem to imply some sort of fun, and a means of entertaining and enjoying oneself. Many definitions have been published in an attempt to explain what play is. Brown & Gottfried (1985, p xix) noted that play is:

> ... related to children's social and emotional development. It is an important indicator of children's language and symbol systems, and of the meanings children give to persons, places and events. It is also an index of children's imagination, curiosity, motivation, preferences, interests and persistence.

According to Quill (2000, p 10), 'play is the fabric of childhood'.

Research has shown that play can be used as a medium to encourage the development of cognitive, social and motor skills, communication and imagination in children. Children begin to integrate the things that they are learning and begin to explore their environment through play. According to Garvey (1977), the key characteristics of play should be:

- intrinsically motivating;
- pleasurable and enjoyable;
- having no extrinsic goals;
- involving active engagement on the part of the player; and
- having certain systematic relations to what is not play.

According to Brofenbrenner (1979) play is essentially *spontaneous* and *voluntary*, undertaken by choice rather than as a result of direction by others. It involves exploration, imagination and motivation and provides a medium for the development of decision making, communication and socialisation skills.

Play is important as it serves as a structure for social interaction with other children and adults. It is through play that young children learn many of their social and communication skills, including co-operating with each other, sharing, taking turns and working collaboratively to achieve a particular goal.

Beyer & Gammeltoft (2000), in the book *Autism and Play*, outline some of the key features of children's play. They suggest that children play solely for play's sake; all children play, regardless of culture or nationality; play provides a platform for the development of imagination and fantasy; play provides opportunities for children to mirror reality and play provides a means for children to express themselves.

Play is an important part of any teaching program involving young children because play activities encourage children to practise their social and communication skills. They can learn to make their own choices, socialise with their peers, share and take turns with others, and communicate their ideas and feelings both verbally and non-verbally. The development of play occurs in stages from solitary play to functional play through symbolic play, constructive play, dramatic play and play involving rules (Piaget 1962). Play forms the foundation for the development of a child's intellect, creativity and imagination, sense of self, resolution of feelings and the capacity to interact with others in positive and appropriate ways (Almy 1984).

What are the developmental stages of play?

Most current early childhood texts discuss numerous theories about how play develops in young children and how important play skills are in children's overall development and skill acquisition.

The foundation for play-based intervention lies in the work of Piaget (1962, 1969, 1991) although the theoretical works of many other researchers also supported the idea of the importance of play in teaching social and communication skills in young children. A number of prominent psychologists have studied the importance of play-based intervention for young children so that the importance of play in the overall development of young children has been well documented.

Parten (1932) formulated a series of stages children normally pass through as their play skills develop. The first stage, referred to as unoccupied play, describes children who are not playing with anything or anyone. During this period, the children are not motivated or interested in either objects or people. The next stage, solitary play, is used to describe very young children who play alone and independently and are focused strictly on their own activity with little or no awareness of others.

Randolph has just started preschool but has no interest or awareness of other children at the centre. He is obsessed with cars and spends most of the day playing alone. If other children approach him to play he cries and grabs all of the cars so that he does not have to share them.

Most children gradually move on to play alongside other children and engage in parallel play. The play is independent but they may show interest by looking at the other children's toys, making eye contact and possibly imitating the actions of another player. Parallel play promotes the emergence of more interactive play development. Once children are comfortable playing alongside other children and have begun to learn some of the skills of social play, they begin to engage more interactively in associative play.

During associative play, children play together at a similar or identical activity with some sharing of equipment and early turn-taking behaviour. The children may interact because of a common interest in the activity but they are not dependent on each other. There is no organisation or taking on of roles. The children still play on their own terms without subordinating their own interests to that of the whole group.

As children develop imaginative or pretend play, they become more social and prefer to play interactively with others in co-operative play.

> When Tim started preschool he used to scream if any of the other children came near him or wanted to play. He enjoys water play and, because he is settled and knows the daily routines, he is happy to let other children play next to him and share the toys and equipment. He waits for his turn and even imitates what the other children are doing.

The children take on pretend roles and introduce taking turns, and some competition, or rules. There is co-operation and dependency between the participants. Play tends to be organised and the children work toward achieving a particular goal. During this stage, children have to subordinate their own interests for the benefit of the whole group.

Boucher (1999) also believes that children advance through a number of developmental stages. He suggests that children advance through the following stages starting with sensory motor play and then advancing through exploratory and manipulative play to focus on physical play. Children enjoy rough and tumble activities and chasing games during this stage but then also move on to more socially oriented play activities. Eventually children develop their pretend play skills and engage in make-believe activities with their peers.

According to Boucher (1999), play encourages children to learn and practise new skills in safe and supportive environments. She also emphasises that play should be fun.

Engaging in play is the norm in early childhood and forms the basis for the development of social awareness and interests that lay the foundation for many later more complex skills. Sensory motor play in very young children teaches toddlers about their own bodies and about objects in their immediate environment. Manipulative and exploratory play teaches children about objects and their properties and also teaches the basics of how they can influence and manipulate the environment around them. Physical play is important because it introduces gross motor skills and provides experiences of physical interaction with objects and other people in their environment. Social play teaches children about social relationships and how to engage in interactions with others.

> Jo and Eddie have learned to share toys and take turns in play. They love to play with bubbles and will take turns to blow the bubbles and to 'pop' them. They will look at each other and wait quietly for their turn.

According to Libby et al (1998) there are different types of pretend play. It is possible to differentiate functional play (such as pushing a toy train along a track and making a 'chchchch' noise) from symbolic play. Symbolic play involves pretending that an object is something else (pretending that a crayon is an aeroplane or an orange is a ball).

Leslie (1987) tried to distinguish sophisticated functional play from symbolic play. True pretence requires two levels of representation. In first-order representation, a child may use a toy as a substitute for the real thing, but not engage in symbolic play because there is a belief in the reality of the object (the orange is believed to be a ball). Second-order representation involves the awareness that the pretend object is not the real thing but is merely being used as a substitute (the crayon is not really an aeroplane) (Williams, Reddy & Costall 2001).

According to Quill (2000, p 10), play is a learning process, a social process and an emotional process and is used by children as a means of learning about the world and people:

Through play, children explore their bodies, toys and objects, as well as learn from adults and peers. Play – which can be a reenactment of previous experiences, a means to try newly acquired skills, or a novel approach to both – is creative. It is the full expression of all learning, relationships and feelings.

According to Restall & Magill-Evans (1994), play provides a medium through which children develop skills, experiment with different roles and interact with others. They found that children with autism were disadvantaged in their use of play for these purposes.

Ungerer & Sigman (1981) suggested that the play behaviours that eventually lead to the development of symbolic play become apparent in young children in the first two years of life. Children with autism, however, do not naturally develop the symbolic play skills that allow them to engage in pretend or imaginative play with other children. Children with autism have to be taught play sequences so that they know what to do in play sessions.

What are the play limitations of children with autism?

Young children with autism have notoriously poor play skills and so do not participate in the natural and meaningful activities associated with play. Their play may be characterized by a fixation on certain objects or rituals and by withdrawal and self-isolation. Though they may eventually develop an interest in a wider range of objects, their play typically remains solitary, with social behaviour restricted to some onlooking or parallel play.

(Clifton & Dodd 1998, p 2)

Autism is a developmental disorder, characterised by difficulties with communication, social understanding, social behaviour and imagination. Children with autism tend to lack the fundamental social skills of joint sharing attention, pointing to communicate, and imitation of actions and sounds that are so obvious in typically developing children. The play skills that form the foundation for later social relating do not develop naturally and children need assistance to master necessary skills, in particular to develop functional play skills.

The play skills of children with autism are different from other children. They do not follow normal patterns of play development — their play, like their other skills, is disordered. There seems to be no correlation between the development of play skills and normal language development, unlike the stages followed by typically developing children. Children with autism spend less time engaged in functional play activities than other children who have been matched for mental age and expressive language. Their play is less varied and integrated and is more likely to be characterised by repetitive actions such as opening and closing the doors or driving a toy car backwards and forwards. Children with autism tend to play with toys in a repetitive, stereotypic way by spinning wheels and sorting and categorising objects. They are more interested in manipulating objects than playing with them in functional ways. They show little interest in playing socially with other children. They have difficulties learning through observation and possess limited or no pretend or imaginative play.

The play of children with autism is primarily solitary and is often characterised by repetitive or obsessive use of a limited number of objects, or exploration of objects at a sensory level. Normally, children develop social play first through interaction with parents in games such as peek-a-boo, and then begin to show an interest in toys. Children with autism develop their play skills differently. Relative to social skills, their motor skills are usually much stronger and they are more interested in objects than people. Children with autism learn to play with objects and particular toys before they learn to play socially with other children or adults.

According to Quill (2000, p 10), 'play is primarily a means to link the emotions of self and others with various social roles and experiences. It has been said that the social skills of life are learned by kindergarten, and, indeed, most are acquired through play.'

The play of children with autism is influenced by their autistic characteristics including:

- restricted interests, such as a fascination with cars or trains;
- repetitive behaviours, such as spinning or lining up objects;
- sensory sensitivities, such as sensitivity to touch of certain textures or a preference for swinging or jumping;
- need for sameness, such as always playing with the same objects, in the same way;
- obsessions, such as wanting to watch a certain video over and over or only playing with toys that focus on numbers or letters;
- disordered communication, such as a lack of functional language and poor comprehension skills; and
- disordered social relating skills, such as preferring to play alone and not sharing or taking turns in play.

According to Jordan & Libby (1997), sensory play in children with autism tends to dominate beyond the age at which it normally declines in children without autism and toys and objects tend to be used in limited and inflexible ways. A child with autism may engage in repetitively opening and closing the doors of a toy car or lining all the cars up in a particular order rather than attempting to drive the car along a road or include other objects such a toy garages, car mats and road signs to play pretend games.

> Samuel loves to spin objects. He likes cars because he spins the wheels and he also likes to watch the clothes spin around in the clothes dryer. He loves to watch ceiling fans and becomes distressed when he is not allowed to go into shops where he knows there are ceiling fans. His mother has made a visual car mat to show Samuel another way to play with cars. He is allowed to spin the wheels for a few minutes after he has played with other toys.

Most children with autism also prefer to play alone without engaging in any sharing or turn-taking activities. Some children, however, would like to play with other children but have little idea how to go about initiating play.

Children with autism have difficulty moving beyond parallel play, without assistance, to develop skills such as:

- sharing toys and play space;
- waiting;
- taking turns;
- using toys and other objects in a functional way; and
- making transitions between activities and play settings.

According to Beyer & Gammeltoft (2000, p 48) the pattern of play in children with autism:

> ... is often described as being mechanical, lacking the natural tendency to explore, with individual activities seeming isolated from any context. Pretend play is rare and when it does occur, it is usually dominated by certain themes, associated with either special interests or specific TV programs that the child is preoccupied with and imitates.

Jarrold, Boucher & Smith (1996) suggested that children with autism are better able to engage in a form of imaginative play if the play is highly structured and prompts (such as visual supports) are included because most of the problems lie in the children's inability to generate spontaneous, pretend play. Most of their play is repetitive, rote-learned and copied from either a video or a sequence that has been taught. A child with autism may act out certain scenes from a favourite video, thus appearing to engage in pretend play, but the same scene is repeated over and over and lacks imagination or originality. According to Harris (1993), children with autism may be prompted into producing genuine make-believe or pretend play by learning certain play sequences, but they continue to have difficulty spontaneously generating and developing their own pretend scenarios or sequences.

Children with autism also have limited experience engaging in either simple manipulation or relational play. They are unable to move on to more complex play actions, such as functional or social play because of a lack of curiosity and interest in exploring. Children with autism tend to engage in stereotyped, repetitive behaviours with certain objects, so there is little interest in playing and interacting socially. They recommend teaching simple manipulative and relational play skills to children with autism. They also suggest that children should be constantly stimulated in their daily lives in a number of different settings to ensure that they are able to generalise any newly acquired play skills.

Unlike most other children who spontaneously and incidentally develop sophisticated and interactive play skills, children with autism have to be taught how to play. By using children's interests and taking into account their individual learning strengths and personal sensory issues, it is possible to engage them in social interactions and work towards developing more advanced communication skills. For young children, play is the most appropriate and effective medium to teach the basic communication and social relating skills that they need to learn. Play does not come naturally to these children and, like so many other skills, has to be taught in a structured and intensive way. Children initially need to be taught how to play in one-to-one sessions with an adult and then encouraged to participate in social play sessions with their peers. During these sessions, children are encouraged to practise their play, communication and social relating skills.

Why teach play?

Play-based intervention is important because it recognises that young children use play to explore their environment, to develop their gross and fine motor skills, to imitate actions, sounds and words, to interact with others through sharing and taking turns with toys, and to manipulate objects. The intervention provides opportunities for children to learn these skills in fun and natural ways that are age-appropriate and across a number of different settings. Play based interventions are extremely important for children with autism because: 'play is a natural activity in which verbal and non-verbal communication, cognitive abilities, and social skills can be taught, practiced and extended' and 'play provides a natural environmental context in which children can learn social and communication skills and how they can have an effect on other people'. (Dodd, Pierce & Webster 2002, p 11).

Structured play-based intervention provides opportunities to learn and practise new skills and enable young children with opportunities to engage in two-way interactions with familiar adults and peers.

Most importantly, however, play-based interventions, if properly structured, well-planned and targeted at appropriate age levels, can show children that playing together with someone else is FUN! Much more fun than playing alone.

Play is important because it is stimulating and challenging for young children and it is the medium through which they learn the skills necessary for their successful inclusion in less restrictive settings such as preschool and school.

Play-based intervention has its foundations in the work of Piaget (1954, 1962, 1969), and has been found to be effective by other researchers including Beyer & Gammeltoft (2000), Linder (1993), Fischer (1980), Vygotsky (1967), Erikson (1950) and Parten (1932).

There is little research available in the area of play-based intervention for children with autism and Wolfberg (1999) wrote that play, especially social play, had played a relatively small part in the education and treatment of children with autism. She failed to find, in her review of current literature, any comprehensive play-based interventions that followed the recognised practices and knowledge of how play occurs and develops in children with autism.

Sherratt (1999) also found little evidence to suggest that teaching children with autism to play was a priority in either the literature or practice. According to Sherratt, the development of symbolic pretend play has much to offer in the remediation of the core difficulties of social relating and communication among children with autism. Symbolic pretend play provides a positive environment for the manipulation of symbolic representations, it also allows children to develop flexibility of thought and offers them opportunities to engage with others in mutually satisfying social play activities.

Teaching spontaneous play skills to children with autism, or even improving existing play skills is not an easy job — if it was easy, it would not be recognised as a core deficit of autism. It is only in the past few years, however, that recognition of the importance of play in the over-all development of children with autism has begun to be accepted more widely.

Despite the difficulties in organising play sessions, teaching play in a structured way, with an emphasis on developing functional and social play skills, can and should be part of any comprehensive educational program for children with autism. One of the most important out-comes from the introduction of structured play sessions for children with autism is that play is so effective in showing children how to enjoy themselves and have fun, especially socially with their peers. Once children know how to play, they are more likely to be asked by their peers to join in play activities and interact socially. Once children begin to interact socially, they also begin to see the benefits of communication and so develop a desire to want to communicate with peers. Play-based interventions encourage children with autism to develop and use their communication and social skills.

How do you teach play skills to children with autism?

A number of important objectives should be considered when designing structured programs to teach play to young children with autism. These objectives should include a focus on:

- ensuring that the child with autism is able to accept partners in play activities and is encouraged to enjoy, rather than just tolerate, the participation of other children in the activities;
- ensuring that the child with autism learns the skills necessary to initiate interaction with others and also the skills necessary to respond to initiations from other children;
- ensuring that the child with autism enjoys the play experience so that the motivation to continue to play develops;
- ensuring that the child with autism learns to play with a range of play materials and is able to use toys functionally;
- ensuring that the child with autism learns to share and take turns with others in play;
- ensuring that the child with autism learns to imitate actions and sounds and eventually words;
- ensuring that the child with autism is able to make choices between objects in play; and
- ensuring that the child with autism can cope with moving on from one activity to another (transitions).

It is important for practitioners to understand that rather than attempting to teach a number of skills through play, it is the play itself that initially has to be taught to children with autism. Once children have been taught how to play with a range of different toys and activities, then play is used as the medium to encourage and teach children with autism how to communicate and interact more effectively

Before developing and implementing a structured play program, children should complete an initial play assessment. A play assessment includes observing children in a structured play situation with an adult and also observing children during free play activities. It may be beneficial to video a child during play. The results of the play assessment help to determine what skills to teach each individual child. The assessment also provides information about each child's play strengths and interests.

A play assessment helps determine at what stage of play development each child is functioning. Children at each stage of play development will require a slightly different approach to intervention. The aim of play-based intervention is to encourage and expand children's interest in playing with a range of different play materials, to develop their play skills, and to motivate them to want to play socially with other children. It is essential to encourage the development of social play, in order to encourage children to want to interact with and communicate with other children and adults. It is through play that children with autism develop the desire to communicate and socialise with others.

There are a number of play assessments available commercially that may be used with young children with autism. A play assessment includes the following sections:
- free play;
- structured play; and
- a play checklist.

Free play session
Provide a range of play materials that includes:
- action-response toys, such as pop-up toys, musical shape sorters, Jack-in-the-Box, spinning top, push button toys;
- sensory toys, such as bubbles, water play, shaving cream, cellophane strips, paint, playdough;
- functional toys, such as cars, blocks, crayons, sorting and matching activities, puzzles;
- gross motor activities, such as balls, slide, mini trampoline; and
- pretend play toys, such as dolls, tea set, car mat, farm animals, dress-up clothes, cooking utensils.

A choice of these materials should be set out for the child in a play area with an adult observing but not leading the play. The adult may join in but only if the child initiates the interaction.

During the play session, the child's behaviour is closely observed with particular attention to what the child chooses to play with, how he/she plays with the different materials and any attempt by the child to engage the adult in social interaction.

Structured play session
After a period of free play, the adult may take the initiative and introduce some structure into the play session. During this period, a number of short play sequences may be introduced that incorporate some of the play materials listed above. For example, the adult may try to engage the child in blowing bubbles, playing with water, completing a puzzle or pushing a car along the road. Visual supports may be introduced into the play activities to assist children to understand what is expected.

During this session, attention should be given to the questions in a play checklist.

Play checklist
A play checklist should include the following questions:
- Is the child's play self-directed?
- Does the child find adult interference in his or her choice of activity distressing?
- Does the child look towards an object held by the adult?
- Does the child tend to use toys to engage in self-stimulation?
- Does the child prefer to play exclusively with one particular toy?
- Does the child prefer to play alone?

- Is the child happy to play alongside other children or adults?
- Does the child show an interest in a range of toys or activities?
- Does the child use toys and equipment in a number of different ways?
- Does the child play mostly on his or her own terms?
- Does the child have skills in sharing toys and activities?
- Does the child cope with a change of activities?
- Does the child interact with an adult in a play situation?
- Does the child take turns with an adult using favoured toys?
- Does the child attempt to imitate the actions and sounds of an adult?
- Does the child have difficulty finishing activities?
- Does the child have difficulty moving from one activity to another?
- Does the child make choices between two different objects or activities?

What play resources should be included in play sessions?

Once children with autism have completed a play assessment to determine their interests and their existing skills, the next step is to determine what toys and activities to introduce into play sessions. Each child will have their own preferences and these preferences should initially be included in individual play sessions. The key to the development of a successful play program is to take into account each child's likes and dislikes and to recognise any existing play skills.

Play resources should include activities that are reinforcing. If the sessions are fun and motivating, the child will enjoy the play experience and want to come back the next day to play again. Toys and activities that are part of a child's obsessions such as cars, trains, numbers or letters should initially be included.

> Andy is obsessed with Thomas the Tank Engine. He has all of the engines and spends hours lining them up. To encourage Andy to extend his play interests, he was given a train track and encouraged to put this together using a visual template. Other trains were also included and then blocks to build a bridge over the tracks. Eventually cars and toy people were added and Andy was shown how to incorporate other objects into his play routine by modelling different ways of playing with trains.

Play resources should include a combination of both open-ended and more structured materials. Open-ended activities, such as water play, sand play, bubbles, blocks, and cause and effect toys, have no real start or finish. They allow children to play for as long as they like and then walk away without having to complete an activity. These toys are highly motivating and are excellent for those children who have poor attending skills and do not tolerate others trying to share or take turns.

Structured materials have a beginning, purpose and end and include toys such as puzzles, books, threading and sorting activities. They provide structure to play sessions and take the emphasis away from playing on children's terms. Structured play encourages children to explore and gradually extend their use of different play materials.

All toys and activities chosen for play sessions should be age appropriate and functional. They should be colourful, recognisable and easy to handle. Toys should, ideally, have more than one use so that they can be played with in a number of different ways. Blocks are used to build towers, to practise turn-taking and fine motor skills; they are used to build roads and bridges to drive cars along; and they are used to sort and match colours and shapes and to teach sequences (see Figure 15.1).

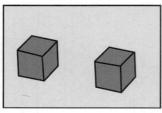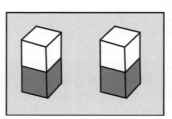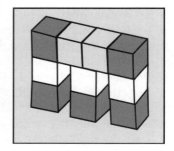

Figure 15.1 *Blocks are versatile toys*

Toys should also be chosen to encourage skills such as waiting, sharing, turn-taking, imitating and following routines. Play sessions may also include dolls, tea sets, dolls' houses, farm animals and dress-up clothes to encourage pretend play and to teach daily routines.

Quill (2000, p 87) recommended a number of play activities for children with autism including:

- exploratory toys and activities including cause-and-effect toys, water, sand, rice, bubbles;
- physical toys and activities including obstacle courses, trampoline, bikes, balls;
- manipulative toys including Duplo, puzzles;
- constructive toys including blocks, road and train tracks;
- art and craft including crayons, paint, playdough;
- books and computer games;
- music activities including music cassettes that encourage dancing and singing, musical instruments;
- socio-dramatic play including doll play, dress-ups, farm animals;
- board games and card games; and
- social activities including ballgames, peek-a-boo, hide-and-seek.

Beyer & Gammeltoft (2000, p 58) claim that there is a connection between cognitive, social and emotional developmental aspects of play and they outline a number of crucial play strategies to work on. They feel that play activities should focus on developing:

- attention, expectation and shared focus;
- imitation and mirroring;
- parallel play and play dialogue;
- script and social stories;
- shifts in taking turns; and
- games and rules in play.

They also state (p 58) that 'setting the stage and visualization can further develop the child's social and instrumental competencies'.

How are structured play sessions set up?

There is a need for structure and careful programming for children with autism. Attention should be given to providing appropriate child-initiated and child-directed activities. It is important to understand the individual differences among children with autism and to take these into account when designing intervention strategies for them. Strategies should be adapted for each child and modified whenever the particular needs of a child require it. Teaching children with autism how to play should therefore be carefully planned and constantly monitored and evaluated.

According to current research, children with autism tend to have difficulty attending to multiple stimuli and respond best to structure and consistency. The skills necessary to promote social and communication abilities should be taught in organised play sessions, with one skill targeted at a time and gradually building on simple activities by adding more complex steps. It is also recommended that play activities are sequenced and that visual strategies are used extensively to support the play.

Many successful social and communication programs have focused on increasing adult and peer interaction through play. Very young children are usually motivated to engage in social interactions with their parents and other familiar adults, and as they grow older they become increasingly competent in their communication skills, both speech and comprehension. Studies of the behaviour of children with autism, however, describe very limited social relating to their parents in terms of initiating interactions through joint sharing of attention. They rarely point to an object, hold an object up for the parents to observe, or bring an object to them. They also rarely share emotion. This joint sharing of attention between young children and their parents is critical for the development of social and communication skills. The ability to share information with another person non-verbally is an important pre-requisite for the development of verbal communication skills and the development of pretend and imaginative play. For many children with autism, the move beyond parallel play is difficult without assistance to develop basic skills such as the sharing of equipment and play space, waiting, taking turns and functional use of play materials. It is important to encourage children with autism to use play materials in a variety of ways, to share and take turns in play and also to begin to relate to peers and siblings during play either verbally or non-verbally.

The ability to play co-operatively with others and to take on alternative roles from everyday life, like pretending to be Mummy or Daddy, is reliant on the ability to take the perspective of others and an appreciation that the thoughts and feelings of others may be different from your own. Similarly, the development of symbolic play is dependent on an ability to understand that one object may be used to represent another — a child may pretend that the banana is a telephone or the spoon is an aeroplane.

The opportunity to observe and interact with others is a basic pre-requisite for the development of reciprocal social interaction and functional communication. Structured play sessions offer a natural situation in which communicative skills, cognitive abilities and social skills can be acquired, practised and extended. Before play sessions can be introduced, some children have to accept or tolerate other people in their immediate environment. They also have to be happy to engage in reciprocal interactions with a familiar adult. As acceptance of adult interaction and intervention increases, children's preference for solitary play begins to decrease.

The *Early Play Program* (Dodd, Pierce & Webster 2001) outlines strategies to organise and implement play sessions with children on a regular basis. The Program suggests three stages of play development.

In *Stage One* of the program, the aim is to increase children's awareness and interest in how they can use and explore a range of different play materials. During this stage, play is very much on the child's terms and all activities are open-ended. The aim is to encourage children to tolerate another person playing alongside and to encourage children to imitate someone else's actions. Among the open-ended activities recommended at this stage are action response toys, pop-up toys, music and craft activities, as well as lots of sensory materials such as water play, sand play, bubbles, and playdough.

Children learn to attend to and become aware of an adult playing alongside. They learn to accept and tolerate an adult following their lead in open-ended play activities. Children also to begin to see the advantages of social interaction with a familiar adult and they begin to realise that playing socially with an adult can be fun.

In *Stage Two* of the program, the aim is to gradually make play more structured and interactive. Children are encouraged to explore and extend their use of play materials. The aim is to extend children's play skills so that they are able to attend to a familiar adult's actions.

Children learn to imitate simple actions and sounds and begin taking turns with an adult in play. They initiate and respond to simple social interactions. As a prelude to coping with change and transition, children are introduced to the concept of 'finish' and to visual supports in play.

In *Stage Three*, play sessions are extended and children are encouraged to play with a range of toys and activities and to play in different ways.

Among the recommended activities to encourage social and pretend play are dolls, tea sets, train tracks, craft activities, gross motor games, puzzles, drawing and dressing up clothes.

The aims of play sessions are to develop an understanding and acceptance of the concepts of 'finish', 'pack away' and 'wait'. Children learn to make choices in play, to transition between activities, people and different settings and to develop turn-taking with peers. They also learn to follow simple comments and directions and to develop their structured play and pretend play skills.

Once these skills have been mastered in a one-to-one situation, they should then be generalised to other natural settings and to other people. Children should be taught skills and given opportunities to practise skills in one-to-one sessions with an adult and then be encouraged to participate in small group activities and finally enrolled in large group activities.

Before exposing children to small or large groups of peers, they should be taught rudimentary social play skills such as waiting, sharing, taking turns and imitating actions and sounds during their one-to-one structured interventions.

How are visual supports incorporated into play activities?

Using visual supports 'mirrors the learning style strengths of children with autism' (Quill 1997, p 699). The use of visual supports provides a bridge towards verbal language acquisition (Bondy & Frost 1994; Schwartz et al 1998). Visual supports assist with transitions, increase children's independence and decrease their frustration during social play (Dettmer et al 2000). The introduction of visual supports in play sessions simplifies activities and therefore increases the likelihood of success.

Visual supports should be introduced gradually and should be pitched at a level the individual understands (see Chapter 12 for information on the hierarchy of visual supports). A child in Stage 1 of the Play Program may be shown an actual toy as an encouragement to 'come and play', while a child in Stage 2 of the program may be introduced to visually augmented toys and encouraged to explore different ways of playing with toys.

Children in Stage 3 of the Play Program may be introduced to visual supports to make choices, take turns, follow simple sequences, engage in simple pretend play and introduce concepts such as matching and sorting. The supports would include a combination of real objects, remnants of packaging, photographs and line drawings.

Visual supports may be introduced to children with autism at an early age. Initially this may include visually augmenting toys and other play activities to make it easier for children to understand what is happening and what is expected of them. Visually augmented toys are used to teach children how to play. Visually augmented toys may include simple car mats, farm templates, block sequence cards and visually augmented songs.

Photographs of favourite toys can be used to develop choice boards and teach play sequences.

What play programs are available?

A number of specifically developed programs teach children with autism, and the people who work with them, how to set up and implement structured play sessions. Among the most popular and widely recognised are the following, which are also discussed further in Appendix 4.

The Early Play Program (2nd Ed) (Dodd, Pierce & Webster 2001)

This program is designed for parents of young children with autism or related language and developmental disorders to help them implement play intervention at home.

The Program offers a step-by-step guide for parents and professionals to teach children social play skills and offers practical suggestions about choices of toys and activities. The guide also provides information about autism, the thinking and learning styles of children with autism, sensory sensitivities, an initial play assessment and how to introduce visual supports.

Hanen Program 'More than Words'

This program trains parents to interact and communicate functionally using opportunities that occur naturally throughout the day. The program is designed for children 0–6 years.

The emphasis is not only on the kinds of difficulties children may have with communication, but also on strategies that can be used to help children. It is written for parents, and teaches them to turn their child's everyday routines and activities into opportunities for communication learning.

In the book, the first two chapters look at what communication is and how it is so much 'more than words'. The remaining chapters offer ideas and suggestions for all stages of communication development.

NAS (London) Early Bird Program

The Program began in 1997 as a pilot project. It has since developed a short-term, focused model of early intervention for families of preschool children with autism, based on a three-month parent program. The program aims to provide parents with effective practical strategies that help them to understand and manage the effects of autism on their child's developing communication and behaviour.

The Early Bird Program works with a group of six families at a time. The program consists of three strands, each of which underpins the others and helps parents to maximise their child's development. Parents learn to understand their child's autism: to appreciate how people with autism experience the world and how the underlying triad of social deficits influences development, thinking and learning. Next, parents learn about communication and how best to build interaction and social communication with their child. Finally, parents are helped to analyse their child's behaviour by examining the underlying triggers and the possible functions of inappropriate behaviours.

TEACCH

North Carolina's program for the Treatment and Education of Autistic and related Communication handicapped Children (TEACCH) is a state-wide, community-based program that includes direct services, consultation, research and professional training. The approach involves a focus on the individual and an understanding of the person's skills, interests and needs. For young children, the primary goal of TEACCH is to help parents work with their children to improve learning, communication and social skills while managing behaviour. This is done by cultivating the strengths and interests of the child and by providing a structured approach to teaching.

The main goal of the TEACCHing Together Group for 2-year-olds is to provide a learning environment adapted to the special needs of young children with autism and related communication disorders.

For detailed information about how to access these programs see Appendix 4.

Summary

Play is a complex skill that impacts greatly on how well children develop many of the skills they require to function socially and communicatively throughout their whole lives. Most play skills are learned incidentally because children are curious, they enjoy socialising and need to be constantly stimulated. Children with autism, however are not naturally curious about their environment, they do not socialise very well and they are usually stimulated in restricted and repetitive ways.

Play is defined as a natural activity that fosters the development of cognitive skills, positive social and emotional behaviours, verbal and non-verbal communication and motor proficiency.

Young children normally move through a number of the stages of play development in order to achieve social and pretend play. These stages include solitary play, parallel play, associative play and cooperative play as outlined many years ago by Parten (1932). Later researchers have refined and modified her findings but the basic concept remains the same. As children develop more complex play behaviours, such as pretend or imaginative play, their play also becomes more social.

While the child with autism is not generally perceived as a child with age-appropriate play skills, it has been shown that children with autism are not totally impaired in play. However, their play differs in both quality and form from their peers and they have major difficulties engaging in any social play activities.

Children with autism need to be taught how to play socially and this is best done through structured play sessions. Unlike most other children who, over time, develop sophisticated and interactive play skills without formal training, children with autism have to be taught how to play. Children with autism have difficulty moving beyond parallel play to develop the skills they need for future communication and social skills acquisition. Play-based interventions provide opportunities for children to learn these skills in natural and fun ways that are age appropriate and also generalised across different settings.

Detailed play assessments should be completed for each child prior to developing and implementing any structured play programs. The assessment helps determine what skills children have, what skills they need to learn and also provides information about each child's play interests so that these may be incorporated into their individual play program.

When developing and implementing structured play interventions, it is important to consider what play resources are most appropriate for each child, and what the interventions are aiming to achieve. It is also essential to plan beforehand and to be well prepared during individual play sessions. Finding out about popular play programs that have been developed for children with autism can provide information about what works and what activities are most effective.

Children with autism are visual learners, so these strategies should be incorporated into children's play sessions.

16

Programming for Change

As children grow up they are expected to become increasingly independent and free from the influence of others while at the same time taking responsibility for their own conduct and obligations. They learn to be flexible, to make decisions, to react to numerous and ever-changing stimuli in socially appropriate ways.

Quill 1995, p 243

In children and adults with autism, the foundation for learning independence and self-responsibility is impaired.

Children and adults with autism are rigid in their way of thinking, have difficulty processing verbal information and do not cope with things that are new and unpredictable. They thrive on routine and prefer to interact with familiar people and objects in a stable, predictable environment. It appears that changes to routine and transitions of any description are unknown, uncontrollable and often frightening events that cause great confusion and anxiety. It is therefore easy to understand why children and adults with autism tend to become distressed and fearful when changes occur without warning.

To understand why change of any sort is a major issue for people with autism, one has to understand the complexities of the disorder. Disordered communication, including speech, comprehension, use of body language, facial expression, tone of voice and gestures make it extremely difficult to be understood by others or to express feelings, likes or dislikes. Disordered social relating abilities make it difficult to mix socially with others. Individuals with autism have difficulty understanding the needs and feelings of others and appear unresponsive and unable to engage in socially accepted behaviours. They have limited ability to read their environment, to understand what is happening and why it is happening. They have limited interests and most behaviour is rigid and repetitive. These deficits serve to make the world appear a scary place where there is no consistency and few rules and routines. Most individuals with autism spend their lives seeking some form of consistency, structure and routine in order to make sense of the world around them.

When addressing the problems encountered by individuals with autism around the concepts of change and transition, a number of common issues appear over and over again. These include:

- difficulties understanding and managing transition;
- insistence on sameness;
- need for routines; and
- benefits of planning for change.

According to Koegel, Egel & Dunlap (1980), people with autism have problems with stimulus overselectivity so that the slightest change to routine may make a situation appear different to them. While most children are able to adapt to minor changes and can be directed verbally, individuals with autism may be so strongly influenced by environmental stimuli that a whole chain of behaviours may be modified by one changed variable. They then lose sight of the original routine and feel totally lost and confused. Autism, therefore, includes a severe deficit in the ability to accept changes to the environment or to process the information coming in from the environment. A person may have difficulty processing new information and may prefer that everything remains constant and unchanged. This insistence on sameness or perseverative behaviour can cause individuals to become very stressed at even minor changes to a familiar routine or activity.

A child, for example, may insist on drinking from the same cup that is filled with a particular drink to a certain level; may eat the same food at every meal; wear the same clothing; and follow a certain route whenever they leave the house. An adult may insist on completing tasks in a certain order; have to sit in the same chair; or wear only clothing that is blue. This insistence on sameness may be an attempt to create order in a changing world because of an inability to read the environment or to pick up clues to help predict what will happen next.

After living in the same house for ten years, Scott's parents are moving to another city. Scott has been distressed ever since the real estate sign was put in the front yard. Even though he cannot read the sign, he realises that things are changing. The furniture has been moved around and many household items are being packed into boxes. Scott keeps putting things back into their regular places and unpacking the boxes. He is distressed because he does not understand what is happening.

People with autism respond to change in different ways: some become silent and withdrawn and others become aggressive. The aggression may be self-directed, such as biting or hitting themselves, or throwing tantrums and lashing out at people or objects.

Individuals with autism also have difficulty coping with transitions and appear unable to move from one activity or area to the next. This relates back to the inability to cope with change and the preference for things to remain the same.

Why is there a need for sameness and routine?

'Children with autism will learn more easily, express more interest and have fewer behaviour problems if there is predictability to their daily and weekly routines' (Olley 1987, p 414).

Even thirty years ago, there was recognition that routines were important for people with autism because they provided predictability and structure to both children and adults who had few skills and little ability to understand and cope with environmental changes.

A routine may be defined as a sequence of actions completed in a regular way or a series of actions completed regularly. When routines are established they foster a feeling of independence and security. These feelings of security lead to a decrease in stress and anxiety as well as a decrease in challenging behaviours. Individuals eventually become more willing to cope with minor change as their self-confidence improves, their learning increases and they tend to spend less time engaged in repetitive behaviours and narrow interests.

Both adults and children who are rigid in their way of thinking need established routines to help them to understand and cope with their environment. They will often build and maintain elaborate routines to provide a feeling of comfort, consistency and order. When things happen in a consistent and regular order the individual feels more confident and in control.

> Over the years, Ryan has introduced a number of rituals and routines into his home that he still religiously follows. When he gets up in the morning he has to be the first person to sit at the table. He has to have his breakfast before he gets dressed and he has to have two pieces of toast, cut into four triangles and spread with honey. He also has a glass of apple juice in his blue cup and only filled to the top of the green stripe.

While many of the rituals and routines may appear odd or bizarre, they serve a purpose. Rituals and routines should only be modified if they interfere with learning, take over the person's life or if they become offensive to others. Sometimes routines become so important that they are hard to break or change. Any attempts to modify them are likely to be met with fierce resistance.

How can routines be modified?

As mentioned in previous chapters, most individuals with autism respond to consistency, structure and visual rules; so the establishment of routines and use of visual supports may be considered as important learning tools in the home, classroom and the general community. However, once routines are in place, they are not easily modified because of this preference for order and consistency. Most people with autism learn rules and establish routines and are comfortable with these. If the routines are changed and the rules are broken, then order no longer prevails and most individuals lose their ability to cope.

Intervention programs aimed at modifying established routines and assisting individuals to cope with change, should take into consideration the specific learning and thinking styles of children and adults with autism. Individuals should not be expected to adapt their ways of learning to fit in with regular teaching approaches. Routines should be presented visually, in a format that is easily understood by the user. Visual routines and sequences can easily be modified to reflect any changes that occur, either expectedly or unexpectedly, so that any distress or anxiety for the user is minimised. Visual supports reflecting change are more easily understood than verbal explanations. They give the person with autism time to process the information they contain because they are non-transient.

Before attempting to change rigid routines, a review of individuals' stress levels should be completed and ways of minimising stress considered as an important part of any program for change. Stress and anxiety about change can be minimised among people with autism. This happens by planning ahead of time for any anticipated changes to regular routines and ensuring that individuals are well informed through the use of visual supports and schedules.

Children and adults are encouraged to become more flexible and spontaneous within their regular home, school and work environments by gradually introducing small changes to routines within these supportive environments. By introducing strategies such as social stories to teach specific concepts, individuals begin to understand that change may not always be a bad thing — some changes are good. For more detailed information about developing and implementing social stories, see Chapter 5.

Change should not be avoided, but rather recognised as a regular part of life. People with autism have to learn to cope with life and the changes that occur within their different environments. However, they need to learn to cope, initially at least, in a supportive environment. The fact that routines and schedules vary from setting to setting and from person to person has to be specifically taught just as, initially, each change to a regular routine has to be recognised and planned for.

Change is an inevitable part of life. For people with autism, adjusting to change is chall-enging. They have difficulties processing information, especially information that is new, not highly relevant to their interests, and unpredictable. They prefer things to remain the same and to be able to interact with people and objects in a stable, predictable environment. For them, changes and transitions are unknown, uncontrollable events that happen, often without adequate warning and little preparation.

What are the problems with transitions and how are they managed?

Transitions are the passing from one condition, stage, activity or place to another. By making transitions predictable, we are able to help people with autism to understand their environments and realise that they do have some control over their lives.

Transitions of different sorts occur throughout life and can create enormous problems for people who do not cope well with change and who depend on routines, rules and structure to make sense of life and the environments in which they live. Transitions vary from the simple change from one activity or task to another, to more complex transitions that occur when individuals have to change from home to school and from school into adult services.

There are a number of techniques that can be used to make transitions more predictable and understandable at home, school, work and in the general community.

The first step to managing transitions is to simplify the transition process and provide a warning before they occur. This allows the person time to prepare for the change. In a group setting, it is important not to rely on giving a group warning, as the person with autism may not comprehend general instructions. People with autism should be given individual instructions, in a format that they understand, such as a visual support. Even for higher functioning individuals, verbal instructions should be accompanied by visual cues. Visual cues assist people to understand changes to rules, routines and transitions and provide them with effective means of understanding the situations where changes occur.

For young children who may be unable to transition from one activity to another without becoming distressed, a visual timer may help them to see when one activity ends and another is due to begin. If a timer is used, it is important to ensure that the transition occurs at the expected time. A visual sequence showing the change from one activity to another should accompany the use of the timer.

At school, Sophie's teacher tries to prepare her for transition from one activity to another by showing her a visual sequence, and giving her a warning that it is nearly time to finish what she is doing and pack away. Sophie knows that she has time to finish her activity while the sequence shows her what will happen next.

A finish box to 'post' the completed activity into may also assist children to understand the concept of finishing one activity before they transition onto another. A modified version of a 'finish box' can be used with adults in the workplace as they move from one task to another (see Figure 16.1).

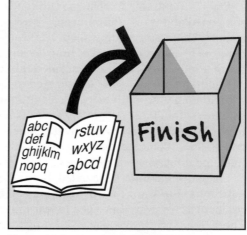

Figure 16.1 *Example of a finish box*

Daily and weekly schedules also provide information about different activities and events that will be happening. Visual timetables and schedules help to make transitions predictable for children and adults.

Timetables may include pictures of routine events as well as the times these events will occur (see Figure 16.2). Timetables can be modified to reflect changes to normal routines but still provide the necessary information to assist with the transition process.

Mon	Tues	Wed	Thurs	Fri	Sat	Sun
work	work	work	work	cook lunch	home	home
work	library	work	shopping	swimming		

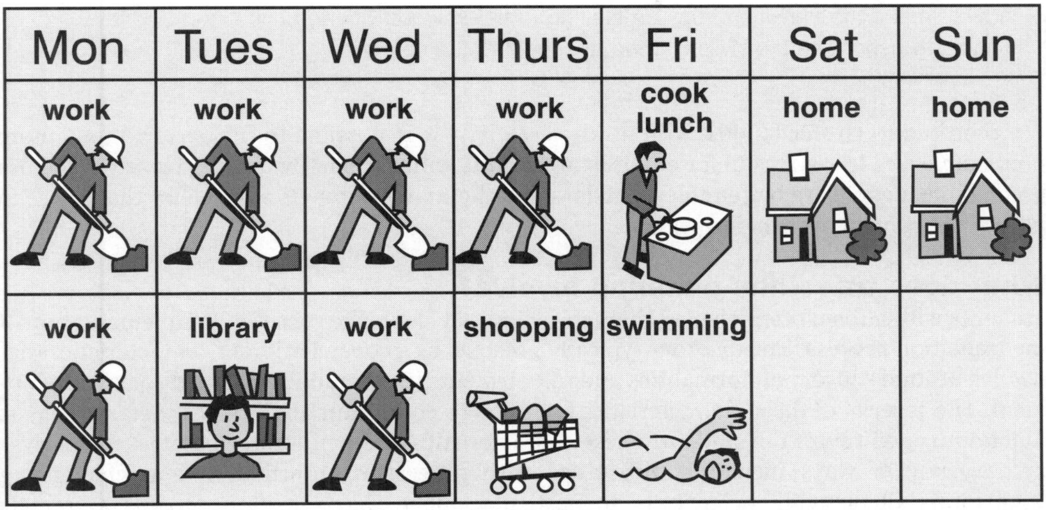

Figure 16.2 *Example of a visual timetable*

Since changes are seen as uncontrollable events in the lives of children and adults with autism, it is a good idea, if possible, to show people that they can have some control over their environments. Allow the person with autism to make choices about transitions. For example, if the timetable indicates that on Thursday morning the usual activity is math followed by reading, the child may be allowed to choose which book to read or where to sit in the classroom during the reading lesson. This will encourage a positive transition from math to reading.

Transitions between different environments may be simplified and seen as positive experiences when there is consistency and communication between the different settings. For example a home/school diary provides information between the home and the school and helps to ensure consistency of ideas, teaching approaches and responses. The diary enables both parents and teachers to know what is happening in the different settings. For example, if the class visited a local museum or library, it is helpful if the parents know so that they can talk with their child about the visit when the child arrives home. Any rules in place at home may be reinforced at school if the teacher is aware of what they are. This helps to minimise confusion and leads to consistent management and assists transition between the different settings.

It is also important that children and adults with autism learn to generalise information across situations in order to make the transition process appear more controllable and predictable. The ability to generalise skills is very limited among individuals with autism and skills learned in one setting are not easily transferred to other environments. New skills should be taught in situ; that is, in all of the different situations that they are most likely to occur. Just because a skill is taught at school, or in the workplace, it should not be assumed that that skill will automatically be transferred to the home or into the general community. The same skill may also have to be taught initially in those other settings as well. The skills needed to cope well with transitions should be taught and practised in a number of different settings, in situations where the transitions occur. If a child has difficulty transitioning from one activity to another, for example, then that skill needs to be practised at home, at school and in the community.

> Julie loves ice-skating and goes skating with her class every Friday afternoon. She gets very excited and has fun on the ice but refuses to stop skating and get changed when it is time to go home. She screams and tantrums and gets really distressed. At school Julie has learned to transition from one activity to another quite successfully. She has to be taught how to make the transition from ice-skating to the next activity at the ice rink. She is unable to generalise the skills learned at school to the new setting.

According to Grofer (1996), with a little creativity it is possible to make transitions more predictable and less stressful for children and adults with autism. By making transitions more predictable, people are better able to understand their environments and realise that they can have some control over their own lives.

What does transition planning involve?

Students with autism often display characteristics that challenge successful implementation of the transition process. The disorder typically presents as a constellation of characteristics that revolve around sensory abnormalities and impairments in communication and social development. The severity of these characteristics falls along a continuum that roughly determines the functioning abilities of the student. These characteristics and limitations manifest themselves in a variety of ways including difficulties with processing information and challenging behaviours. Challenging behaviours in particular make the transition process extremely difficult and often unsuccessful for some students. Although students with autism have many characteristics in common, they all have unique needs that must be evaluated to determine the best course of action. While there are a number of general strategies to assist transition for both children and adults with autism, it is important to remember that each person is unique. Each person has different strengths and needs that they bring to the transition planning process. Transition planning processes must therefore be individualised to meet these unique needs and ensure that each person is able to successfully make a transition from one activity, event or condition to another.

There are some simple guidelines to follow to plan for successful transitions between activities, classes, schools or even different work programs.

Children should be introduced to supports at an early age to assist them to transition from one activity to another. Strategies include visual timetables and sequences, finish boxes, providing information, planning ahead for change and providing choices. The supports should remain available throughout life, in one format or another, whenever they are needed by an individual to assist them to transition from one activity to another. These supports are useful for the small, everyday transitions that occur. It is also important to recognise those times in life when major transitions occur that impact on the general lifestyle and living arrangements of the person with autism. Among specific changes that occur throughout life for everyone are the transitions that occur from one program to another. The most obvious of these transitions include starting school, changing classes, changing from primary to high school, leaving school to join the workforce, work programs, friendships and family changes, and eventually moving into retirement. These major life changes require careful planning if they are to be achieved with the minimum of stress.

Begin to prepare for transition in advance. Try to meet relevant people in the new setting and identify key personnel who will have primary responsibility for the student.

Organise visits to the new setting prior to placement and locate bathrooms, classroom, lockers, offices and playground areas. Organise for the student to meet new teachers.

Encourage the student to walk through the new setting several times before starting. Take photographs of the school, the new teachers, the classroom, the playground and any other relevant areas. Make a photo album that the student can refer back to over the holidays or prior to starting.

Once the new teacher is identified, organise a case conference or team meeting to provide the teacher with information about the student including their current level of functioning. A meeting also gives the teacher an opportunity to provide input into the new goals and objectives.

If possible, include the person with autism in the transition planning process.

Develop a written plan to assist in facilitating the transition. This should be a summary of decisions made at the planning meeting and outline the responsibilities of each person involved in the transition process. Responsibilities and timelines for each person involved in the process should be clearly stated in the written plan.

A package of information about the student should be provided to relevant people in the new setting and should include:

- personal information about the student including their likes and dislikes, motivators, strengths and weaknesses;
- information about the student's current communication system including examples of visual supports that are being used;
- information about the student's disability and general teaching strategies for students with autism;
- information about any modifications and adaptations to the new environment that may be necessary before the student can start;
- information about any positive behaviour supports already being implemented that can be transitioned to the new setting; and
- suggestions on how to maintain lines of communication between the home and the new setting.

Organise for the new teacher to observe the student in the current setting or provide a videotape of the student. Arrange for some consultation support from an autism specialist to assist with the transition process.

Prepare material for the other students in the class to assist them to understand the person with autism. Encourage other students to ask questions and learn how they can help and support the student with autism. If other students are aware and involved in the transition process, they will form the basis of a social support group, in the classroom and the playground. One way of introducing the student with autism to new classmates before starting the program is through a book that is created about the student. The book may include information about the student, including likes and dislikes. The book should emphasise the similarities with peers, with autism being just one of many attributes.

It is especially important that the teacher has information about any current strategies in place for the student that are working (or not working) so that these can be carried over to new settings to minimise the student's distress and anxiety.

Often, the first major transition difficulties occur around starting preschool and transitioning from preschool to school. Students also change class every year and they must adjust to changes in staff, schedules, routines, peers, programs, building, teaching approaches and expectations. In order to maximise a person's success, everyone involved needs to work together to facilitate smooth transitions.

How are children prepared for preschool?

One of the first major transition events that face young children with autism is leaving the security of parents and home to face the unknown challenges of preschool. Preschool is important for children with autism because it provides an environment where they can safely learn and practise their communication, social and play skills. Preschool also provides opportunities for children to learn the basic rules and routines that are necessary for their successful transition into the school environment. They also learn that things are no longer completed 'on their own terms'. To facilitate children's transition into preschool, the following suggestions may be helpful:

- Visit the preschool prior to enrolment to meet with staff members to discuss the child's needs. Children should be encouraged to visit their new preschool a few times prior to enrolment to familiarise them with the new setting.
- Take children for a walk/drive past the preschool a few times prior to enrolment to point out their 'new school' so that they become familiar with the route, and will be more aware of where they are going when they first start preschool.
- If permission is given to visit the centre, initially visit during indoor or outdoor play times so that children can see the toys and play equipment and maybe have time to play. Avoid quiet structured times such as rest time or group time, as these periods may be overwhelming for some children. Keep visits short and positive to begin with.
- During the initial visits, staff members should try to make contact with new children to encourage them to join in the play activities and become less dependent on their parent or other familiar adult. Parents may be encouraged to join in the play activities, either with their child or with another child, to demonstrate how to play and how much fun preschool is. If children see their parents are enjoying the activities and are relaxed, then they will feel less threatened and overwhelmed by the new situation.
- Encourage parents to take photos of the preschool, especially areas such as the toilets, outdoor playground, indoor areas and bag storage area, staff members, their child's school bag and some of the most popular toys and activities. Place the pictures in a mini album and encourage parents to look through the photographs together with their child.
- Prepare a package of information about the disorder and about individual children's strengths and needs for staff members and ensure that this information is available prior to enrolment. Encourage staff members to consult with someone from the nearest specialist autism service for advice and support. They may also provide information about specific training workshops, information packages and resources that are available and provide regular consultation and support to the centre.
- Initially, send a favourite toy or 'obsession' to preschool with a child as something familiar to help them feel more comfortable and settled. If a particular centre does not encourage children to bring personal belongings, explain why this may help the child and set limits about what to bring and for how long an item may accompany a child.

Kristy is starting preschool next month and her mother is worried that she will not cope with the program. Kristy has never been separated from her Mum, because she screamed whenever her mother tried to leave her with other family members or friends. Kristy has visited the preschool with her mother and she has a photo album of photographs taken at the centre. When Kristy first starts she will only go to preschool for a few hours per day and, as she becomes more familiar with the routines, the staff will gradually increase her time until she is able to stay a full day. Kristy's mother is happy with that arrangement.

How are children prepared for school?
Preparing young children for school is both an anxious and an exciting time for most parents. For parents who have a child with autism however, the anxieties far outweigh the excitement.

Most parents are proud of the fact that they, and their child, have come so far, but they are also anxious about the next step along the road to independence. School is a place where children no longer do things on their own terms, a place where they must conform to rules, a social place where they must learn to get on with their peers and a place of overwhelming sensory stimuli. No wonder parents feel anxious and afraid. This is one reason why the transition process is so important, for both students and for parents.

Transition is an important aspect of education, with all students being expected to adjust to changes in teachers, classmates, schedules, buildings and routines. These transitions can be extremely difficult and challenging for the student with autism. Both parents and teaching staff need to be aware of potential problems that may arise when children first make the transition from preschool to school. Children with autism can, however, cope with changes to their normal routines if these changes are handled sensitively, if careful planning and preparation occurs and if the individual needs of each child are considered.

Children with autism are rigid in their way of thinking and rely on structure and routine to cope in different situations. It is when unexpected changes to their routines occur that children become anxious and distressed and challenging behaviour occurs. The transition from pre-school to school is a major change for all children, but especially so for children with autism.

The first step in the transition process from preschool to school is for parents to find the most appropriate school setting for their child. If more than one option is available, parents should look carefully at each of the possible options to find the one that will best meet the needs of their child.

Once a school has been selected, both parents and professionals currently working with the child can begin to consult with the staff at the new school to ensure the transition from preschool to school proceeds as smoothly as possible. A number of changes to the classroom and a few additional routines may minimise the stress and anxiety of the children and ensure a successful transition to school.

> Kyle has just started school and seems to be coping very well. His teacher has a large visual timetable on the wall at the front of the class and every morning when the children first arrive she helps them to complete the timetable for the day's activities. All of the children discuss the day's events and so everyone knows what will happen during the day. Sometimes the teacher leaves a small space on the timetable for a surprise activity. Kyle is learning to cope with surprises.

Provide each child with a copy of the classroom routine (in a suitable format), to take home and discuss with parents. Parents can help their child to learn the regular classroom timetable. Where possible, any changes to the regular routines should be provided in advance and presented to the child in an appropriate format. Advance warning gives children information that will assist them to cope with the change. If unexpected events happen, tell children what is happening calmly, in simple, clear language to minimise their anxiety. *The Transition to School Manual* (Brennan, Dodd & Fryer 2002) published by the Autism Association of NSW may be a valuable resource for parents starting their young child at school.

What should parents look for in a school?

Parents should consider their child's placement in school at least six to twelve months before the child is due to start. They should find out what school programs are appropriate for their child and what options are available locally. Parents should then visit each of the prospective schools with a list of questions and a number of expectations. There are a number of things that parents need to consider in both the classroom and the playground. Key issues may include:

- The size of the school and the number of children in each class is important. Children with autism tend to prefer smaller schools with smaller classes that are well structured, less noisy and not cluttered.
- The configuration of the playground is also important as well as the level of teacher supervision. Children with autism tend to have limited awareness of danger; they can also become the victims of bullying; and have trouble understanding social rules. They therefore need to be closely supervised in the playground.
- The philosophy of the school towards children with special needs should be considered. Are all staff members familiar with the needs of children with autism and do the school policies reflect a commitment to the development of each child regardless of their academic ability?
- Has the school been recommended by other parents or by professionals working locally?
- Check the location of the school, its accessibility and the level of security provided.
- Assess the level of remedial support available for each child with a disability. This may include staffing levels, funding support, special equipment and teaching resources.
- Is there availability and commitment to the use of visual supports throughout the school to augment communication and support behaviour?
- Assess the attitude of all staff members, from the Principal through to support staff, to having a child with autism in the school.

These are just some of the issues that parents have to address when they are going through the process of finding the most appropriate educational placement for their child. Parents should check all possible schooling options from a regular placement, with or without additional support, through to support classes and specialised schools.

The Department of Education in each state will provide parents with information about state schooling options, as well as information about the transition process for children with disabilities. There are also guidelines available for parents about choosing a school and the resources available to assist children to transition from preschool into school. It is recommended that parents contact their district/area Department of Education office at least six to nine months before their child is due to start school.

How are children prepared for high school?

According to Janzen (1999), 'researchers and practitioners recognize that although the vast majority of students with Asperger Syndrome have average to above-average intellectual abilities and are included in general education classrooms, they experience academic problems'. It is extremely difficult for students with Asperger's syndrome to integrate into regular classrooms and to follow normal school rules and routines because of 'social and communication deficits combined with obsessive and narrowly defined interests, concrete and literal thinking, inflexibility, poor problem-solving and organisational skills, difficulty in discerning relevant from irrelevant stimuli, and weak social standing.

The move from primary to secondary school is a challenge for all students, but especially for students with autism. There are a number of factors to take into consideration when a child is transitioning from primary school into secondary school. These factors place children with autism under pressure because of the nature of their disability. For example:

- having to cope with a larger school environment with more students and a less structured and noisy atmosphere;
- bigger school grounds and playgrounds with older students to have to interact with, unfamiliar surroundings and lack of knowledge about the different school rules that apply in the playground and in the classrooms;

- having to cope with different teachers and different classrooms for each school subject, fear of getting lost in the larger school and being late for class;
- increased levels of anxiety about the changes to routines and sensory arousal from the larger, less structured environment. Anxiety from the higher expectations and increased need for independence paired with the difficulties associated with having to be better organised and having to remember separate books, materials, teachers and classrooms for each subject;
- having to meet the individual expectations of each teacher concerning discipline, homework, quality of work and class participation but with limited time to build rapport with teachers;
- increased amounts of homework and increased numbers of subjects to understand and be knowledgeable about;
- awareness of being different from the other students along with increased peer pressure to conform and to be socially competent. Fear of being ostracised by peers;
- anxiety about the increased workload and academic requirements. The need to engage in socially acceptable behaviours and manage sensory overload;
- having to deal with increased possibility of being bullied and teased by peers and not understood by teachers. This often leads to poor self-esteem, depression, anxiety and challenging behaviour; and
- having to cope with normal physical changes associated with puberty and adolescence.

To assist children to minimise the stress and anxiety associated with the transition from primary to high school, there are a number of strategies that can be implemented. For example, there should be a planning meeting held prior to the transition to discuss the process. This meeting should involve parents, primary school staff and high school staff and should discuss the individual needs of the student involved as well as collecting information about the student.

Opportunities should be provided for the student to become familiar with the new setting, teaching staff and the new routines. A visit to the new high school should be part of the orientation process for all students leaving primary school. Visual supports should be included as part of this process. Remember that people with autism do not cope well with change unless they are prepared and forewarned.

Teaching staff should be offered training in autism to improve their empathy and understanding of the problems associated with the disorder as well as its impact on learning and behaviour. This training will assist them to understand the particular learning styles of children with autism and ensure that each students' individual needs are met both in the classroom and in the playground.

Classes need to have a clearly defined structure with rules and routines in place to minimise chaos and disruptions. Students should be provided with a map of the school with particular classrooms highlighted as well as the routes between classrooms.

Students may be given a five-minute warning before the end of class to help them to prepare for the transition to the next class. It may be a verbal signal or a short alarm.

Pre-warn students of any major changes in order to minimise stress around change to routine. Have the secretary call the student's home if it is known that one of the student's teachers will be absent. This will enable parents to prepare the student for the change to their daily timetable.

An additional strategy is to introduce the student to a mentor or coach, perhaps an older student, to assist with any difficulties encountered during the transition period and to provide the student with a social role model to assist their social integration in the playground. A staff member could also be assigned to assist the student with any organisational difficulties, to provide emotional and social support and act as a confidante if the student is not coping or is being bullied.

Visual supports should remain an integral part of each student's program and these should be used in each classroom as appropriate. Social skills training as part of the regular curriculum or in specialised social skills groups should also be available to individual students with special needs. Give the student positive self-talk phrases to help him/her cope during times of change or stress. For example, the student may be encouraged to repeat phrases such as 'it is different today' or 'there is another way of doing things today that will be OK' to help cope with change to routine. Social stories are also a positive method of teaching students to self-manage.

Students may also be allowed to submit homework and assignments in different formats that may be better suited to their individual learning styles. Some students may not be able to cope with the normal workload and may need to enrol in fewer subjects and have more 'free periods' or 'study time'.

Some students will also benefit from having a room or home base set aside as a resource, or safe room that they can go to during the day when they are overwhelmed by noise, social interaction, sensory overload or peer pressure.

How can young adults manage their differences?

So you shouldn't always think a person who is different gets the same balanced information from the world that you do. His eyes and ears can be focused on the same things yours are, but once that information gets onto the pathways to his brain, it can go off in wrong directions or get changed or faded or scrambled or confused. So the information might not get to his brain in the same condition the information arrived at your brain. (Brad Rand, p 3)

Brad Rand has written a booklet about Asperger's syndrome called *How to Understand People Who are Different*. He describes how different it feels be have autism and then outlines some of the experiences individuals face in coping with these differences. Unlike Rand, however, most young adults with autism are not able to articulate their experiences, interests, and preferences or needs in a way that is generally understood. They rely on their behaviour to provide the messages about their special needs; behaviour that requires interpretation from those people who live and work with them. When these needs are addressed in a systematic way, it is more likely that their desired goals will be achieved and their particular interests, preferences and needs addressed.

Students with disabilities should have an individual transition plan to guide them through the transition process from school to adulthood. This plan should address a job, a home, family, leisure and recreation opportunities, and long-term life planning. The desired outcome is to assist young adults with autism to enjoy a reasonable quality of life. However, how one defines a quality of life is subject to individual interpretation. According to Pratt (2002, p 1):

To avoid determining a life, which does not reflect the individual's goals, the most important participant in the planning process is the person with autism spectrum disorder. Each person should have the opportunity to choose leisure activities, job opportunities, personal schedules, living arrangements, and so on. Involving the person with autism in his/her own transition planning is called self-determination. Self-determination refers to the obvious step of making one's own life choices, setting personal goals, and initiating a plan of action.

Among the suggestions to consider when preparing a young person with autism for adulthood are:

■ use the person's interests and try to offer choices when looking at work or study options;

- ensure that some of the necessary skills for adulthood are taught within the school curriculum to allow plenty of time and opportunity for the student to master them. For example, skills such as being organised, being prepared, completing assigned tasks, following directions, and interacting with others are important work skills;
- introduce other curriculum options to teach life skills such as cooking, cleaning, shopping and budgeting;
- encourage the involvement of students in extracurricular activities such as school clubs, sport and other social events or special interest groups to build a support network;
- during school years, encourage work experience programs and volunteer positions to obtain experience in a real work environment;
- teach behaviours that are appropriate to specific work environment in natural settings; and
- ensure that the student has appropriate hygiene and dress habits that are suitable for the work environment and teach individuals the skills to socialise and participate in general work-related discussions with colleagues during work hours.

> Ryan is an 18-year-old young adult with Asperger's syndrome. He has left school and is currently looking for a job. He likes numbers and math and has an excellent memory. During the Olympics, Ryan worked for the Transport Department advising people what buses and trains to catch. He had memorised all of the bus and train timetables and routes and was able to answer any questions about what train or bus to catch and the times they ran. He would like to have a similar position on a full-time basis.

How may young adults be assisted to enter the workforce?

Every year, thousands of students prepare to leave school in search of the perfect job, place to live, relationships, and lifestyle. The transition from school to adulthood is pivotal in the lives of all students. For a person without a disability, this dramatic change from the secure world of school to the uncertainty of adulthood can be stressful and challenging. For the person with autism, the shift is even more overwhelming and daunting. For the person with autism, transition of any kind can be challenging and the transition from school to the workplace may seem even more so. Many individuals with disabilities such as autism experience high drop-out rates, high unemployment, low wages, few job choices, limited relationships, and restricted living options. Most of these students leave school unprepared to handle simple daily routines such as paying bills, balancing a budget, or completing the basic tasks required for independent living. And these are the more mildly affected students.

The options for young adults with more significant or severe forms of autism are even more limited. There is little ongoing support and training available to assist these young people to integrate into the general community in any form of supported employment. This bleak outlook is devastating for parents and individuals and highlights the need for those involved in the education of individuals with autism to begin to systematically and seriously pursue effective transition planning (Pratt 2002). With thoughtful planning, the transition process for the student with autism can be less disorienting and confusing and infinitely more successful. Planning includes using proactive and creative strategies that specifically address the behavioural and educational needs of these students.

According to Osborn & Wilcox (1992), transition planning for young adults serves several important functions because it:

- introduces the family and the student to adult service systems;
- determines the level of support the student requires to live, work, and recreate in the community as an adult;

- identifies adult service system gaps and inadequacies, and advocates for more appropriate services;
- provides information to adult service providers about individual needs so that service providers will not assume that all people with disabilities have identical needs when planning services and implementing programs; and
- provides information critical to determining appropriate Individual Educational Plan (IEP) goals. Through the IEP, parents and educators can target skill development necessary for a smooth transition.

Temple Grandin, (1996b, p 1) a young woman with Asperger's syndrome, and a strong advocate for people with autism, has written about her experiences in making the transition from the world of school to the world of work. She stresses the importance 'of a gradual transition from an educational setting into a career'. She also talks about the importance of encouraging people with autism to use their interests or obsessions as the basis for a career if possible. Grandin offers a number of suggestions to assist the person with autism to transition successfully into the workplace. These include:

- Making the transition from school to workplace a gradual move by introducing work for short periods while the student is still at school — this is an extension of the work experience model. She recommends finding supportive employers and providing them with information about the person and also about the disability.
- Encouraging the person to develop a relationship with someone who can act as a mentor, be a special friend but also teach social skills. The most successful mentors have interests in common with the person with autism. By educating employers and employees about the person's strengths and limitations, cognitively, communicatively and socially, it may be possible to avoid situations that could cost the person with autism their job.
- Thinking about the option of freelance work, especially for people with special skills in computers, music or art and creating a portfolio to sell skills rather than personality. Since people with autism do not perform well at interviews, they often need to find work via the 'back door'. Technical people respect talent, and a person with autism needs to sell their talent to a prospective employer (p 4).

According to Grandin, transition from school to post-school activity can be a challenging and exciting time in a student's life. A well thought out and carefully orchestrated transition plan for a student with autism will augment strengths and deal productively with challenges in a way that will enhance the life of the student and support and assist them to achieve a seamless transition to desired post-school outcomes. Patience and an ability to think 'outside the box' will ensure success.

Pratt (2002, p 3) also suggests that:

People with autism spectrum disorder can make an important contribution to society. Unfortunately this contribution is not capitalized on when the person is not prepared or supported. As family members and professionals, our job is to guide the person in determining a future, which is both meaningful and realistic. With careful planning, people can leave school prepared for a lifetime of struggles and successes.

What are the benefits of planning ahead for any change?

Planned change refers to a systematic way of altering familiar social and physical environments. Events, people and their environments are constantly changing and, with assistance, individuals with autism can learn to become more adaptable and able to cope with change. Support in the form of clear, understandable information that is presented in a familiar format and is presented ahead of time helps the person to predict what will happen, thereby minimising distress and encouraging flexibility (Powers 1992).

Planned change uses visual forewarning and provides a vehicle to explain unexpected changes to regular routines. Prior to the introduction of planned change strategies, routines and visual supports should be established and consistently used. Most planned change strategies involve substituting activities according to the person's preferences.

A normal routine at school may include a music lesson before visiting the local library every Wednesday for storytime. However, one Wednesday the routine may be changed to accommodate a special visitor to the classroom. This change in routine may be presented visually to children with autism to forewarn them and to minimise stress or anxiety due to the change in routine.

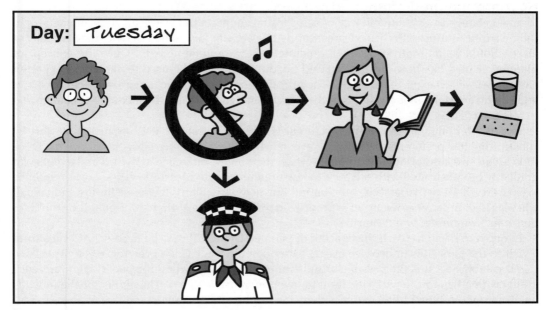

Figure 16.3 *Example of a visual planned change strategy*

Quill (1995, p 248) says:

Because children with autism might react to changes by becoming agitated and upset doesn't mean that they can't learn to accept change. The important factors are to identify what environmental stimuli a child relies on for stability, to provide accurate information about the change prior to the event, to offer choices about alternatives to the change when possible, and to elicit the child's involvement in the change when appropriate.

It is far easier to explain changes to a normal routine if visual strategies are already in place rather than trying to rely on verbal explanations. If changes are explained verbally, there is no guarantee that the person with autism has understood the change until the change actually occurs. The individual's reaction to the change will be an indication of whether they understood and accepted the verbal explanation. If the person is not able to understand the change, he may expect to proceed as normal and become very distressed when the change occurs.

A child who is told that he will not be going to the park after his swimming lesson may have a huge tantrum when he gets in the car and is driven past the local park on the way to Grandma's house. He needs to see the picture of the park crossed out or removed from his visual sequence and replaced with a picture of Grandma. Seeing the sequence changed visually and even participating in the change may help him to understand what is happening and be more willing to accept that change.

An adult working in a supported employment program was told by his supervisor that the following Monday was a public holiday. He still became very distressed and anxious on the Monday morning when his regular driver did not turn up to take him to work. He did not fully comprehend the verbal information and needed to see a visual strategy explaining that his workplace was closed and explaining why he did not have to go to work on the Monday. The visual strategy could also have offered him an alternative option, such as a visit to his favourite museum or park.

How are planned change strategies introduced?

Planned change is a systematic way of using visual supports to forewarn people of changes to their current routines. It relies on substituting one activity for another activity that, initially at least, should be as motivating for the person as the original activity. Once the concept of planned change has been introduced and taught, it can then be used to explain unexpected changes as well as expected changes. The introduction of planned change assists children and adults who are rigid about routines and environments to recognise the meaning of change and to tolerate change.

In order for changes to routines to be successful and accepted, it is important to start by substituting low preference activities or events with high preference activities or events. Once individuals are comfortable with this process, then high preference activities and events can gradually be substituted with medium to low preference activities and events. Low preference events are those activities that are routine but not particularly favoured by the individual, whereas high preference events are favourite activities such as a trip to McDonalds or the train museum, swimming, or a train ride.

In order to begin to teach the concept of planned change, it may be necessary to substitute a visit to the park (low preference event) with pizza for lunch (high preference activity). Once this is established, it is the possible to substitute a trip to the swimming pool (high preference event) with a trip to the park (medium to low preference activity). The aim is for the individual to accept the substitution of one activity for another and to understand that changes to regular routines are acceptable and to move away from having to use highly motivating activities as substitutes. Eventually it should be possible to substitute a high preference activity with even a low preference activity if the process is explained beforehand (see Figure 16.4)

step 1

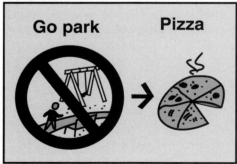

step 2

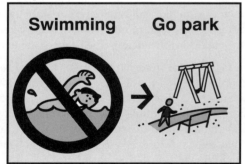

Figure 16.4 *Planned change*

When working with individuals with autism any planned change strategy should be presented visually to assist children and adults to understand what is happening. Visual symbols should be used consistently across all settings to avoid confusion.

Widely accepted planned change symbols include symbols for 'no', arrows and borders.

International symbols for 'no' indicate that the event/activity will not happen. The symbols may be coloured red for 'no' and placed over the image of an event or activity that will not occur because of a change of circumstances. The original image should still be quite visible under the symbol.

The arrow may be coloured green for 'yes' and indicates that the event or activity following the arrow will happen as a consequence of the preceding activity.

Borders are used to highlight certain images and assist the child to focus on what is important. A variety of different colours may be used for the borders.

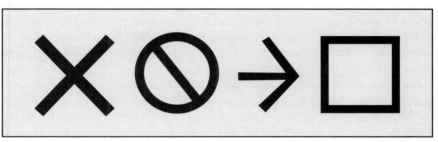

Figure 16.5 *Shows four widely accepted change symbols*

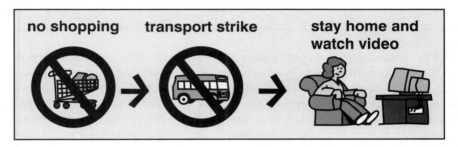

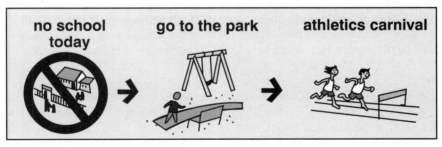

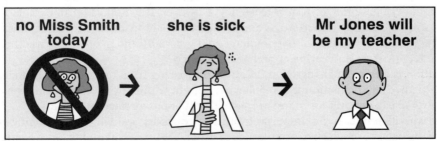

Figure 16.6 *Shows examples of planned change strategies*

What happens if unexpected changes occur?

It is not always possible to predict changes ahead of time as changes sometimes occur that are unforeseen. If the teacher becomes sick and has to leave class, if it starts to rain and there is no outdoor play, if Mum runs out of chocolate chip cookies, or if there is a power failure and the workplace has to close down, there may be no warning. Unexpected changes are just as distressing, if not more so, for the person with autism. It is at times like this that the importance of having visual sequences in place is realised. If possible, a substitute may be put into the normal visual sequence before the individual becomes too distressed or anxious, and a choice of alternative activity or object can be offered.

According to Quill (1995), dwelling on the change is not beneficial but supporting the person to understand the change by presenting information visually and immediately changing the visual sequence may help to minimise stress. Whenever it is possible to solve the problem with visual supports, the changes seem to be accepted more readily, with less fuss and less anxiety.

> Patrick managed a change when the teacher was sick and his 12.00 pm class was cancelled. Initially he became quite agitated because he did not know what he should do during that period and how he would be able to manage for the remainder of his regular classes that day. Once he was shown a visual support explaining the change to his routine and offering him a couple of alternatives, he decided to go to the school library and read his textbook for the period and then proceed with the rest of his classes as normal.

All of the strategies outlined above have been developed to assist and accommodate the needs of children and adults with autism who, as part of their everyday lives, have to cope with numerous changes to their normal routines. It is important to recognise the difficulties these individuals face daily as they struggle to make sense of a world that is usually disordered and generally chaotic. Most people struggle to understand basic rules and regulations and to cope with life changes. It is so much harder for people with autism who do not read environmental cues or understand general social expectations.

However, with a recognition of their strengths and needs and an understanding of their limitations and particular learning styles, there is no reason why individuals with autism cannot achieve their goals and, at the very least, some degree of independence.

Summary

Children and adults with autism, because of their unique characteristics, have difficulty coping with change to their regular routines. They spend their lives seeking consistency and structure from the world around them.

Routines are crucial for people with autism because they provide order and structure to daily lives and offer some form of consistency. However, it is important to be able to modify routines without causing undue stress and anxiety to the individuals with autism who rely on them. If possible, changes should be implemented gradually and people prepared beforehand for them. A consistent and caring approach is required.

Transition is a form of change that involves the passing from one condition, stage, activity or place to another. Transition is a regular part of life within a community but is something that is particularly difficult for many people with autism to manage successfully.

Transition planning is an important process to assist individuals in coping with the transition from one event, activity or place to another. Transition planning, once again requires careful preparation and provision of information in an appropriate format.

There are certain transition periods that are recognised as being difficult for the person with autism and these include starting preschool, starting school, moving from primary to high school and then leaving school for the workplace or other post school options. Each of these periods can cause distress and anxiety for individuals with autism unless strategies are in place to prepare children and young adults for these particular events.

The importance of planning ahead for change is well researched and documented. Planned change procedures include introducing warning ahead of any changes, making extensive use of visual supports, and providing acceptable alternative activities, events or objects to the person with autism. Examples of visual supports to minimise stress associated with change have been provided throughout the chapter.

Sometimes it is not possible to forewarn people of change, but individuals can still be assisted to cope in these situations if there are clear and appropriate visual sequences in place that can be quickly modified.

CHAPTER

17

Teaching Strategies

Students with autism spectrum disorders present a unique challenge to educators. There is considerable heterogeneity among this population, which means that each individual may need qualitatively and quantitatively different levels of educational and behavioural support. As a result of this variability, students with autism spectrum disorders are educated anywhere along the placement continuum from specialised programs to general education classrooms.

Pratt, Lantz & Loftin, p 1

Dr Bryna Siegal of the University of California, San Fransisco, estimates that approximately 25% of classically autistic children respond to intensive interventions and that about 7% do well enough to attend mainstream schools, and lead normal lives. The response rates are much higher among more able children with mild autism and experts agree that early intervention is the key to success. The earlier intervention begins, the better the longer-term prognosis for most children.

What strategies can be introduced to teach skills?

Some of the commonly used teaching strategies for children with learning difficulties occur quite naturally in most families. These include providing verbal cues, modelling appropriate behaviours and using visual supports to assist communication and social interaction. Other strategies, such as physical or verbal prompting, fading, shaping, and chaining do not come as easily to parents and may require more effort and patience to master. These concepts are explored in more detail in this chapter.

When teaching any new skills, or even reinforcing previously learned skills, it is important to start by obtaining the person's attention. This may involve showing a visual support such as a photograph or written list. Once they are attending, they still need to be told or shown what to do. It may be beneficial to demonstrate by modelling an appropriate response. As soon as the task is successfully completed or even attempted, it is important to provide some form of reinforcement for work well done.

There are several ways to assist children and adults to learn new behaviours and skills. These include:

- verbal/visual cues;
- modelling;
- visual supports;
- prompting;
- fading;
- shaping; and
- chaining.

Verbal/visual cues

Verbal/visual cues (telling and showing) are the instructions that are given to children or adults to assist them to complete a desired task. Tell the person how to respond appropriately in a given situation. This may be done verbally, or non-verbally using a manual sign or a visual strategy. Sometimes people with autism require prompts to assist them to complete an activity even though they know what to do. When giving verbal cues, language should remain as simple and consistent as possible. Individuals should be given ample time to consider and process each instruction and formulate a response. A response time of between 10 and 30 seconds is usually more than enough but longer time should be available if necessary. No response or an incorrect response may mean a lack of understanding of the instruction, or an inability to know how to respond correctly. When this occurs, it may be necessary to give further prompting to provide further information.

For example, if you are feeding a child and want him to participate by holding the spoon and scooping up some food, then you may need to remind him with 'hold spoon'. You may sign 'eat' or show the child a picture of someone feeding themselves. You may follow a similar process to encourage a child to help dress himself.

> Johnny is learning to dress himself but prefers not to wear trousers. He has to be reminded to put on his trousers and to pull them up. He still requires a verbal prompt such as 'pant up' to pull up his pants but will usually respond correctly if he is allowed to play a video game or play outside once he is dressed.

Modelling

Modelling involves showing the person what to do in a particular situation. Most children learn by imitating the behaviours of others, especially parents, siblings and peers. Modelling often provides the most appropriate means of teaching new skills. For example, showing a child how to bathe, dress and feed a doll by modelling the different steps or teaching an adult how to make a cup of coffee or a sandwich by modelling the steps are effective ways of teaching these functional skills.

If you want a child to complete a puzzle, you may start by telling the child, 'put in'. Always wait at least 5–10 seconds to allow the child time to process the request before repeating it. If he or she does not seem to understand the request, you should repeat it and model the correct response by putting one piece in the puzzle yourself.

Successful teaching programs have shown the effectiveness of using peers as models to teach communication and social interaction skills. Individuals with autism may initially need to be taught how to observe others and to copy what they are doing. Peer models may need instruction and support to learn techniques to work with a child with autism and to encourage appropriate responses.

Visual supports

Visual supports are used to enhance communication, transfer information, support behaviour and develop independence. They include visual timetables, sequences, reminders, forewarning, augmentation of the environment, choice boards, contingency contracts as well as gestures, facial expressions and body language. Visual strategies, or visual supports, assist people to communicate and to understand what is happening around them. For example, visually showing a child each step of a sequence will assist in the teaching of new skills such as toileting, dressing or washing hands and also explain a bedtime routine to a person with poor sleeping habits (see Figures 17.1 and 17.2).

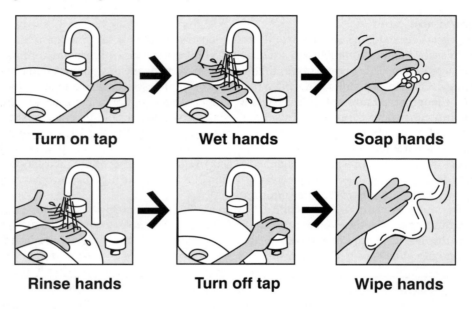

Figure 17.1   *Example of a visual sequence to teach a person to wash hands*

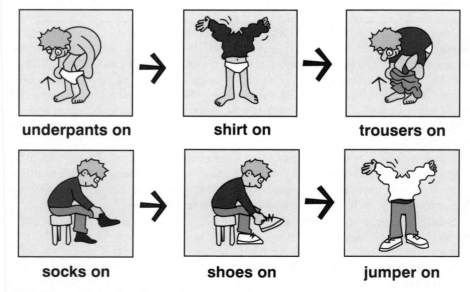

Figure 17.2   *Example of a dressing routine presented visually*

People with severe comprehension difficulties may continue to rely on visual cues indefinitely to support their poor auditory processing skills. It should not be assumed that the ultimate goal for all individuals is to be able to respond solely to verbal prompts. Even high functioning children and adults with autism benefit from using visual supports throughout their lives to augment communication, assist self-organisation and teach social skills.

Prompting

Prompting is an additional cue to help facilitate a correct response. Individuals may initially need to be physically guided to complete a task. Offer the least amount of guidance necessary while encouraging the person to complete as much of the activity as possible without physical assistance. Providing a physical prompt will often ensure a successful outcome for the individual.

The most common physical prompt involves full hand over hand assistance to help complete a given task. Reinforcement should follow immediately, just as if the person had completed the task independently. As competence in the task increases, the amount of physical assistance is withdrawn. This may mean a change from hand over hand prompting to a light touch on the arm to encourage an attempt at the required action. Alternately, a person may attempt the initial action independently, but require some gentle assistance to complete it successfully.

> James loves peanut butter sandwiches and is learning to make a sandwich for himself at home. He initially needed help to spread the butter and peanut butter on the bread but now requires only a light touch on his arm by his Mum to complete the task independently.

The following are some of the established guidelines for using prompts:
- *Prompts should focus the person's attention* on the task, item or activity being taught and not distract from it.
- *Prompts should be as weak as possible.* The use of strong prompts when weak will do is inefficient and may delay children's mastery of the skill being taught. Use the least intrusive prompt possible to elicit a correct response. Verbal and gestural prompts are less intrusive than modelling and all are less intrusive than physical guidance.
- *Prompts should be faded as quickly as possible.* Continuing to prompt longer than necessary may result in dependence on the prompts.
- *Unplanned prompts should be avoided.* Sometimes individuals may be unknowingly prompted by involuntary facial expression or hand gestures. Both of these are useful prompts as long as their use is controlled.

Fading

Fading is the systematic reduction of a prompt. It is simply the gradual reduction of any physical assistance. When fading assistance, do it gradually and continue to reward improvements in skills as they occur. This technique is most successful in teaching new tasks, as the individual always achieves success and is reinforced for it. The ability to successfully fade prompts requires sensitivity, which is gained through experience. It requires practice and experience to know how much assistance to give and when to begin to slowly withdraw that assistance. It is important to fade assistance so that people do not become dependent on the prompts and cues.

Shaping

Shaping involves reinforcing successive approximations of a desired behaviour. Sometimes behaviour can be shaped to an appropriate response. Shaping is a procedure used to develop a skill or behaviour that does not already exist in a person's repertoire.

Because it is a more time-intensive process than prompting, shaping is only used when there are no prompts that can be successfully employed to obtain a correct response. When shaping, it is necessary to work towards an appropriate response by initially reinforcing responses that even vaguely resemble the correct response. It is used in teaching quite complicated skills such as dressing, feeding and socialising with others. For example, parents may praise young children the first time they dress themselves, even if the shirt is on inside out and the shorts are on back to front. Later, children may only be complimented if the clothes are on properly with the buttons fastened and shoelaces tied.

> Isobel's parents started to teach her to feed herself by initially praising her whenever she picked up a spoon and held it. Eventually they showed her how to scoop up soft food on to the spoon, to take the spoon to her mouth and then to put the spoonful of food into her mouth and eat it. Isobel learned the sequence one step at a time.

Chaining

Chaining involves the creation of a complex behaviour by combining simple behaviours that are already part of a person's repertoire, into a sequence of behaviours called a chain. This is the instructional procedure in which a task is broken down into smaller steps and each step of the 'chain' is taught in correct sequence. The chaining procedure involves the linking together and reinforcement of several simple learned behaviours to form more complex behaviour.

For example, teaching a child to clean his teeth involves initially rewarding him for each small step of the process. The steps may include putting paste on the brush, putting the brush in the mouth, moving the brush up and down, spitting out, rinsing the mouth and rinsing the brush. It then becomes possible to put all of these steps together in sequence to achieve the more complex procedure of teeth cleaning.

The procedure of teaching a person to perform a sequence of small actions as one single task is a chaining procedure. A distinction may be made between *forward and backward chaining*.

Forward chaining involves starting with the first step of the chain of behaviours, and teaching that step before moving on to the next step and so on until the final step.

Backward chaining involves starting with the last step of the chain of behaviours and working from the last back to the first. For example, teaching the necessary steps to independent toileting may first of all involve breaking the toileting sequence down into small steps and then teaching children the last step in the sequence first. The parent may initially help the child complete all of the toileting steps and only expect them to complete the last step independently (for example, to pull up the pants). Once this is mastered, the second-last step in the procedure is taught, and so on until all steps in the sequence have been taught and the child is able to use the toilet independently. A visual sequence should also be prepared and used as a part of this process.

What teaching practices benefit students with autism?

When teaching children and adults with autism, it is important to teach to their strengths while acknowledging and understanding their deficits. Their strengths generally include superior visual abilities and rote learning skills relative to their other skills while deficits include a limited ability to process language for meaning and an inability to self-regulate or organise themselves.

Among the recommended strategies to use when teaching students with autism are to:

- keep language simple and avoid verbal overload irrespective of the person's communicative abilities;

- introduce visual supports into all teaching sessions and use visual cues and prompts;
- use planned change strategies including visual supports to prepare students for changes to routines;
- introduce structure and organisation into daily programs and maintain a consistent approach to teaching new skills;
- understand the tendency to focus on detail and the inability to understand the bigger picture;
- provide positive feedback and encourage successful outcomes for all students;
- understand the nature of autism and recognise the stress and anxiety that is commonly associated with the disorder;
- take time to know each student and recognise each person's individual needs; and
- recognise the importance of consistency and routines in assisting individuals with autism to cope with life on a daily basis.

The role of the teacher is:
- to maximise the use of visual supports and minimise dependence on abstract thinking;
- to reduce factors that cause stress including waiting, physical contact, ambiguity and overload;
- to be aware and sympathetic toward sensory difficulties (including sensory overload);
- to examine messages behind challenging behaviour rather than taking the behaviour personally;
- to be as concrete and literal as possible when giving instructions or providing information to students;
- to avoid complex verbal instructions and keep language simple and free from idioms, double meanings, teasing or sarcasm;
- to prepare students in advance for any changes to regular routines and use visual supports to ensure that the message is received; and
- to be consistent in teaching methods, expectations of students and management approaches.

Individuals learn better if their teachers are *organised*, *consistent* and *positive*. Following are some strategies for both parents and professionals to help make learning more effective and enjoyable.

Be organised and prepared

Be organised and prepared and set realistic, achievable goals. In an educational setting, all teachers responsible for the provision of services should be aware of each individual's educational goals and programs and should work together to ensure goals are achieved. All activities should be planned and teaching materials prepared before starting a lesson. Structured routines should be maintained until they are familiar — then settings may be changed or modified to help individuals adapt to change and generalise their skills to other settings.

Be consistent

Be consistent, teach rules and generalise these to larger groups and other settings. Design rules in such a way that they apply to all members of the group, not just the person with autism. Ensure that messages are understood and achievable. It is important to take small manageable steps to begin with. Remain realistic about a child's social ability and gradually extend the length of time the child is expected to stay with the other children during group activities. It is also important to recognise that an adult may be uncomfortable in a social situation and therefore expect them to participate in certain activities for a short time only.

Use simple language

Use simple language to provide clear directions that recognise the problems with auditory processing and allow adequate response time. Wait at least 10–30 seconds (or longer if necessary) before repeating an instruction. Don't phrase something as a question when it should be presented as a direction. For example if you are requesting that a young adult complete their allocated chores at home, don't ask: 'Will you help me clean-up the kitchen and prepare dinner?' when what you really mean is 'It is your job to help clean the kitchen and prepare dinner.'

Be positive and offer praise

Be positive and offer praise by reinforcing appropriate responses with positive attention. This includes offering verbal praise, smiles, touches, tickles or tangible rewards for appropriate behaviour. Reinforce language by giving attention and responding to any attempts that the individual makes to communicate either verbally or non-verbally. Offer encouragement and praise to individuals who attempt a task or activity.

Program brief periods of work without interruption

Program brief periods of work without interruption and prioritise tasks. Gradually increase the amount of time spent on each activity. It may only be possible to program for a few minutes work to begin with and gradually increase the time as the individual learns what is expected of the task. Timetable for periods of free time during the day to enable individuals to pursue their own activities. People with autism may have difficulty attending and remaining focused for long periods and may require regular short breaks with no pressure.

Elizabeth Moon, in her book *Speed of Dark* (2002, p 8), a futuristic novel about a man with autism, describes how Lou, the protagonist, copes at work in his job as a computer analyst:

> When the edges blur, I shake myself and sit back. It has been five hours and I did not notice. Above my workstation, a pinwheel spins lazily in the draft of the ventilation system. I blow at it, and after a moment — 1.3 seconds, actually — it spins faster, twinkling purple-and-silver in the light. I decide to turn on my swivelling fan so all the pinwheels and spin-spirals can spin together, filling my office with twinkling light.

Ellie attends a work program for people with disabilities. She works in the mail room preparing letters for mailing. Ellie enjoys the work but can only attend and concentrate for short periods of time. Ellie works for 20 minutes and then is allowed to listen to her Walkman and read a magazine for 10 minutes. She has earphones and does not disturb the other workers. Ellie is much more relaxed and calm after she has a break.

Prioritise problems

Prioritise problems and work as a team to develop and implement teaching strategies to address problem areas. Use a consistent approach and provide clear messages.

Be flexible

Be flexible and try not to become too directive. Show people what to do rather than tell them because most individuals with autism are visual learners. If a person is not responsive, try to redirect them to something of more interest but keep the activity short. If still unsuccessful at engaging a person's interest, try again later.

Be aware of obsessive behaviour

Be aware of obsessive behaviour and try to ignore it unless it is interfering with learning or is socially inappropriate. If necessary, redirect the person to alternative activities. Use obsessions as rewards.

Try to complete activities

Always try to complete activities to show that there is a beginning and an end to most activities, routines etc. Initially make each activity short, and easily achievable.

Create a positive environment

Create a positive environment to encourage active participation in tasks and activities. A positive attitude to learning assists individuals to improve their motivation and self-image.

Provide opportunities to teach basic social skills

Provide opportunities to teach basic social skills by encouraging children and adults to become involved in several group activities even if only for very short periods of time. Encourage sharing and waiting. Teach play skills to young children and encourage them to play socially with their peers. Use social stories to teach children social skills and then provide structured opportunities to practise these skills. Teach social rules and routines and expect these to be followed. The rules should be displayed in visual formats using simple, clear language.

> James and Georgie live in a supported residence with three other young adults. They have several jobs that they have to complete each day but they also have opportunities to complete some activities together. James and Georgie also go horseriding with the other residents and every Friday evening they go to the movies together. They are learning how to socialise and make friends.

Small groups to practise skills

Introduce the idea of small groups to practice skills. Small groups are less threatening to people with autism than larger groups. Encourage interactions with peers. Initially introduce one other person into an activity and gradually extend the number of people in the group.

Introduce rules and routines

Introduce rules and routines and present these visually. Use visual supports to indicate changes to normal routines, be flexible and give the person time to learn new rules and to cope with changes to regular routines.

What strategies support the development of communication skills?

Special care should be taken to establish what children and adults understand and what form of communication they respond to. Messages may be conveyed through tone of voice, gestures, body language, pictures and words. It is important to establish a relationship of mutual respect by introducing communication systems that people are comfortable with. Consider using visual means to convey information wherever possible.

A number of techniques have been successful in encouraging individuals with autism to be more effective communicators. These include the following strategies:

- try to remain positive;
- demonstrate what to do;
- teach how to listen and attend to others;
- have clear expectations and clarify these;
- prepare for changes;
- keep language simple and relevant;
- remain positive;
- avoid ambiguity in messages;

- avoid confusing statements and questions;
- expect appropriate responses but allow time for processing;
- discuss and label emotions;
- exaggerate feelings and emotions; and
- avoid negative actions and statements.

Try to remain positive

Be positive and model appropriate language — praise often and honestly and be specific when praising. 'Good talking' is better than 'Well done' at providing appropriate feedback to the person with autism.

Demonstrate what to do

Remember that visual skills are often superior to auditory skills. It is important to maximise visual information. Many people with autism 'think in pictures' rather than in words and have highly developed visual skills relative to their auditory processing abilities. By modelling what a person should do, they receive a very clear message that is easily understood.

Teach how to listen and attend to others

Teach listening skills — when giving a direction, obtain the person's attention and ensure that they have understood the message. People do not follow directions if they do not understand the meaning of what is said. Obtain the person's attention first. This may involve getting down to that person's eye level, and perhaps touching him or her. It is important to be consistent and expect a response when the message is simple and understandable. Initially, it may be necessary to support a request with some form of visual augmentation and either physical or verbal prompts.

Have clear expectations and clarify these

Ensure requests are reasonable — be very clear about what is expected of individuals and why. All requests should be made in an appropriate format, be reasonable, relevant and within the person's capabilities.

Prepare for changes

Provide adequate information to forewarn of changes — tell people in advance what is going to happen next. This may be done verbally (if appropriate) or visually. Inform them of any changes, involve them in plans and explain what behaviour is expected. Use simple language, pictures and gestures, daily schedule boards, visual timetables, sequences routines and picture wallets to provide information.

Keep language simple and relevant

Use language that is simple, clear and concise — giving too much verbal information or too many directions may lead to frustration and confusion. Many children and adults with autism comprehend only a limited amount of verbal information. Use a calm clear voice. Loud, excited voices are difficult to listen to. Do not engage in baby talk or use an unnaturally high-pitched voice with young children. Remember that language does not always need to be presented verbally. Many requests can also be made non-verbally. Pointing or gesturing or showing a photograph of what is expected provides a very clear message.

Remain positive

Tell people what to do and avoid telling what not to do — use statements that will provide information about what is acceptable behaviour. Negative statements only tell a person what is unacceptable and do not provide relevant information to help them understand what to do differently and more appropriately.

Avoid ambiguity in messages
Be as neutral as possible when giving directions — the tone of the voice, facial expressions or the ambiguity of a word can change the meaning of a question, direction or statement.

Avoid confusing statements and questions
Avoid asking questions with a choice — unless a person is actually being given a choice. Directions should be given to be followed or to provide information. Do not ask a child if they want to do something unless it is acceptable for them to say 'no'. Avoid using questions unless absolutely necessary as they are particularly difficult to interpret. For example, it is better for a child with autism to be told 'It is time to come inside when the bell rings' rather than 'Are you ready to come inside now?'

Expect appropriate responses but allow time for processing
Teach children and adults to respond immediately — to certain words, phrases, environmental cues or questions. For example, teaching the words 'stop' or 'help' can assist young children to learn rules and provide them with the means of asking for assistance. However it is also important to remember that people with autism may require up to 15–30 seconds to process information and formulate a response.

Discuss and label emotions
Label feelings — children and adults with autism have difficulty recognising the feelings of others and expressing their own feelings. Use photos, books and social stories for older children. Introduce visual supports and discuss emotions in the context in which they may occur with children and adults (see Figure 17.3). This should never be done in a negative way. Criticising or attaching negative labels to children and adults only reduces their self-esteem and self-confidence.

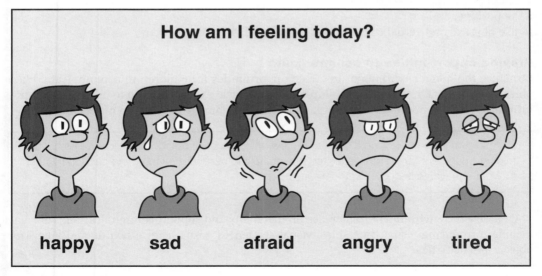

Figure 17.3 *Visual support showing emotions*

Exaggerate feelings and emotions

Exaggerate facial expressions — children with autism often fail to use facial expression as a means of communication and their expressions may not match their thoughts. Use exaggerated expressions to model feelings and thoughts in different situations. For example, a child with autism may laugh and giggle when another child falls and hurts himself. In that situation, it is important to model an animated response such as frowning and looking concerned: 'Oh dear, you fell and hurt your knee'. At other times a more natural (not exaggerated) facial expression may accompany a verbal explanation to ensure the person is focusing on the verbal directions rather than concentrating on reading and interpreting facial expressions.

Avoid negative actions and statements

Avoid reprimands — use rules that are consistent and neutral. Reprimands do not benefit anyone. Rules may be presented in a variety of different ways depending on the form of communication each person responds to. Support words with visual cues. Present important information visually by drawing pictures, pointing to real objects or photos and using gestures.

What can parents do to help young children at home?

Parents and professionals may need to modify the environment in order to facilitate communication and social development. Families play a major role in the development of their children's functional skills. When children are very young, parents should ensure that they have their children's attention before speaking; simplify language; allow their children time to reply; and reward all attempts to communicate.

In addition, it is important that parents should to the following:

- provide opportunities to communicate;
- respond to communication attempts;
- motivate children by using their interests and obsessions;
- encourage imitation;
- try to interact by following child's lead;
- model and shape appropriate responses;
- avoid giving directions and model appropriate behaviour;
- simplify language and use visuals;
- be positive; and
- use physical and verbal cues to assist with meaning.

Provide opportunities to communicate

Structure the home environment to create opportunities for children to communicate. Place objects out of reach to encourage children to have to ask, expect children to use skills at home, introduce visual supports to augment language and encourage children to make choices.

Lucy's mum puts her favourite objects in view, though out of reach, and encourages her to take her hand and point to the desired object. Taking her mum by the hand and leading her to what she wants is Lucy's way of requesting.

Organise the environment to increase predictability and support communication. This may include introducing visual timetables, visual sequences, visual choice boards and labels for objects and activities.

Respond to communication attempts

Initially accept any attempt to communicate including screaming, gestures, moving toward the desired objects or even looking. Model appropriate requesting and encourage children to imitate actions and sounds. Respond to any attempts by a child to communicate by giving them attention and interpreting what they want.

Motivate children by using their interests and obsessions

Be aware of, and responsive to, children's interests. One of the most effective ways of obtaining and keeping a child's attention is to use their interests or obsessions to capture their interest. Individual interests and obsessions will be most motivating for children with autism.

Encourage imitation

Encourage children to imitate actions and sounds, and also to accept and respond to comments from others. For example if children enjoy 'Wiggles' on video, dance with them and encourage them to imitate the actions, providing some physical prompts as necessary. If children enjoy playing with trains, join in their play and make appropriate sounds such as 'choo, choo'.

Try to interact by following child's lead

Follow children's lead by responding to events and activities of interest to them.

> Amie's mum set up water play in the yard with lots of toys to encourage Amie to play alongside her. Amie loves water and is more likely to tolerate her mother playing near her during her favourite activities.

Model and shape appropriate responses

Build upon utterances made by children and gradually shape these into more effective communication. For example if children repeatedly say the sound, 'b, b, b', 'b, b, b' model a more effective form of communication such as, 'brmm, brmm' and use it in context. Additionally, if children say a single word utterance to request, such as 'ball', model a descriptive word to extend the language such as, 'big ball' or 'red ball'.

> Whenever Raymond started to push his cars along the floor, his Dad would imitate his actions with another car and make the sounds 'brmm, brmm'. Raymond enjoyed playing with his father and started to imitate the same sounds.

Avoid giving directions and model appropriate behaviour

Talk with children in an interactive not directive way. Emphasis should be placed on sharing information rather than on giving directions. Augment verbal information with visual supports. Show children what you want them to do as well as telling them.

> When it is time for Ellen to get out of the sandpit and put on her shoes, the teacher asks her to finish playing and she takes Ellen's shoes over to her as a visual prompt or shows her a photo of shoes. The visual prompt helps Ellen to understand what the teacher wants.

Simplify language and use visuals

Avoid abstract concepts and confusing words with more than one meaning. Keep language simple and concrete when communicating with children and add visual supports as appropriate to assist understanding.

Be positive

Be positive rather than negative and always frame requests or directions in a positive way. For example, instead of saying 'no flapping' you might say 'hands down', or instead of telling a child not to do something ('don't touch the television', 'don't jump on the lounge') it will be more effective to suggest something positive to do ('let's play outside' or 'let's jump on the trampoline').

> Jack loves to jump and always jumps on his bed or on the lounge. Whenever he starts jumping, his mum reminds him, 'we **sit** on the lounge and we **jump** on the trampoline. Do you want to go outside and jump?' She lets Jack go outside to jump on his trampoline.

Use physical and verbal cues to assist with meaning

Provide cues to assist children to respond correctly. Cues should be given when needed to encourage independence. Cues may include physical prompts (such as putting their hands on a crayon and physically assisting them to draw a line), environmental cues (such as sitting children at the table in front of food at mealtimes as a prompt to eat) or verbal cues that are learned over time. In addition, gestures, photographs and written words may be used to cue children and adults to a particular response. We all rely on visual cues throughout our daily life to help us to organise our thoughts and activities.

Why should children be taught to make choices?

Making choices is an important skill that helps to promote independence. Initially children learn to request, which helps them to understand that they can have an impact on what happens in their lives.

Once children have developed simple requesting behaviours (such as taking a person by the hand to what they want, bringing a desired object to a person, pointing to, or standing in front of a particular object), they can learn to make a choice between objects. Young children usually demonstrate that they are ready to learn choice making by indicating preferences for certain people, food and toys and refusing other things. Children with autism have to be taught how to choose between objects and be given the opportunity to make choices in everyday, functional situations. Children need to understand that the ability to request and make choices allows them to make decisions about what they want and don't want. It is important to give clear messages when offering choices and to accept children's decisions once they have made a choice. Children also need to be taught how to refuse a choice of objects or activities by indicating 'no' either verbally or non-verbally.

People should be taught to make choices in real situations using real objects. When working with children and adults with autism, the emphasis is on developing functional skills that will enable individuals to become more independent and participate in decision making processes.

What strategies are effective in teaching choices?

When first introducing choices, start with two objects that the child recognises; one that is a favourite and one that they do not like. By initially offering a choice of one preferred and one non-preferred item, the choice becomes a simple one. The first few times the idea is introduced, the child may need to be prompted to make a response. Once they learn that they will be given whichever object is chosen (by looking, pointing, touching, grabbing or labelling), the process may be extended to other situations. Eventually a choice between two preferred items can be offered. This decision may be difficult for the child initially as they will probably want both items even though they have learned that they are supposed to choose only one.

Present two objects — favourite toys or foods are usually good to begin with. Say clearly 'what do you want'. If the non-preferred is chosen and it is clear that it is not wanted, say and model 'no', use gesture and show visual 'no' sign if a child is non-verbal. If the preferred item is chosen, then give the child the item and say, 'good boy, you want _____ (name of item chosen)'. Present choices often during play, at snack time, during meals, at free time, and when dressing or bathing young children. Assist children to understand by praising them for making choices. Reinforce choice making by carrying through with the children's choice. Start by offering a choice of two real objects, then introduce photos of objects and gradually add additional items over time. Provide individual choice boards that act as visual reminders for children and adults of the choices available (see Figure 17.4).

Once children have grasped the idea of making a choice between two objects, the lesson can then be expanded to include additional objects and activities. In order to make an informed choice, children should experience the activity, object or person. So often, rejection comes from lack of knowledge and the preference to stick with what is familiar. Only when they know what — for example, bushwalking is from their own experience — can they choose to walk, choose something else, or refuse to walk at all. Being spontaneous and able to change plans, being asked to join in and deciding whether to do so, are all part of decision making and choice. Children need to learn how to communicate 'yes' and 'no' if they are to have a say in what they want and any control over their own lives.

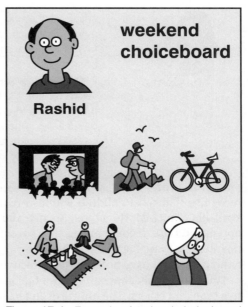

Figure 17.4 *Example of a visual choiceboard*

How can children be taught to indicate 'yes' and 'no'?

Some children with autism answer 'yes' to everything. This may be because the children do not understand that they really have a choice. It may be a learned response to all questions, or a general desire to comply with what others say.

Correctly using 'yes' responses and 'no' responses are important skills that need to be mastered if a child is to become independent. In order to make decisions, 'yes' and 'no' responses should be acknowledged and encouraged.

When initially teaching children to say 'no', intentionally offer them a less preferred food. When they push it away, they are communicating 'no' in a non-verbal way. Their non-verbal response can be imitated and extended to include the verbal 'no' and a shake of the head to teach the appropriate response. The visual sign for 'no' may also be shown (see Figure 17.5).

When a favoured object or food item is unavailable it is important to demonstrate this by

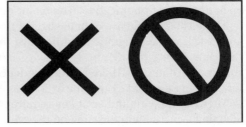

Figure 17.5 *Examples of visuals used to illustrate 'no'*

presenting the message visually. In order to avoid confusion, it is best to show only the choices that are available at the time. It is important to remain alert and keep choice boards 'up to date'. Check before offering a choice that everything on the board is available. If children or adults independently request something that is not available, then show the 'no' sign and offer an alternative. Place a 'no' sign on top or next to the unavailable picture on the choice board (see Figure 17.6).

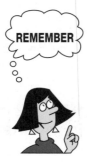

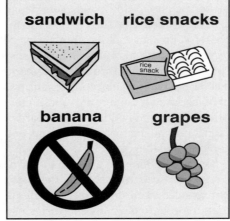

- Constantly update choice boards so that only available options are displayed. If an item is not available, remove it from the board or cover with a 'no' sign to avoid confusion and distress if it is chosen. Choice boards are most effective if they can be modified. Use Velcro to attach pictures to the board so that they can be easily changed or removed if not available.

Figure 17.6 *Visual choice board for food*

The teaching strategies mentioned above provide parents and professionals with some ideas on how to work with, and stimulate, individuals with autism. However, it is also important to recognise that most children will also require specialist intervention, and the sooner this is available to a child, the more effective and successful it is likely to be. There are a number of options and it is recommended that parents do their research about the different approaches that may be available to them. All of the approaches listed below have been widely recognised, although not all have been proven effective.

Different approaches suit different people and no one approach has been proven more effective than any others. The only proven fact is that early intervention is crucial — whatever it is!

What teaching approaches are available and effective?

There are a number of different teaching approaches and methods of working with children and adults with autism that have been independently evaluated over the past few years. It is important that parents and professionals involved with individuals with autism understand the different approaches so that they can make informed choices.

Among the most popular programs that offer intensive early intervention, including applied behavioural analysis, discrete trial training, structured teaching, interactive play strategies and the picture exchange communication system (PECS), all use simple conditioning exercises to open lines of communication. The major differences lie in how the exercises are implemented.

There is no conclusive data to suggest that any one educational methodology, philosophy or model will make a significant difference to every child with autism. According to Dawson & Osterling (1997, p 308), in a survey of nationally recognised early intervention services for children with autism, there is 'little evidence that the philosophy of a given program is critical for ensuring a positive outcome as long as certain fundamental program features are present'

They outlined a number of key requirements for effective early intervention programs that included a curriculum focusing on the strengths and deficits of autism, an environment that is highly structured with high levels of one-to-one support, an acknowledgement of the need for predictability and routine, an emphasis on teaching functional skills, a collaborative approach between parents and teachers, and a program that supports transitions and is intensive.

During the past few years, the focus of intervention with children has moved away from an emphasis on the acquisition of cognitive and language skills using discrete trials in a highly organised and precise style of instruction. Some researchers have suggested that typical characteristics of discrete-trial behavioural approaches may not be the most effective means of facilitating the development of social-communication skills (Wetherby 1986; Seibert & Oller 1981).

The current focus has moved towards developing teaching strategies that accommodate the individual learning styles of children, encourage exploration of both objects and people, encourage social initiation, and emphasise functional communication and social interaction in real-life situations (Janzen 1996; Attwood 2000; Quill 2000).

Pratt, Lantz & Loftin (p 6) are of this view:

The skill and ability to merge effective practices to benefit children with autism spectrum disorders in the general education setting is the art of good teaching. And many of the strategies promoted for students across the autism spectrum, will benefit other children as well.

Children with autism usually demonstrate an uneven pattern of development with verbal and non-verbal communication skills and social skills being limited but visual spatial skills a relative strength. Teaching activities, therefore, are most successful when they are matched to each child's current developmental level, individual learning style, strengths and interests.

Summary

This chapter explores some of the most commonly used approaches to teaching children and adults with autism.

Children and adults with autism think and learn differently from their regular peers and therefore require different approaches to teaching new skills and supporting their social and community integration.

According to research, there is no one method that works definitively for all people with autism. The most effective approach is one that accommodates the particular strengths and deficits of individuals with autism, is highly structured and individualised, provides predictability and routine, teaches functional skills and provides consistency across different settings and teaching methods. Among the most popular strategies used to teach skills are providing visual and verbal cues, prompting, modelling, shaping and chaining. Effective teaching practices are also important to consider.

Individuals with autism learn best in a positive environment where teachers are organised and consistent in their teaching approaches. Specific teaching strategies may be implemented in the classroom, home or work environment to encourage optimal learning but also to ensure that the learning experiences are positive and enjoyable to both teacher and student.

Children and adults should be able to request and to make choices if they are to develop independence. Most individuals need to be motivated to learn these skills, to work towards independence and to understand concepts such as choice making and 'yes' and 'no'. A number of successful approaches have been developed to teach children and adults with autism. It is recommended that these approaches are reviewed by teachers, parents and other professionals working closely with children and adults with autism before they introduce new strategies.

18

Programming Ideas

A good level of skill in one area does not mean an equally good level in another. Pressing someone with an autistic disorder to attempt a task beyond their ability is a sure way of inducing inappropriate behaviour. On the other hand, no progress is made unless new things are tried. Parents and teachers tread a narrow line between too many demands and too few.

Wing 1996, p 128

There are a number of behaviours that cause problems for children and adults with autism and for the people who care for them. This chapter contains practical suggestions on how to handle some of the most common problems that occur at different points of a person's life. Some of the issues may cause concern during the early periods, at home and at preschool, while other behaviours become more problematic at school. Certain behaviours cause concern right through the life of an individual with autism.

How is aggression managed?

Aggression in any environment is of serious concern. Aggressive children and adults may display behaviours such as biting, hitting, pulling hair, kicking or pinching. These behaviours may be self-injurious and also pose a danger to others. They should, therefore, be dealt with swiftly and consistently.

Strategies

Strategies to combat aggression should focus on promoting long-term adaptive alternatives for the individual and also provide immediate strategies to prevent the behaviour from recurring. Aggressive behaviours often occur out of frustration at not being able to communicate effectively or at not being able to understand the communication attempts of others. The following are suggestions to assist parents and teachers to manage and eventually eliminate aggressive behaviours.

- *Remember* that all behaviour is communication — difficult behaviour is often a most effective way of communicating what is wanted or not wanted.
- Begin by looking carefully at the environment. Is there a specific time, place or situation where aggression regularly occurs? Modify the environment to remove any antecedents

(possible causes) that may trigger aggression. This may help prevent the behaviour from occurring again.

- Aggression may continue because of the reinforcement that is inadvertently given when problem behaviour occurs. Children and adults are reinforced when they are given attention, such as when they are given long explanations about why a particular behaviour is not appropriate. Attention is reinforcing even if it is negative attention. If aggressive behaviours are to be reduced, there should be no reinforcing consequence when the behaviour occurs. People with delayed communication skills are unlikely to understand lengthy explanations anyway and so it is more appropriate to merely give a very clear message that the behaviour is not acceptable (a loud and firm 'NO').

- Try to put intervention strategies into effect immediately after aggression occurs and try to avoid reinforcing the behaviour. Give no eye contact, state briefly and firmly 'no hitting/biting/kicking etc', remove the person from the situation and then give attention to the injured party.

- The serious nature of aggressive behaviour means that it cannot be ignored. Such behaviour is not acceptable and should not be tolerated.

- There needs to be a consistent approach to dealing with aggression. All people should follow the same strategies and be very firm in their approach to avoid confusing messages.

- Look carefully at the possible function of the behaviour. What purpose does it serve for an individual? Is the behaviour used to avoid unwanted situations, to obtain attention, or as a means of requesting. For example, does a child bite another child to obtain a toy she wants, or does a young adult hit one of his peers to obtain his attention.

- Whatever the communicative intent of the behaviour, it is important to teach more effective and appropriate ways of communicating and socialising. Introducing visual supports including visual timetables, choice boards, sequences and social stories works for people with autism who are primarily visual learners.

- Acknowledge and respond immediately to any attempts to communicate. This should help to minimise frustration.

- Autism is a social communication disorder, which includes poor comprehension as well as disordered expressive language. When giving information or directions, remember to keep language simple and use visual supports.

- Teach children basic social play skills. If children do not understand turn-taking, waiting or sharing, then they are more likely to become angry and frustrated if other children get too close. This frustration or anxiety may lead to aggression.

- If appropriate, a short period in time-out may be necessary to calm children down. Time-out, however, is not usually recommended as a

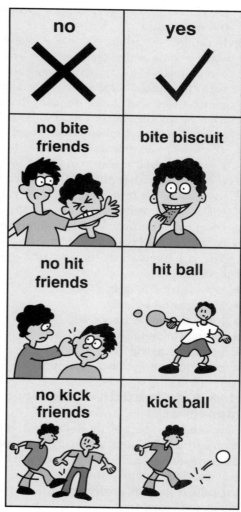

Figure 18.1 *An example of an alternatives board*

management strategy when difficult behaviour occurs. If a person is aggressive to avoid an unwanted situation, then using time-out achieves what the person wants, and the inappropriate behaviour is then reinforced. Time-out is only ever a short-term solution that enables an individual to be removed from a difficult situation and ensures a safe environment for the person to calm down. Time-out should be introduced in a safe place for 2–3 minutes only. With young children, a large beanbag may be an effective time-out option as it is comfortable, safe and difficult to climb out of.

- Emphasis should be placed on teaching more functional and appropriate skills to enable individuals to communicate and socialise more effectively.
- Redirecting people to other activities may avoid an aggressive action if they appear to be getting agitated or frustrated.
- Always reinforce appropriate behaviour. It is important to teach the idea that certain behaviours are unacceptable but it is also important to let individuals know what behaviours are acceptable and appropriate.
- Teach basic survival phrases to help regulate the behaviour of others, such as 'go away', 'give me' or 'my turn'.
- If children or adults are being aggressive to avoid certain activities, it may be possible to compromise. For example, allow a child to play with favourite objects or toys only after completing a short task. Gradually increase the time spent on the 'unwanted' activity and reduce the time spent on preferred activities.
- Teach more acceptable alternatives to aggressive behaviours, as shown in Figure 18.1.
- If appropriate, introduce visual 'Rules Boards' to provide clear messages about rules and routines for different settings. The boards should state clearly what behaviour is accepted, as is shown in Figure 18.2.

The key approaches to managing aggressive behaviours are to:

- provide consistency;
- give clear messages;
- teach alternative responses;
- redirect to more appropriate activities;
- remain firm; and
- reinforce appropriate behaviours.

How are destructive behaviours managed?

Children who engage in destructive behaviour such as throwing toys, emptying out equipment, destroying other children's work or tearing books may have few appropriate play skills and may be frustrated by their environment. They may not understand what is expected of them in a particular play situation, they may not know how to play

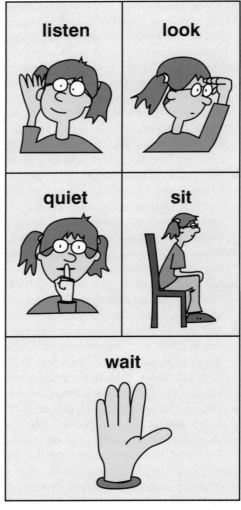

Figure 18.2 *Example of a visual rules board*

with particular toys. They may find throwing, tearing, breaking toys and destroying children's work quite stimulating.

Strategies

Children and adults with autism engage in destructive behaviours because they are frustrated or angry, do not understand what is expected of them in a particular situation, or do not have the necessary skills to respond appropriately.

These children and adults are certainly conveying a message that they are not coping. It may therefore be necessary to modify the environment, but also to teach new skills and alternative responses. Remember that all behaviour serves a purpose and so the first step in any management plan is to determine the function of the behaviour; that is, what the behaviour achieves for an individual.

Destructive behaviour may be a form of sensory stimulation. For example, children who enjoy tearing paper and knocking over other children's constructions may be looking at the effects of their actions. They may like the sound of the ripping paper or enjoy watching the blocks falling. They may be unaware of the consequences of their actions and unsympathetic to the feelings of the other children.

Destructive behaviours also occur because children do not know how to play in any other way. They are unaware of the functions of toys and other play materials, and do not know how to use them appropriately. They may need to be taught appropriate ways of playing with equipment.

Teach appropriate skills in the situations in which they will occur. Emphasis should be placed on teaching social skills to assist children and adults to interact more appropriately.

Determine what purpose a particular behaviour serves for a person and develop strategies to teach alternative, more appropriate responses that will serve the same purpose.

Teach children and adults to understand the consequences of their actions. If appropriate, assist a person to repair any damage, such as picking up any thrown toys, repairing broken equipment or wiping up spills, and then redirect them to something else.

Give a clear message when destructive behaviour occurs. This may be a firm 'NO'. It is important to keep verbal language simple, direct and clear when communicating to avoid giving confusing messages. Trying to reason with individuals with autism will not work. They learn rules and so should be given consistent messages when they break these rules. A firm, clear 'NO' is much more effective and appropriate than a drawn out verbal explanation when an inappro-

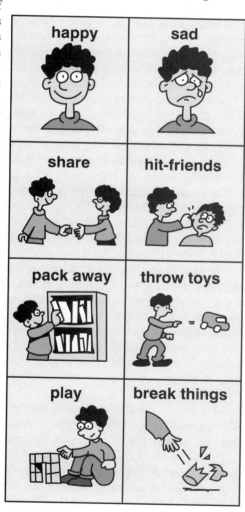

Figure 18.3 *Example of a visual rules board for preschool*

priate behaviour occurs. They should be redirected to another activity, given assistance to complete the task and then given positive feedback for remaining on task.

Rules for behaviour may be established in each setting, discussed, presented visually, and left on display as a constant reminder for everyone involved. Figure 18.3 shows a visual rules board.

A person may be looking for a reaction and may target passive peers who are easily distressed by acts of aggression. Encourage passive individuals to be more assertive — teach them to say 'no'. At the same time, it is also important to teach aggressive individuals to tolerate waiting, sharing and taking turns with others

How can group times be managed in preschool?

Group times are usually difficult sessions to manage at preschool when there is a child with autism in the group. Children with autism do not tend to relate socially to others and prefer to play alone rather than participate in or interact with the other children in group activities.

Strategies

If a child is unable to remain seated with other children during group activities, it may be necessary to modify the session and change expectations. Allow the child time to learn the social rules and gradually be introduced to group time routines.

Initially it may be necessary to simplify expectations. Expecting children to sit for the duration of group time may cause stress and frustration for everyone. Children should be introduced to the group gradually and the length of time spent at group activities slowly increased.

Encourage children to sit for the introduction. Begin the session with an activity that will attract their attention such as bubbles, puppets, balloons, Jack-in-the-Box, pictures, visually augmented songs (see Figure 18.4), musical instrument or taped music.

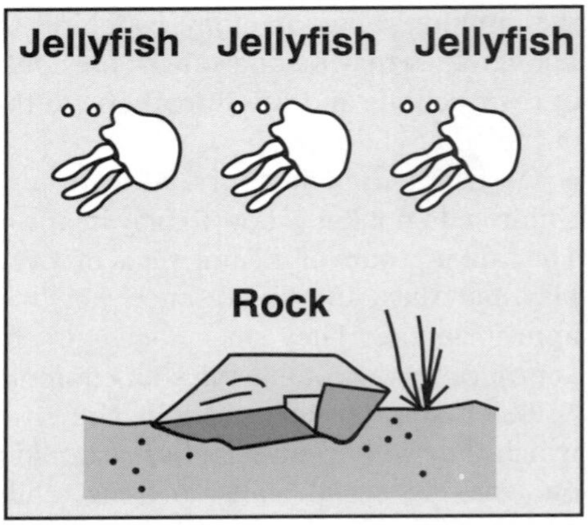

Figure 18.4 *Example of a visually augmented song 'Three Jellyfish'*

Praise children for 'good sitting' and encourage them to remain with the group for as long as possible. If a child is only able to tolerate sitting for short periods, reinforce the good sitting but allow the child to leave the group and go to a quiet area such as book corner before they become disruptive. The objective is to gradually extend the length of time that a child is able to remain with the group and participate in the group activities.

Provide children with information about what will be happening during group time so that they know what to expect. This may be shown as a visual sequence that is discussed with the children at the beginning of the session. Sometimes, children may be offered a choice of activities (see Figure 18.5).

Introduce a visual choice board during singing activities so that children are able to choose what songs to sing (see Figure 18.6). A visual choice board allows the child with autism to participate with the other children, make choices and also understand what is happening in the session.

If children leave the group during the session it is important to remember to bring them back into the group before the end so that they can be a part of the transition to the next activity.

Gradually extend the amount of time that children spend with the group. Initially they may prefer to be seated near the teacher. If resources are available, a member of staff should sit with the children to prompt them through the group activities, to imitate actions, to assist them to remain seated and also to praise them for 'good sitting'.

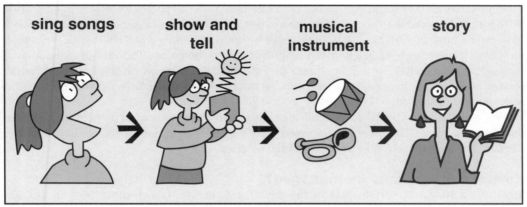

Figure 18.5 *Example of a visual sequence for group time*

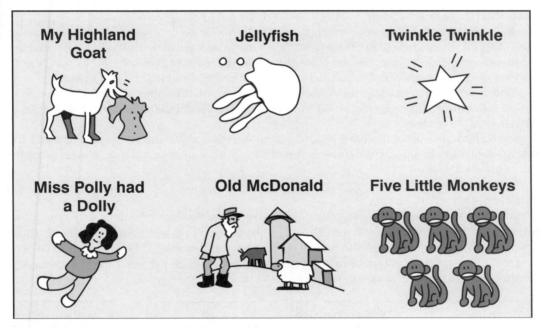

Figure 18.6 *Example of a visual choice board for songs at group time*

Sometimes children may remain calm if they are allowed to hold a favourite object during the session. This should only be allowed while children remain seated and the particular object kept for group time only. If they get up to leave the group, the object may be taken away. Gradually children can be reinforced with a stamp or a sticker for remaining with the group.

If a child becomes distressed by the other children or disrupts the group session, they may be removed to the edge of the mat or even away from the group. One staff member should sit with the child and prompt him or her through the activities while giving little attention or eye contact. The child may be brought back to the group as behaviour improves.

Occasionally children may be too stressed or anxious to participate in large group situations and it may be necessary to provide alternative activities during this period. For example, children may assist a staff member to prepare for the next session or help set the tables for morning tea/lunch. They should not be offered an alternative *fun* activity, as the aim is to eventually encourage them to participate with the other children as their anxiety levels decrease.

Some children find it difficult to sit on a large mat or floor space with no confined seating. Without set boundaries, they may be encouraged to roll around or lay on the floor. Initially they can be prompted to remain in their space by offering them a small chair with their photo on it or a small carpet square that can be positioned in the group. The idea of using a visual support such as a chair or carpet square may assist children to sit on the floor and remain relaxed. Eventually the visual support may be removed and the children seated on the floor with the other children.

Use a visual rules board to remind all children in the group what is expected of them during group time. This may be discussed briefly at the beginning of the session and then displayed as a visual reminder throughout the session.

How can meal times be managed?

Meal times are an important part of the day. They provide opportunities for children and adults to practise social and communication skills as well as the skills necessary to sit and eat independently. Meal times, however, may be difficult for individuals with autism who are not interested in, or motivated by, food.

Some individuals have a sensory impairment. They may be very sensitive to certain tastes and smells or the texture of different foods. They may also have difficulty coping with changes to their routines or the introduction of anything new (including new foods). Many people with autism are fussy eaters with limited diets and/or obsessions around food and eating.

They may not have an appropriate social awareness of what belongs to them and what food belongs to others. They may steal food from to their peers without understanding the distress this may cause to others.

Most children and adults have limited communication skills and do not understand the established, but often unspoken, rules and routines that are an essential part of meal times for most people.

Strategies

Establish a few simple rules to simplify mealtime routines. For example, individuals should sit at the table to eat and drink and they should not be allowed to take other people's food. These rules may be presented visually to ensure that they are understood. It is important to be consistent in the implementation of these routines if they are to be achieved and maintained. A routine for mealtimes is shown in Figure 18.7.

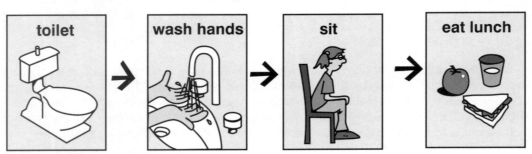

Figure 18.7 *Example of a visual routine for mealtimes*

Provide consistency during meal times by allowing individuals to have a regular place at the table. For example, a placemat with a child's photograph on the front is a visual reminder of where they should be sitting (see Figure 18.8).

Use peers as role models and seat a person with autism near a peer who has good table manners and is able to model appropriate eating skills.

Remember to reinforce appropriate sitting by providing positive feedback to individuals when they are sitting at the table as part of the group.

If necessary, encourage an adult to sit next to, or just behind the individual with autism to prompt him/her to sit and then to remain seated throughout the mealtime. The adult can also keep the person focused on his or her own food and prevent them from stealing other's food.

Do not force people to eat. If a person does not eat, continue to offer them a small portion of food that they usually enjoy. Some individuals with autism have taste and smell sensitivities that limit the type and amount of food they will eat. It is important not to become frustrated with them but to remain positive and continue to offer favoured food. Reinforce for eating. A visual reward strategy, as shown in Figure 18.9, may be used to encourage them to try new foods by offering favoured activities as a reward for trying something new.

Ensure that mealtimes are not stressful times and that everyone recognises and understands simple mealtime routines.

Concentrate on encouraging individuals to sit, even if they do not participate in eating. Initially this may only be for very short periods of time but do try to set some limits on what they are allowed to do during mealtimes if they leave the table.

Parents may be able to offer advice on food preferences and mealtime routines that are in place at home. It is important to work closely with everyone involved with an individual so that information is available across services to ensure a consistent approach. A major aim when working with children and adults with autism is to generalise skills, behaviours, rules and routines across different settings to minimise confusion and anxiety.

Establish a consistent routine for mealtimes. Let individuals know when it is time to pack away, go to the toilet, wash hands and sit at the table. If children or adults are non-verbal or have difficulty processing verbal information, use a visual sequence to show them what is required.

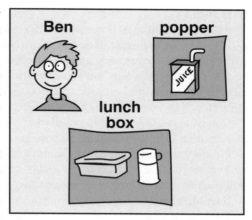

Figure 18.8 *Example of a visual placemat*

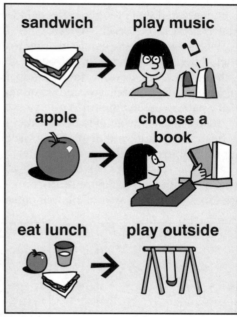

Figure 18.9 *Example of a visual reward strategy for mealtimes*

How are undressing problems managed?

Many children with autism like to strip off clothing. Some children prefer to run around naked or without shoes and socks. It is important to try to determine why a particular behaviour occurs. Children may strip-off because certain textures against their skin feel uncomfortable. They may enjoy the sensation of being naked or may enjoy the fuss and attention received when they remove clothing. Many children with autism have a sensory impairment that may vary from hyper-sensitivity to hypo-sensitivity to different sounds, sights, tastes, touch, movements and smells.

Strategies

The important thing to remember is to remain calm and in control when a child begins to strip off. Have rules in place but do not try to chase the child around forcing them to replace clothing. It all then becomes a game and everyone becomes angry and frustrated.

Discuss the problem with parents to determine possible causes. Do children remove clothing at home and what strategies do parents use to discourage this? Try to introduce a consistent procedure for home and preschool or school.

It may be possible to dress children in difficult to remove clothing such as overalls, playsuits, jeans with a belt, dresses with zippers at back or shorts with buttons.

Whenever children begin to remove clothing, immediately redirect them to a structured activity giving minimal attention to the undressing. Choose an activity that they enjoy and that will occupy their attention for some time.

If children remove clothing, make no comment, give no eye contact, replace the clothing and redirect them quietly and firmly to a more appropriate activity.

If children run away, do *not* chase them. This may be misconstrued as a game and the inappropriate behaviour is then reinforced by lots of attention. If other children make comments, tell them to ignore the behaviour. Try to minimise the fuss and your reactions as well as those of the other children.

Develop some tactile games in order to desensitise children to different textures and the feel of clothing against the skin. Introduce children to different fabrics such as rough towelling, cotton wool, satin, lycra, feathers, sandpaper, and so on. Introduce tickle games, touch games, finger painting, soft scarves, and wrapping children in blankets, for example.

If children continually strip, begin by expecting them to wear one article of clothing and gradually increase the number of items that they must keep on.

Introduce a rule, and display this visually, that children are not allowed outside without a hat (in Summer) or a jumper (in Winter).

A similar rules board can be used to show children that they are not allowed to play outside when it is raining (see Figure 18.10). Some children find it difficult to accept the fact that there are times when they are not allowed outside.

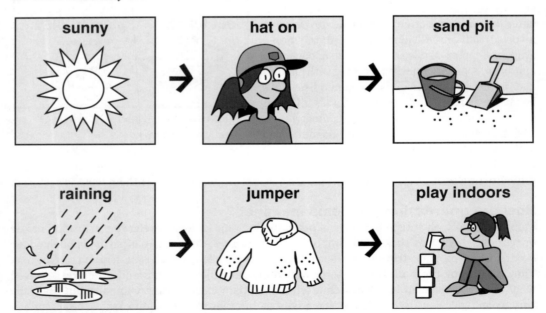

Figure 18.10 *Example of a visual rules board for outdoor play*

A favourite cartoon character or TV personality on an article of clothing may draw children's attention away from the sensitivity issue; for example, Thomas the Tank Engine, Bananas in Pyjamas.

Introduce some contingencies to children such as 'You can play outside if you wear your shoes' as shown in Figure 18.11.

Consistency is important. Any rules that are introduced must also be reinforced in other settings. For example, at home and at preschool, if children strip off they are immediately handed pants and told 'Pants on'. Physical assistance to replace pants may be initially required but keep eye contact and attention to a minimum.

Reinforce children for wearing clothing. If necessary, introduce a reward chart where they are rewarded for keeping clothing on (see Figure 18.12).

Sometimes in hot weather children may be allowed to strip off to play under the sprinkler or in a wading pool. This may be confusing for some children so it is important that the rules are clearly defined. Children need to be shown when stripping is appropriate and when it is not. This may be done visually using photographs.

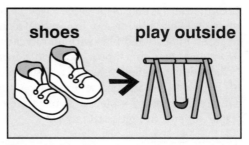

Figure 18.11 *Example of a visual rules board for outdoor play*

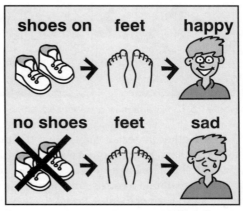

Figure 18.12 *Example of a visual reward chart for wearing shoes*

How is rest time managed at preschool?

Rest time for some children may be a most difficult time of the day. If children are not in the habit of having an afternoon nap at home, it may be hard for them to adapt to a different preschool routine. However, it is important for children to cope with different situations and to learn to follow the general rules and routines of their particular preschool centre. The following suggestions may help make rest time peaceful and stress-free.

Strategies

If children are not accustomed to resting during the day, initially shorten the expected rest period. Gradually increase the time and provide the children with some clear rules to follow. If children are unable to remain on their bed, provide them with a quiet activity away from the other children.

Make the classroom environment more conducive to sleeping/resting. For example, dim the lights, place toys and equipment out of sight, play some restful music, and have teachers sit quietly with the children.

Keep verbal commands to a minimum, and only pat children if they are lying down on their bed. Do not give eye contact to children if they are sitting up or if they attempt to get off their bed.

If children are disruptive, move their bed away from the rest of the group and reinforce them for lying quietly; for example, 'Good resting'.

In some situations it may be necessary for children to rest in another room until they are able to lie quietly on their bed with the other children. This will require adult supervision.

Ask parents for any ideas they use to help settle their child at home at bedtime.

Sometimes it may be possible to use children's interests or obsessions as a motivator to keep them quiet and resting. For example, if a child is interested in numbers, he may be quite happy to sit on his bed and play with an old calculator. If a child is interested in music, she may lie down and listen to a tape of favourite songs on a small Walkman with headset.

Introduce a visual system to reassure children that rest time does not last forever. A picture of them lying on the bed followed by a picture of them reading a favourite book or doing an activity followed by a picture of playtime may help convey this message. This is shown in the visual support in Figure 18.13.

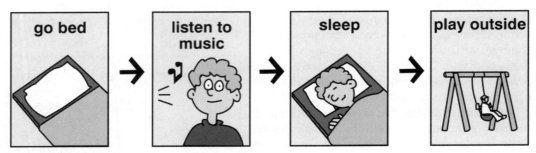

Figure 18.13 *Example of a visual sequence for rest time at preschool*

Some other materials may help settle individual children. Books, a comfort toy, teddy bear, toy car, mazes, puzzles, quiet activities, headphones with a favourite tape or story, sand timers, and liquid timers have all been effective ways to help settle children during rest periods.

Try to maintain a consistent approach in the rest time routine. This will help children to learn what is expected of them. A visual strategy to show children the rest time sequence will be of benefit to all children. Another example of a visual strategy for rest time is shown in Figure 18.14

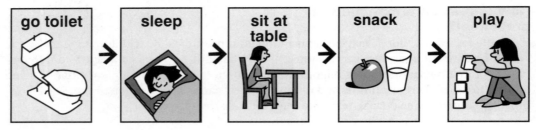

Figure 18.14 *Example of a visual sequence for rest time*

Some children may prefer to bring a favourite bedtime toy from home to make them more comfortable. These toys should only be used at rest time and then put back in the schoolbag to go home.

Introduce a visual reward system for children if they remain quiet during rest period, such as that illustrated in Figure 18.15.

How can sharing and turn-taking be taught?

Sharing is a major concern for both parents and professional workers as children who find it difficult to share and take turns come into conflict with their peers. Children can only be expected to share objects and information with others when they are developmentally ready and when they have been taught the necessary skills.

Children who are willing to share objects with others have generally progressed through three important stages of play and social development:

1. solitary play (no reference to others);
2. onlooker play (observing but not participating); and
3. parallel play (playing alongside other children using similar materials but without interaction).

Once children have moved through parallel play, they are generally more willing to share and take turns with other children. Sharing and taking turns are social activities that form the basis of social interaction and social development in all children.

Strategies

Children with autism have difficulty with many aspects of social development, so sharing and taking turns are skills that must be taught in structured ways. Initially, with young children, it is most appropriate to begin by encouraging them to share with one adult who can model the behaviour and guide them to participate in social activities.

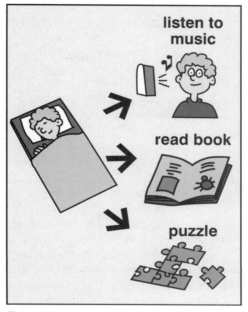

Figure 18.15 *Example of a visual reward system for rest time*

As children become comfortable sharing and taking turns with a familiar adult, another child may be introduced into the activity with additional peers added gradually to make up a small group. All sharing and turn-taking activities involving children with autism should initially be adult directed.

Sharing and turn-taking involves children having to wait. In the beginning, children should be expected to wait only a very short time for another person, preferably a familiar adult, to have one quick turn. Waiting time may gradually be extended as the turns become more equitable and other children are included to share the toys and take turns in the activities. A visual strategy may be employed to assist children to take turns with other children. A small photograph of a child may be glued to one side of a paddle pop stick and a photograph of a familiar adult glued to the other side (see Figure 18.16). The stick may be rotated to indicate whose turn it is at a particular activity.

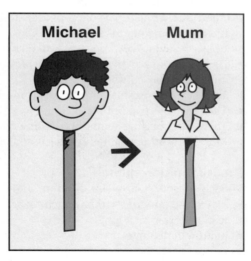

Figure 18.16 *Example of visual turn-taking sticks to teach children to take turns in play*

A visual turn-taking board may be introduced to assist children to wait for their turn as a member of a small group, especially when it involves a preferred activity. Having a visual representation on view allows children to see when their turn is. Children should not have to wait too long for their turn when the turn-taking board is first introduced. Ensure that children's photographs and/or names are clearly displayed on the board (see Figure 18.17). Each child's name and photograph is then removed when their turn is finished.

Social play activities may be introduced at preschool to encourage sharing and turn-taking among young children. More able children should be encouraged to act as role models for children who have difficulty sharing and playing together with other children.

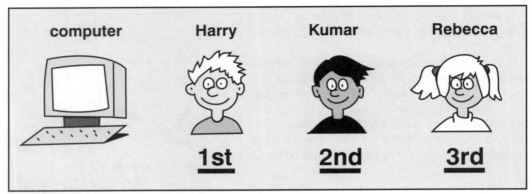

Figure 18.17 *Example of a visual turn-taking sequence board*

During group time at preschool, children should be encouraged to participate in different activities that promote waiting, turn-taking and sharing toys and information.

Suggested activities to promote sharing and turn-taking may include:

- Peek-a-boo games. Hide your face with a scarf. Pull it off and say 'Boo'. Play a turn-taking game and cover each child's head with the scarf and sing 'Where is _____(child's name)'. Children have to wait for their turn.
- Roll a ball, throw a beanbag or push a car to children. Encourage them to return the object.
- In peg board games, take pegs from a container one by one and put into board saying 'My turn, your turn'. Encourage children to have their turn.
- Build a tower using wooden blocks. Take turns with children to put each block on. When tower is complete take turns to knock over 'Ready, set, ... crash'. Extend the waiting time between saying 'set' and 'crash' to encourage children to wait.
- Gross motor activities may include taking turns on swings, slides, tunnels, mini trampolines and other play equipment.
- Take turns threading large beads or macaroni on to a string.
- Take turns to pop bubbles.
- Take turns putting shapes into a shape sorter or box.

More turn-taking games are discussed below.

Discrimination games

Make a sensory board. Use different materials to make a sensory 'feely' board and take turns to match the material. Other matching activities that may involve turn-taking include:

- leaf or flower matching;
- picture matching;
- colour matching;
- lotto card games; and
- picture dominoes.

Listening skills

Ideas to promote listening skills include:

- sounds lotto game — play the tape and take turns identifying the sound;
- follow the noise — take turns when blindfolded to identify which direction a particular sound is coming from;
- hide a noisy toy, such as a ticking clock, wind-up musical toy or radio and encourage children to find it;

- 'Simon says'; and
- whisper games.

Memory games
Encourage the development of concentration by using pairs of picture cards placed face down on the table. Take it in turns to turn over two cards at a time. If a pair is found, it is kept by the person who turned it over.

Fine motor activities
Some fine motor activities include:
- washing — take turns to hang dolls clothes on a clothesline;
- peg design — take turns to follow a pattern to make a design using coloured pegs, beads or blocks;
- fishing game — take turns to fish with a magnet on a piece of string. The 'fish' are paper cut outs with paper clips attached; and
- put pegs onto a container and sort them by colour.

Art and craft activities
Some good art and craft ideas are:
- threading beads;
- nailing wooden shapes into a cork board;
- making a collage by taking turns to paste items on coloured paper; and
- drawing pictures or making patterns sharing different materials including crayons, chalk, Textas, paint, coloured water and paintbrush or wet sand and paddle pop sticks.

Gross motor activities
You can also try the following gross motor activities:
- quoits — take turns to throw rings onto a stick;
- follow the leader, taking turns to be the leader;
- sandpit play — digging and building and sharing utensils;
- outside equipment — walking along a balance beam, climbing through a tunnel, climbing over boards.

How can children be encouraged to interact socially?
Children with autism have difficulty processing information and playing socially with other children. These skills are delayed and disordered in comparison to their peers. Communication is also limited and attempts to communicate may include inappropriate behaviours such as screaming, hitting or pushing other children. Skills required to interact and relate to other children on a social level are also poor. Children with autism have difficulty taking turns, waiting and sharing as these are all 'social' behaviours requiring skills in social interaction.

Strategies
Intervention strategies to encourage children to participate in small and larger group activities and to feel more comfortable around other children, should focus on teaching appropriate social interaction and play skills and providing a means of functional communication.

Engage children with autism in structured play sessions with a familiar adult and guide them through these sessions. Reinforce good playing. A few minutes is enough to begin with. This can be extended to include other children as a child learns to tolerate higher levels of interaction.

Introduce a parallel play activity where the teacher or another child is playing alongside with no demands put on the child with autism. Sharing and turn-taking activities may be gradually introduced into the play activity choosing toys that the child with autism is familiar with and enjoys.

Comment on activities other children are engaged in. Keep the language simple but animated.

Teach children with autism the necessary play skills to interact socially with their peers.

During group time, ensure all children participate in the first and last activities of a session. The entire session may be too long to cope with initially. This way each child starts and finishes the session. Children with autism should be allowed to leave the group and be provided with another activity during the middle section of the session if they are unable to cope with the other children for long periods of time. Gradually extend the time the children stay with the group until they are able to remain for the entire session. Remain positive and verbally reinforce at all times.

It may also be necessary to modify the content of group time to make it more appropriate for children with autism. This may include introducing visual supports such as choice boards, visually augmented songs and stories and simplifying language (see Figure 18.18).

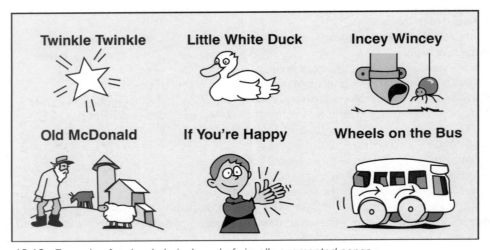

Figure 18.18 *Example of a visual choiceboard of visually augmented songs*

Start by introducing a child into a small group. Introducing a child to small groups of peers is less intrusive and will be less confronting than expecting him or her to cope in a large group without any support. Introduction of activities requiring peer interaction, sharing, turn-taking and communication can help develop play and social skills but only if phased in gradually when the child is settled and comfortable.

Take photographs of children playing with or near the other children in the centre. Use these photographs to make stories that may be used to rehearse social play. Write the child's name and a brief comment under each picture.

Children can take social stories home. Parents can read the stories and talk about their child's friends. Social stories not only provide opportunities for social discussion and for teaching social rules, but also allow parents to see what is happening and to reinforce what is being taught in situations outside the home. See Figures 18.19 and 18.20 for examples of simple social stories.

Introduce the idea of home/school diaries to help children. They also provide information about the day at school that parents can discuss with their child when they arrive home. Pictures of activities that a child completes, examples of completed work, ticket stubs from

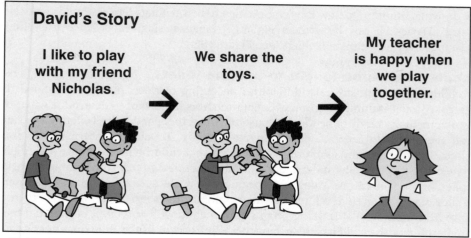

Figure 18.19 *Example of a simple social story that encourages children to share toys*

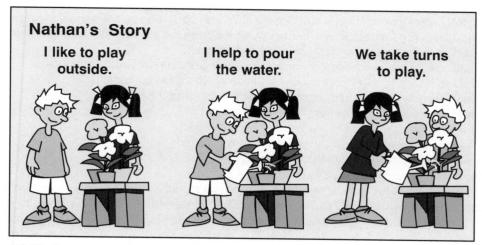

Figure 18.20 *Example of a simple social story that encourages children to take turns in play*

excursions, remnants of packaging from special foods or treats, or the handprint of a friend may be placed in a special folder or book and sent home at the end of the day. This is then used to remind children of their day and provides a prompt for parents in any discussion about the day's events. Home/ school diaries assist children to initiate social conversation with their parents.

Teach children basic survival phrases such as 'my turn', 'your turn', greetings and farewell, 'stop', 'more' and 'help, please' and encourage children to use these in social situations.

Assist children to read other people's body language, including facial expressions. Commenting on other children's emotions and feelings is one

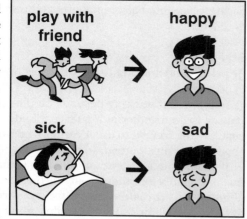

Figure 18.21 *Example of a visual feelings board*

way of drawing attention to how they communicate their feelings. For example 'Jane fell over, she is sad', 'David is happy, he wants a hug'. Keep language simple and, if necessary, introduce visual supports to help explain feelings (see Figure 18.21).

How can children be taught to use the toilet?

Many children with autism have difficulties becoming bladder and bowel trained. Before initiating any toilet training program with children, it is important to determine whether they are developmentally ready to be taught to use the toilet independently. Toileting is a skill that children acquire when they are developmentally ready. Toileting is not usually a problem behaviour. There are a number of prerequisite skills that children must acquire before they are able to learn to use the toilet independently. They also need to feel comfortable about sitting on a toilet before they can be expected to begin using it. Because toileting is a developmental skill, children with delayed development will usually acquire these skills later than their peers.

Before beginning a toilet training program for a child with autism, it is essential to firstly determine whether the child has the necessary skills to begin. If the child does not understand what is required, it is better to place the child back in nappies for a month or two and then try again.

The following signs will help you decide if a child is ready to begin a toilet training program:
- a child stays dry for at least two hours at a time during the day or is dry after their nap;
- a child has regular and predictable bowel movements;
- a child notices that something is happening when urinating without a nappy on;
- a child indicates by words or actions that he or she needs to go to the toilet;
- a child starts to watch other members of the family using the toilet;
- a child is able to take his or her pants on and off;
- a child indicates when his or her nappy is wet or soiled;
- a child indicates when he or she wants a nappy changed;
- a child is comfortable about sitting on a potty or toilet; and
- a child refuses to wear a nappy any longer.

In order to check for signs of readiness, it is often recommended that parents remove their child's nappy. Allow the child to run around naked (preferably outside on a warm day) and watch what happens when they urinate. Because children do not get a sensation of voiding with a nappy on, they will tend to notice that something is happening. If they become distressed and attempt to stop the flow, this indicates an awareness of the process. Parents can then proceed with toilet training. If the child appears unaware of the fact that he or she is urinating, place him back in nappies and wait a little longer. The child is probably not yet ready to toilet train.

Strategies

Be patient and don't try to force the pace. Wait until children are ready and be prepared for lots of accidents.

Independent toileting depends on the acquisition of a number of different skills and then putting them together in sequence. Children have to feel comfortable about sitting on a toilet before being trained to use it regularly. Parents should check that their child feels comfortable about sitting on a potty or toilet without becoming distressed.

If a child refuses to sit on the toilet without becoming distressed, parents need to work on this problem before they go any further. Successful toileting actually involves mastery of two different skills. Children have to feel comfortable about sitting on a toilet or potty and then they have to know how to use the toilet. Finally they also need to learn how to generalise their toileting skills so that they can use a number of different toilets in a range of different settings.

To assist children to overcome any anxiety about sitting on the toilet, parents should:

- Introduce a reward (such as a lolly for sitting); the reward should be given if a child sits down on the potty or toilet (even for 1 or 2 seconds).
- Teach children to sit on the potty as one part of a regular nappy-changing routine. Change children's nappies near the potty and when the soiled nappy is removed, sit the child on the potty for a few seconds before replacing the nappy. No comment about the toilet should be made at this time.
- Do this every time the child's nappy is changed so that it becomes part of a regular routine. Gradually extend the amount of time sitting on the toilet and distract the child with a favourite toy or activity (Thomas the Tank Engine, book, bubbles, calculator or sing a song). This special reward is kept near the toilet or potty and only given when the child sits. The aim is to have children feel comfortable about sitting on the toilet for 3–4 minutes without becoming distressed by pairing something positive with sitting. At this time there is no expectation from the parents that the child will do anything on the toilet except sit happily.

The next step is to determine how a child reacts when they are wet or soiled. Is the child aware that he or she is soiled? Children indicate awareness when they pull at their pants, look down and frown and appear to notice if they are urinating, take off soiled nappies, go off to a particular room or corner to defecate, and become agitated if they need to toilet. Once parents notice these signs in their child, and the child seems comfortable with sitting on a potty or toilet, parents should proceed.

If possible, chart the pattern of a child's toileting habits to provide information about how often the child voids. This indicates how often they will need to be taken to the toilet.

Try to control the child's drinking by offering drinks at set times. Controlling the input of drinks will help to control the child's urinary output.

Remove children's nappy so that they feel and see what is happening when they urinate. This is best done during summer months when the weather is warm and they can play outside. There is minimal mess if accidents happen. Once the nappy is removed, it becomes easier to find a pattern in each child's toileting behaviour. It may be necessary to keep a record at home and at preschool for a few days to determine how often a child urinates. A general rule is to encourage a child to sit on the toilet or potty for 2–3 minutes, about 15–20 minutes after having a drink.

Introduce training pants or pull-ups once children are ready to begin toilet training.

Advise any other services involved that the child is starting a toileting program and ask them to follow through on the program in the other settings. They should use the same strategies and similar visuals and reinforcers.

If children wet or soil their pants, immediately change them without fuss. Do not scold and keep verbal interaction to the minimum. A brief comment such as 'do wee in toilet' acts as a reminder for children. Encourage children to assist with the cleaning up process by giving them a washcloth to help clean themselves or encourage them to put the faeces in the toilet if they have opened their bowels.

Be positive. Praise every little accomplishment and build children's confidence. Ignore accidents and have some tangible rewards ready for when children successfully use the toilet. Keep some special treats in a bag in the cupboard for when a child first uses the toilet. Make a big fuss and immediately offer a reward.

By this time, children should be comfortable about sitting on the toilet for 2–3 minutes with a favourite toy. Use a toilet insert for greater comfort and buy a toilet step to assist with later independence. Make this a fun, positive time so that children stay relaxed.

Play tickle games, blow bubbles and run water to encourage children to urinate on the toilet or potty.

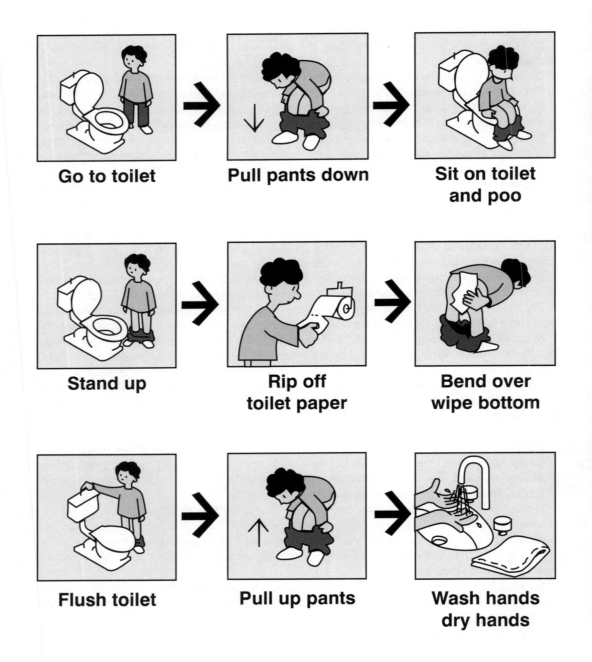

Figure 18.22 *Example of a visual toileting sequence*

Children should be taken to the toilet at regular intervals throughout the day depending on how frequently they usually urinate. This is known as 'toilet timing' and is the first step in the process towards total toileting independence. Children should be toileted on waking in the morning, half an hour after food or drink, at hourly intervals during the day, before bathtime and before bedtime.

Let children set the pace. It is important to remember that complete dryness may take anywhere from a few days to several months. Try not to compare one child with another child. Every child is different and unique and will develop at his or her own individual pace.

Be consistent. Once children are out of nappies, stick with pull-up pant/nappies or training pants and don't go back to nappies unless a child is having lots of accidents and is really not ready to continue the toilet training process. Mixed signals will only lead to confusion.

Use visual representations such as a photographic sequence or a series of line drawings to teach the toileting sequence (see Figure 18.22). Depending on children's comprehension level, either use a single photograph of the toilet or prepare photos of the toileting sequence. These should be placed on the wall near the toilet and children shown each step in the sequence every time they are toileted.

Even if children do not use the toilet successfully every time, still follow the steps of the toileting sequence, including flushing the toilet and washing and drying hands. This is less confusing and helps to teach the whole toileting routine.

Be alert to 'holding' of urine or faeces. Seek immediate medical advice if this occurs. Some children with autism, because of their poor diet and fears, may become constipated. If this occurs, it is worth seeking medical advice early before it becomes chronic.

Use the visual toileting sequence to encourage children to complete all steps involved in the toileting process. Initially, an adult will be required to take children through the sequence and provide physical prompts where necessary. These physical and verbal prompts should be faded as children become more skilled. They should eventually be able to go to the toilet independently.

Generalise children's toileting program to other settings including preschool, grandparents and friends' places and eventually public toilets. Use the visual supports to provide consistency and routine.

Consistency is important during the toileting process, so the same set of visuals should be on the wall at home and at preschool and both parents and preschool staff should use the same approach to toileting.

Try to remain relaxed about the toileting program. Progress may be slow and changes to regular routines may cause occasional setbacks. Success is guaranteed, however, if a consistent approach is maintained and parents remain relaxed and confident.

Summary

A number of behaviours in particular interfere with children's ability to participate in different activities, to integrate successfully into group settings and to behave appropriately in the community. Most of the problems stem back to the core deficits of autism. These deficits affect how individuals with autism read their environment, determine what is important and respond to different stimuli.

Individuals can learn how to behave and respond appropriately in different situations if they are taught the necessary skills, if they are given adequate supports and if the expectations of other people are reasonable. It is important to remain positive, consistent and very structured when working with children and adults to develop their skills and to manage their behaviour.

Appendices

Appendix 1 The False Belief Test (Baron-Cohen, Leslie & Frith, 1985)

In the test, a child observes two dolls — Sally and Anne. Sally has a basket and Anne has a box. Sally and Anne act out a scenario where Sally has a marble that she places in her basket and then leaves the scene. While she is absent, Anne moves the marble from Sally's basket into her own box. And then she also leaves the room. Sally returns and wants to play with her marble. At this point the child is asked the test question: 'Where will Sally look for her marble?' The answer, of course, is 'in the basket'. This answer is correct because Sally has put the marble in her basket and has not seen it being moved. She believes the marble is still where she put it originally. Most of the non-autistic children gave the correct answer by pointing to the basket and showing an understanding that Sally would look in her own basket. However, 80 per cent of the children with autism said that she would look in the box where they knew the marble to be. The findings suggest that, in autism, there is a genuine inability to understand other people's minds.

This is Sally.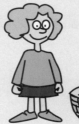

Sally has a basket.

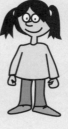 This is Anne.

Anne has a box.

Sally has a marble.

She puts the marble into the basket.

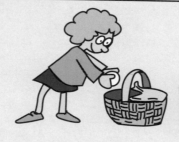 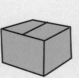 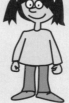

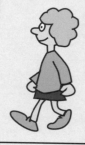 Sally goes out for a walk.

 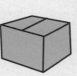 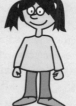

Anne takes the marble out of the basket and puts it in the box.

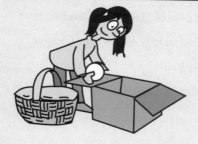

Now Sally comes back.

She wants to play with her marble.

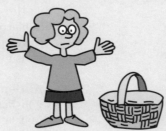

Where will Sally look for her marble?

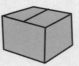

The Sally-Anne Experiment

Appendix 2 Autism in Children Under the Age of 3 Years

Autism is likely when at least 15 of the following 22 symptoms are present:

1. Does not play like other children	☆
2. Appears to be isolated from surroundings	☆
3. There is (or has been) a suspicion of deafness	☆
4. Over-excited when tickled	
5. Difficulties imitating movements	
6. 'Empty' gaze	☆
7. Does not try to attract adults' attention to own activity	☆
8. Plays only with hard objects	☆
9. Occupies self only when alone	☆
10. Does not smile when expected to	
11. Late speech development	
12. Does not point to objects	
13. There is something strange about his/her gaze	☆
14. Late development	
15. Does not understand what people say to him/her	
16. Difficulties getting eye contact	☆
17. Interested only in certain parts of objects	
18. Cannot indicate his/her wishes	
19. It does not matter if there are people around or not	☆
20. There was something the matter already before age 1 year	
21. Exceptionally interested in things that move	
22. Does not listen when spoken to	

☆ = Key Items

Source : C Gillberg et al (1990) 'Autism under age 3 years'. *Journal of Child Psychology and Psychiatry* 31:921–934

Appendix 3 National Contacts

Autism Spectrum Australia (Aspect)
41 Cook St
Forestville NSW 2087
(02) 8977 8300
Infoline: (02) 8977 8377
info@autismnsw.com.au

Autism Association of Qld
437 Hellawell Rd
Sunnybank Hills, Qld 4109
(07) 3273 2222
Infoline: 1800 657 077
mailbox@autism.qld.asn.au

Autism Victoria
PO Box 235
Ashburton Vic 3147
(03) 9885 0533
admin@autismvictoria.org.au

Autism Tasmania
PO Box 1552
Launceston Tas 7250
(03) 6423 1086
www.autismtas.org.au
autism@autismtas.org.au

Autism Association of WA
37 Hay St
Subiaco W Perth 6872
(08) 9489 8900
autismwa@autism.org.au

Autism Association of SA
3 Fisher St
Myrtle Bank SA 5064
(08) 8379 6976
aasa@autismsa.org.au

Autism Association of ACT
PO Box 717
Mawson ACT 2607
(02) 6290 1984
autismact@homemail.com.au

The Hanen Centre
Suite 403–1075 Bay St
Toronto ON M5S 2B1
Canada
(416) 921 1073
info@hanen.org

The Centre for Autism and Related Disabilities (CARD)
Louis de la Parte Florida Mental Health Institute
University of South Florida
13301 Bruce B. Downs Blvd
Tampa Florida 33612-3899
(813) 974 2532
card-usf@fmhi.usf.edu

Appendix 4 Information about Play Programs

Autism Spectrum Australia (Aspect): Early Play Program
Currently available through Autism Spectrum Australia (Aspect):
PO Box 361
Forestville 2087 NSW
(02) 8977 8377
helpdesk@autismnsw.com.au
The *Early Play Manual* is being published in 2004 by Jessica Kingsley Publishers.

Hanen Program: More Than Words
The Hanen Program is available in most states of Australia. Information about the program is available through the Hanen Centre:
Suite 403-1075 Bay St
Toronto ON M5S 2B1
Canada
info@hanen.org
The *More Than Words Manual* is also available through the Hanen Centre.

National Autism Society (London): Early Bird Program
Information about the services run by the National Autism Society (London) is available by contacting the NAS in London:
393 City Road
London EC1V 1NG
The Early Bird Program also has a parent training manual. For more information about the Manual and the Parent Training Program contact the NAS in London.

Treatment and Education of Autistic and related Communication handicapped Children (TEACCH): Together Group
University of North Carolina
Chapel Hill NC 27599-7180
(919) 966 2174

Appendix 5 Suggested Reading Materials

For parents
Attwood T 1998 *Asperger's Syndrome: A Guide for Parents and Professionals*. London, Jessica Kingsley Publishers

Bailey M 1998 *Toilet Training Program*. Sydney, Autism Association of NSW

Brennan L, Dodd S & Fryer M 2002 *Transition to School Program*. Sydney, Autism Association of NSW

Dodd S 1994 *Managing Problem Behaviours: A Guide for Parents and Preschools*. Sydney, MacLennan & Petty

Dodd S, Pierce E & Webster S 2001 *Early Play Program* 2nd Ed. Sydney, Autism Association of NSW

Hodgdon LA 1995 *Visual Strategies For Improving Communication*. Michigan, Quirk Roberts Publishing

Holliday Willey L 1999 *Pretending to be Normal*. London, Jessica Kingsley Publishers

Holliday Willey L 2001 *Asperger Syndrome in the Family*. London, Jesica Kingsley Publishers.

Howlin P, Baron-Cohen S & Hadwin J 2000 *Teaching Children with Autism to Mind-Read*. NY, Wiley

Jackson, J 2003 *Multicoloured Mayhem: Parenting the Many Shades of Adolescence*. London, Jessica Kingsley Publishers

Janzen J E 1999 Autism. *Facts and Strategies for Parents*. USA, Therapy Skill Builders

McAfee J 2002 *Navigating the Social World. Arlington*, Future Horizons

Quill KA 2000 *Do-Watch-Listen-Say*. Baltimore, Paul H. Brookes

Sussman F 1999 *More Than Words*. Ontario, The Hanen Program

Yapko D 2003 *Understanding Autism Spectrum Disorders*. London, Jessica Kingsley Publishers

For young children
Amenta CA 1992 *Russell is Extra Special*. New York, Magination Press

Davies J 1997 *Able Autistic Children — Children with Asperger's Syndrome*. Nottingham, Child Development Research Unit, University of Nottingham

Lears L 1998 *Ian's Walk, A Story about Autism*. Illinois, Albert Whitman & Co

Vermeulen P 2000 *I am Special. Introducing Children and Young People to their Autistic Spectrum Disorder*. London, Jessica Kingsley Publishers

For adolescents
Holliday Willey L 2003 *Living with the Ups, the Downs and Things in Between*. London. Jessica Kingsley Publishers

Hoopman K 2001 *Of Mice and Aliens*. London, Jessica Kingsley Publishers

Jackson L 2002 *Freaks, Geeks and Asperger Syndrome*. London, Jessica Kingsley Publishers

For adults
Aston MC 2001 *The Other Half of Asperger Syndrome*. London, The National Autistic Society

Aston M 2003 *Asperger's in Love*. London, Jessica Kingsley Publishers

Datlow Smith M, Belcher RG & Juhrs PD 1995 *A Guide to Successful Employment for Individuals with Autism*. Baltimore, Paul H. Brookes

Meyer RN 2001 *Asperger Syndrome Employment Workbook*. London, Jessica Kingsley Publishers

Appendix 6 What to Look for in a Preschool

The following questions may assist parents to choose a preschool that will benefit their child and meet their child's particular needs:

- Do staff members have experience working with children with special needs, especially children with autism and related disorders?
- What access does the preschool have to additional help and support for children with disabilities that they can call on if necessary?
- Does the preschool develop and implement individualised programs for each child and cater to their particular needs and strengths?
- How structured is the preschool and does it have a regular daily routine that is followed?
- Do the preschool staff members encourage consultation with other agencies and seem happy to share information and ideas?
- Are there policies and procedures in place at the preschool that are based on specific government standards and protect the rights of each child?
- Are family members encouraged to participate in regular sessions, visit the preschool and have regular consultation with their child's teacher?
- Are the toys and teaching materials well looked after, complete and challenging for the children?
- Are the toys and teaching materials set out in such a way to encourage children to explore new activities and interact with their peers?
- Is there a range of toys and teaching materials available to cater for children's different learning styles and ability levels?
- Is there a policy in place that encourages all staff members to work with the special needs children so that children learn to generalise skills?
- Are visual supports used in the preschool for all children as part of their daily routines?
- Are the visual supports age-appropriate, easily accessible and used widely throughout all of the different activities? Supports may include visual timetables, choice boards, augmented songs and sequences.
- Do the staff members keep records on each child's progress, regularly send information home and have written programs for each child?
- Is there an emphasis on individual, small group and large group instruction throughout the day?
- Does the preschool have a structured transition process for children who will be starting school?
- Is the preschool centre a nationally accredited service?

Day care centres/ child care centres/ long day care centres

These centres provide intervention and support for children from birth to 6 years. Long day care operates for extended hours, usually between 8 and 12 hours daily for at least 48 weeks per year. Because the centres accommodate babies and toddlers, they require trained staff members to be present. Meals are often provided.

Preschool centres

Provide structured educational programs and care for children over 3 years. Most centres require children to be toilet trained (or toilet timed) prior to enrolment. Most centres operate during school hours and follow normal school terms. Meals are not generally provided.

Occasional child care centres

Provide education and care for children aged birth to 6 years. The centres tend to offer short-term care and usually have limits on the amount of time parents can access the program each month. Tend to be used more as babysitting services and are not usually structured enough for children with autism. Meals are not generally provided.

Glossary

Abstract reasoning: the ability to think in terms of ideas and general concepts rather than only in concrete facts.

Affect: the emotional tone a person expresses. A person's affect may be appropriate or inappropriate to the situation. Individuals with autism may be described as having a flat affect.

Antecedent conditions: conditions that occur just prior to problem behaviour that may impact on why the behaviour occurs.

Applied behaviour analysis (ABA) therapy: psychological teaching method that relies on the use of shaping and positive reinforcement to replace dysfunctional behaviours with functional skills.

Attention deficit/hyperactivity disorder (AD/HD): neurological disorder characterised by deficits in attention and/or hyperactivity/compulsivity.

Auditory discrimination: the ability to discriminate between words that are similar or different in the way they sound.

Auditory memory: the ability to remember accurately an auditory stimulus.

Auditory processing: the ability to recognise and identify sounds and words and to understand what they mean.

Autism spectrum: refers to all of the different autism diagnoses along a continuum.

Casein-free diet: a diet that is free from any animal milk or milk products.

Central coherence: is the ability to focus on both details as well as wholes. People with autism appear to have a heightened focus on details rather than on wholes, a cognitive style termed 'weak central coherence'. This accounts for why some individuals with autism have hypersensitive sensory perceptions.

Chaining: a behavioural technique in which a complex skill is broken down into its separate components and taught step by step. The last step in the sequence is usually taught first because it is followed by immediate reinforcement (backward chaining).

Chunking: breaking down a complex task into smaller incremental steps or chunks. The complete task is eventually mastered by firstly mastering each small step individually.

Cognition: pertains to the mental processes of thinking, knowing, and reasoning.

Cognitive: relates to intelligence or the ability to think abstractly, to reason and to problem solve.

Comic strip conversation: is a conversation between two or more people that incorporates the use of simple drawings. These drawings serve to illustrate an ongoing communication providing additional support to individuals who struggle to comprehend the quick exchange of information that occurs in a conversation.

Co-morbid disorders: the co-existence of two or more disease processes or disorders.

Concrete thinking: thinking that focuses on facts, figures and details rather than on concepts, ideas or theories.

Consequences: what happens after problem behaviour occurs that influences the likelihood that the behaviour will occur again in the future.

Contingency management: operant or instrumental conditioning ensuring that a desired behaviour is followed by positive consequences and that undesired behaviour is not rewarded.

Contract: formal or informal written or verbal agreement between two or more parties on a specific course of action. Contracts may be presented in a visual format.

Desensitisation: treatment used to reduce anxiety by making a previously threatening stimulus innocuous by repeated and guided exposure to the stimulus under non-threatening circumstances.

Didactic: intended to convey instruction or factual information.

Discrete trial training: a method of teaching new skills based on the applied behaviour analysis model. Each new skill is taught in small and brief units called trials. Each trial consists of an instruction, a prompt, an opportunity/response and feedback.

Dyspraxia: difficulties associated with motor planning.

Echolalia: The repetition of speech produced by others. The echoed words or phrases can include the same words and exact inflections as originally heard, or may be slightly modified.

Empathy: the ability to understand the thoughts and emotions of another person.

Etiology: the study or science of the causes of specific diseases or disorders.

Executive function: the ability to plan and organise tasks, monitor one's own performance, inhibit inappropriate responses, utilise feedback, and suppress distracting stimuli.

Fade: to gradually withdraw either prompts or reinforcers to encourage the completion of a task without the need for outside influence.

Flat affect: a severe reduction in emotional expressiveness, the individual may not show signs of normal emotion, perhaps may speak in a monotonous voice and have diminished facial expression.

Fluctuation: the change or movement in skills over time so that they do not remain constant.

Generalisation: the transfer of skills learned in one context to different contexts, including the ability to use the skills in different locations, with different people and at different times.

Genome: the total genetic material of an organism, comprising the genes contained in its chromosomes. The human genome comprises 23 pairs of chromosomes.

Gestalt processing: the distinct information processing mode common to individuals with autism. Information is taken in, recorded, and stored quickly in whole units, or 'chunks', without analis for meaning.

Gluten-free diet: a diet that is free from wheat, rye, barley and oats or any products containing these grains.

Gustatory: relating to the sense of taste or to the organs of taste.

Hierarchy of visual representation: a graded list of visual supports that may be introduced to individuals according to their ability to understand that the visual represents the real object.

Hyperlexia: a preoccupation with letters and words at an early age, and exceptional word-recognition skills with delayed comprehension of meaning.

Hypersensitivity: reflects a heightened response to a particular sensory experience, as the sensations are registered too intensely.

Hyposensitivity: reflects a dampened response to a particular sensory experience, as the sensations are registered less intensely than normal.

Incidence: measures the development of 'new' cases and is usually studied for cases with clear onset.

Individual education plan (IEP): a written plan describing the special education program and/or services required by a particular student. It identifies learning expectations that are modified from or alternative to the expectations given in the curriculum. It also documents any accommodations and special education services needed to assist the student in achieving his or her learning expectations.

Inhibition: the process of concentrating on what are important and ignoring meaningless sensations.

Jargon: a form of speech that is made up of unintelligible sounds without meaning.

Joint attention: the social act of obtaining someone's attention in order to share either information or an object.

Kanner autism: so-called 'classic' autism as described by Leo Kanner in 1943.

Kinaesthesia: the sense that enables the brain to be constantly aware of the position and movement of muscles in different parts of the body.

Literal thinking: adhering to facts or to the ordinary construction or primary meaning of a term or expression that is free from exaggeration or embellishment.

Mastery: the point at which a task is completed correctly nine times out of ten or three times in a row.

Metabolic disorders: relating to metabolism, the range of biochemical processes that occur within all living organisms.

Mitigated echolalia: is a form of echolalia where some changes occur either in the form or intonation of an echolalic utterance demonstrating a more creative use of language.

Modulation: the process of balancing incoming sensory information to function efficiently.

Neuro-typical population: refers to the general population with no known disabilities.

Olfactory: pertaining to the sense of smell.

Overload: an inability to filter out what is not important or to selectively attend to things.

Perseveration: The redundant repetition of words, thought or motor movements without the ability to stop or move on.

Pervasive developmental disorders (PDD): an umbrella term that refers to the spectrum of disorders that includes autism, Asperger's syndrome, pervasive developmental disorder not otherwise specified (PDD-NOS), Rett's disorder and childhood disintegrative disorder. Individuals have severe impairments in reciprocal social interactions and communication skills and frequently have stereotyped behaviour, interests and activities.

Pica: from the Latin word for 'magpie'. An eating disorder typically defined as the persistent eating of non-nutritive substances.

Picture exchange communication system (PECS): is a unique augmentative alternative training package that allows children and adults with autism and other communication deficits to initiate communication. First used at the Delaware Autistic Program, PECS has received worldwide recognition for focusing on the initiation component of communication. PECS does not require complex or expensive materials. It was created with educators, resident care providers and families in mind, and so it is readily used in a variety of settings.

Prader-Willi syndrome: a congenital condition in which obesity is associated with mental retardation and small genitalia; diabetes mellitus frequently develops in affected individuals.

Pragmatics: the social use of language.

Praxis or motor planning: the ability to plan and execute different motor tasks.

Prevalence: measures the number of individuals with a condition at a point in time or over a defined period.

Prompt: to encourage, remind or cue someone to do something. Prompts may take several forms from physical prompts to verbal prompts. Prompts should be faded gradually as skills are learned.

Proprioceptive sense: assists in the processing and understanding of information relating to gravity, the positioning and movement of the body, the movement that is perceived in the local environment and the full range of internal sensation.

Prosody: as it applies to speech, prosody is comprised of the pitch/intonation, loudness and tempo of the spoken words.

Protodeclarative pointing: pointing as a means of sharing information and attention with another person.

Protoimperative pointing: pointing as a means of communicating a desire for a particular object.

Savant: individuals who have extraordinary, or splinter, skills not usually seen in the general population.

Semantics: the meanings of words and expressions.

Sensory integration: refers to the process of creating efficient sensory pathways and connections in the central nervous system.

Sensory processing: includes an ability to register, decode, comprehend and categorise sensory information from a number of different sources. The ability to organise and interpret information that is received through the senses.

Sequencing: arrangement that follows a particular hierarchical order.

Shaping: a method of teaching new behaviour in a graded step-by-step way by reinforcing the individual for a close approximation of the target behaviour. Successively closer approximations to the target behaviour are then reinforced/rewarded until it is mastered.

Social stories: are a tool for teaching social skills to children with autism and related disabilities. Social stories provide an individual with accurate information about those situations that he or she may find difficult or confusing.

Stereotypic behaviours: the constant repetition of a complex action, which is carried out in the same way each time.

Structured teaching: Structured teaching is an intervention philosophy developed by the University of North Carolina, Division TEACCH (Treatment and Education of Autistic and related Communication Handicapped Children). Structured teaching is an approach in instructing children with autism. It allows for implementation of a variety of instructional methods (e.g., visual support strategies, picture exchange communication system (PECS), sensory integration strategies, discrete trial, music/rhythm intervention strategies.

Syntax: the study of the rules whereby words or other elements of sentence structure are combined to form grammatical sentences.

Tactile: relating to or affecting the sense of touch.

Theory of mind: the ability to understand or predict what another person thinks, feels, desires, intends or believes about something.

Triggers: an event that precipitates a certain behaviour or response.

Vestibular: senses that convey information about the body's posture and movements in space and allow coordination and balance.

Visual discrimination: the ability to discern similarities and differences visually.

Visual figure ground: the ability to visually attend to the designated stimulus and not be distracted by the background.

Visual memory: the ability to store and retrieve information that has been given with a visual stimulus.

Visual motor: the ability to relate visual stimuli to motor responses in an appropriate way.

Visual tracking: the ability to track one's eyes from left to right in an efficient manner to enable a task to be completed quickly.

WISC-R: a Wechsler intelligence scale for children (WISC) is a test used by psychologists to identify learning disabilities. The WISC-R (R=Revised) is an intelligence test that can be administered only by a licensed psychologist or tester.

References

Aarons, M. & Gittens, T. (1992). *Autism. A Guide for Parents and Professionals.* London, Tavistock/Routledge.

Adrien, J. L., Barthelemy, C., Perrot, A., Roux, S., Lenoir, P., Hameury, L., & Sauvage, D. (1992). 'Validity and Reliability of the Infant Behavioural Summarized Evaluation (IBSE): A Rating scale for the Assessment of Young Children with Autism and Developmental Disorders.' *Journal of Autism and Developmental Disorders* 22(3): 375–94.

Adrien, J. L., Faure, M., Perrot, A, Hameury, L., Garreau, B., Barthélémy, C., & Sauvage, D. (1991). 'Autism and Family Home Movies: Preliminary Findings.' *Journal of Autism and Developmental Disorders* 21(1): 43–9.

Adrien, J. L., Lenoir, P., Martineau, J., Perrot, A., Hameury, L, Larmande, C., & Sauvage, D. (1993). 'Blind Ratings of Early Symptoms of Autism Based Upon Family Home Movies.' *Journal of the American Academy of Child and Adolescent Psychiatry* 32(3): 617–26.

Almy, M., Monighan, P., Scales, B., & Van Horn, J., Ed. (1984). *Recent research on play: The teachers perspective. Current topics in early childhood education.* Norwood, N.J., Ablex.

Amenta, C. A. (1992). *Russell is Extra Special.* New York, Magination Press.

American Journal of Orthopsychiatry 26: 55–65.

American Psychological Association (1994). *Diagnostic and Statistical Manual of Mental Disorders.* Washington D.C., American Psychiatric Association, 4th edition (DSM-IV).

Andron, L. (Ed.) (2001). *Our Journey Through High Functioning Autism and Asperger's Syndrome.* London, Jessica Kingsley Publishers.

Arkwright, N. (1995). *An Introduction to Sensory Integration.* Arizona, Therapy Skill Builders.

Asperger, H. (1944). 'Die "Autistichen Psychopathen" im Kindersalter'. *Archive fur Psychiatrie und Nervenkrankheiten.* 117: 76–136.

Asperger, H. (1991). 'Autistic psychopathology in childhood.' *Autism and Asperger syndrome.* Cambridge, England, Cambridge University Press: 37–92.

Aston, M. C. (2001). *The Other Half of Asperger Syndrome.* London, The National Autistic Society.

Attwood, T. (1993). 'Unusual behaviours associated with autism'. *Health Visit* 66(11):402–3.

Attwood, T. (1998). *Asperger's Syndrome. A Guide for Parents and Professionals.* London, Jessica Kingsley Publishers.

Attwood, T. (2000). 'Strategies for Improving the Social Integration of Children with Autism.' *Autism* 4(1): 85–100.

Autism Society of America. *Next Steps: A Guide for Families New to Autism.* Autism Society of America Publication. Seattle, Washington.

Ayres, A. J. (1972). *Sensory Integration and Learning Disabilities.* Los Angeles, Western Psychological Services.

Ayres, A. J. (1979). *Sensory Integration and the Child.* Los Angeles, Western Psychological Services.

Ayres, A.J. (1989). *Sensory Integration and Praxis Tests.* Los Angelos, Western Psychological Services.

Bailey, A. (1995). 'Autism as a strongly genetic disorder: evidence from a British twin study.' *Journal of Psychological Medicine* 25: 63–77.

Baird, S. & Peterson, J. (1997). 'Seeking a Comfortable Fit Between Family-Centred Philosophy and Infant-Parent Interaction in Early Intervention: Time for a Paradigm Shift?' *Topics in Early Childhood Special Education* 17(2): 139.

Bandura, A. (1969). *Principles of Behaviour Modification.* San Fransisco, CA: Holt, Rinehart & Winston.

Bandura, A. (1993). 'Perceived self-efficacy in cognitive development and functioning'. *Educational Psychologist.* 28(2):117–48.

Baron-Cohen, S. & Bolton, P. (1993). *Autism: The Facts.* Oxford University.

Baron-Cohen, S. (1987). 'Autism and Symbolic Play.' *British Journal of Developmental Psychology* 5: 139–48.

Baron-Cohen, S. (1988). 'Social and Pragmatic Deficits in Autism: Cognitive or Affective.' *Journal of Autism and Developmental Disorders* 18(3): 370–402.

Baron-Cohen, S. (1989). 'Perceptual role-taking and protodeclarative pointing on autism'. *British Journal of Developmental Psychology* 7: 113–27.

Baron-Cohen, S. (1991). 'The theory of mind deficit in autism: how specific is it? *British Journal of Developmental Psychology* 9: 310–14.

Baron-Cohen, S. (1995). *Mindblindness: An Essay on Autism and Theory of Mind.* MIT Press/Bradford Books.

Baron-Cohen, S. (2000). 'Early identification of autism: the Checklist for Autism in Toddlers (CHAT).' *Journal of the Royal Society of Medicine* 93: 521–25.

Baron-Cohen, S. (2003). *The Essential Difference: The Truth about the Male and Female Brain.* Perseus Publishing, U.K.

Baron-Cohen, S., Allen, J. & Gillberg, C. (1992) 'Can autism be detected at 18 months? The needle, the haystack and the CHAT.' *British Journal of Psychiatry.* 161: 839–43.

Baron-Cohen, S., Leslie, A. M., & Frith, U. (1985). 'Does the autistic child have a "theory of mind"?.' *Cognition* 21: 37–46.

Barron, J. & Barron, S (1992). *There's A Boy In Here.* New York, Simon & Schuster.

Bauman, M. & Kemper, T. (1994). *Neurobiology of Autism.* Baltimore, Johns Hopkins.

Belser, R. & Sudhalter, V. (1995). 'Arousal difficulties in males with Fragile-X Syndrome: a preliminary report'. *Developmental Brain Dysfunction.* 8: 270–9.

Berk, L. (2002). 'Cognitive Development in Early Childhood.' *Infants and Children: Prenatal through Middle Childhood.* Boston, MA, Allyn & Bacon: 323–63.

Bettelheim, B. (1956). 'Childhood schizophrenia as a reaction to extreme situations.' *Journal of Orthopsychiatry* 26: 507–18.

Bettelheim, B. (1967). *The Empty Fortress.* Free Press, N.Y.

Bettison, S. (1996). 'The long-term effects of auditory training on children with autism' *Journal of Autism and Developmental Disorders.* 26(3):361–74.

Beyer, J. & Gammeltoft, L. (2000). *Autism and Play.* London, Jessica Kingsley Publishers.

Blakemore-Brown, L. (2002). *Reweaving the Autistic Tapestry.* London, Jessica Kingsley Publishers.

Boardmaker (2001). *Spectronics.* California, Mayer-Johnson Inc. Version 5.

Bondy, A. & Frost, L. (1994). 'The Picture Exchange Communication System.' *Focus on Autistic Behaviour* 9(3): 1–19.

Bondy, A. & Frost, L. (1998). 'The picture exchange communication system.' *Advocate* 30(5): 7–9.

Bondy, A. (2001). 'PECS: Potential benefits and risks.' *The Behaviour Analyst Today* 2: 127–32

Boon Hong, T. 'Coping with Bullying.' *Arc Newsletter* 3(4): 2–9.

Boucher, J. (1999). 'Editorial: interventions with children with autism — methods based on play.' *Child Language Teaching and Therapy* 15(1): 1–5.

Bovee, J., P. (1999). 'My experiences with autism and how it related to Theory of Mind — Part 1.' *Advocate* 32(5): 18–19.

Brennan, L., Dodd, S., & Fryer, M. (2002). *Transition to School Program.* Sydney, Autism Association of NSW.

Brofenbrenner, U. (1979). *The Ecology of Human Development.* Cambridge, MA, Harvard University Press.

Brown, C.C. & Gottfried, A.W. (1985). *Play Interactions: The Role of Toys and Parental Involvement in Children's Development.* Skillman, N.J.: Johnson & Johnson Baby Products.

Buggey, T. (1995). 'Video-taped self-modeling: The next step in modeled instruction'. *Early Education and Development* 6: 39–51.

Buggey, T. (1999). 'Using videotaped self-modeling to change behaviour'. *Teaching Exceptional Children.* March/April, 27–30.

Buggey, T., Toombs, K., Gardener, P., & Cervetti, M. (1999). 'Training responding behaviours in students with autism: Using videotaped self-modeling'. *Journal of Positive Behavioural Intervention.* 1: 205–14.

Burgoine, E. & Wing, L. (1983). 'Identical Triplets with Asperger's Syndrome.' *British Journal of Psychiatry* 143: 261–5.

Carr, E. & Darcy, M. (1990). 'Setting Generality of Peer Modeling in Children with Autism.' *Journal of Autism and Developmental Disorders:* 45–59.

Carr, E., & Dores, P. (1981). 'Patterns of language acquisition following simultaneous communication with autistic children.' *Analysis and Intervention in Developmental Disabilities* 1: 1–15.

Carr, E., Pridal, C., & Dores, P. (1984). 'Speech versus sign comprehension in autistic children. Analysis and prediction.' *Journal of Experimental Child Psychology* 37: 587–97.

Charlop-Christy, M.H. (2000). 'Assessment of emerging speech and social behaviours and problem behaviour reduction as a function of PECS.' Paper presented at the first annual PECS Expo. San Diego, CA.

Charlop-Christy, M.H., Carpenter, M., Le Loc, LeBlanc, L., & Kellet, K. (2002). 'Using the Picture Exchange Communication System (PECS) with Children with Autism: Assessment of PECS Acquisition, Speech, Social-Communicative Behaviour and Problem Behaviour.' *Journal of Applied Behaviour Analysis* 35: 213–31.

Charlop-Christy, M.H., Le, Loc, & Freeman, K.A. (2000). 'A comparison of video modeling with in vivo modeling for teaching children with autism'. *Journal of Autism and Developmental Disorders.* 30, 532–7.

Charman, T. & Baron-Cohen, S. (1997). 'Brief Report: Prompted Pretend Play in Autism.' *Journal of Autism and Developmental Disorders* 27(3): 325–32.

Corbett, B. (2003). 'Video Modeling: Applications for children with autism spectrum disorders'. M.I.N.D. Institute, Dept Psychiatry and Behavioural Sciences.

Courchesne, E. (1995). 'New evidence of cerebellar and brainstem hypoplasia in autistic infants, children and adolescents: the MR imaging study by Hashimoto and colleagues.' *Journal of Autism and Developmental Disorders.* 25(1): 19–22.

Courchesne, E. (2002). 'Abnormal early brain development in autism.' *Molecular Psychiatry.* 2: 521–3.

Courchesne, E., Carper, R. & Akshoomoff, N. (2003). 'Evidence of Brain Overgrowth in the First Year of Life in Autism.' *Journal of the American Medical Association* 290: 337–44.

Courchesne, E., Towsend, J., Akshoomoff, N., et al (1994). 'Impairment in shifting attention in autistic and cerebellar patients.' *Behavioural Neuroscience* 108: 848–65.

D'Souza, R., Campbel-Lloyd, S., Isaacs, D., Gold, M., Burgess, M., Turnbull, T., & O'Brien, E. (2000). 'Adverse events following immunization associated with the 1998 Australian Measles Control Campaign'. *Communicable Diseases Intelligence*. 24(2).

Dahlgren, S.O. & Gillberg, C. (1989). 'Symptoms in the first 2 years of life. A preliminary population study of infantile autism.' *European Arch. Psychiatry Neurological Science*. 238(3): 169–74.

Dales, L., Smith et al (2001). 'Time trends in autism and in MMR immunisation coverage in California.' *JAMA* 285: 1183–5.

Datlow Smith, M., Belcher, R.G. & Juhrs, P.D. (1995). *A Guide to Successful Employment for Individuals with Autism*. Baltimore, Paul H. Brookes.

Davies, J. *Able Autistic Children — Children with Asperger's Syndrome*. Nottingham, Child Development Research Unit, University of Nottingham.

Dawson, G. & Osterling, J. (1997). 'Early intervention in autism: Effectiveness and common elements of current approaches.' *The effectiveness of early intervention: Second generation research.* M. J. Guralnick. Baltimore, Paul H. Brookes: 307–26.

Dawson, G. E. (1989). *Autism: Nature, Diagnosis and Treatment*. New York and London, Guildford Press.

Dawson, G., Meltzoff, A. N., Osterling, J., Rinaldi, J., & Brown, E. (1998). 'Children with Autism Fail to Orient to Naturally Occurring Social Stimuli.' *Journal of Autism and Developmental Disorders* 28(6): 479–85.

DeMyer, M. K. (1975). 'The nature of neuropsychological disability in autistic children.' *Journal of Autism and Childhood Schizophrenia* 8: 109–28.

Department of Education and Training. (1997). The transition to school for young children with special learning needs. Guidelines for families, early childhood services and schools. NSW, Department of Education.

Department of Education and Training. (2001). *Who's going to teach my child? A guide for parents of children with special learning needs*. Sydney, Dept of Education.

Dettmer, S., Simpson, R. L., Smith-Myles, B. & Ganz, J. B. (2000). 'The use of visual supports to fascilitate transitions of students with autism.' *Focus on Autism and Other Disabilities* 15(3): 163–72.

Dodd, S. (1994). *Managing Problem Behaviours: A Guide for Parents and Preschools*. Sydney, MacLennan & Petty.

Dodd, S., Pierce, E. & Webster, S. (2002). *Early Play Program* 2nd Ed. Sydney, Autism Association of NSW.

Dowty, T. & Cowlishaw, K. (2002). *Home Educating our Autistic Spectrum Children*. London, Jessica Kingsley Publishers.

Dunn, W. (1999). *Sensory Profile. User's Manual*. USA, The Psychological Corporation.

Dunn, W. (2001). 'The sensations of everyday life: Empirical, theoretical and pragmatic considerations'. *American Journal of Occupational Therapy*. 55(6): 608–20.

Durand, V.M. (1992). *Motivation Assessment Scale*. Topeka, KS: Monaco & Associates.

Eaves, L.C., Ho, H.H., & Eaves, D.M. (1994). 'Subtypes of autism by cluster analysis'. *Journal of Autism and Developmental Disorders*. 24(1):3–22.

Edelson, S. (1995). *Theory of Mind*. The Center for the Study of Autism.

Edelson, S.M., Rimland, B. & Grandin, T. (2003). 'Response to Goldstein's commentary: Intervention to facilitate auditory, visual, and motor integration: "show me the data"'. *Journal of Autism and Developmental Disorders*. 33(5): 551–2.

Erikson, E.H. (1950). *Childhood and Society*. New York: Norton.

Everard, M. P. (1976). Mildly autistic young people and their problems. International Symposium on Autism, St. Gallen, Switzerland.

Fenske, E. C., Zalenski, C., Krantz, P. J. & McClannahan, L. E. (1985). 'Age at Intervention and Treatment Outcome for Autistic Children in a Comprehensive Intervention Program.' *Analysis and Intervention in Developmental Disabilities* 5: 7–31.

Fischer, K. W. (1980). 'The theory of cognitive development: the control and construction of hierarchical skills' *Psychological Review*. 87: 477–31.

Folstein, S. (1977). 'Infantile autism: a genetic study of 21 twin pairs.' *Journal of Child Psychology and Psychiatry* 18: 297–321.

Freeman, B. J. & Ritvo, E. R. (1984). 'The syndrome of autism: establishing the diagnosis and principles of management.' *Paediatric Annual*. 13(4): 284–90.

Freeman, B. J. (1997). 'Guidelines for Evaluating Intervention Programs for Children with Autism.' *Journal of Autism and Developmental Disorders* 27(6): 641–51.

Frith, U. (1989). *Autism — Explaining the Enigma*. Oxford, Basil Blackwell Ltd.

Frith, U. (1991). *Autism and Asperger Syndrome*. Cambridge University Press, London.

Frith,U. (2004). Emanuel Miller lecture: confusions and controversies about Asperger syndrome. *Journal of Child Psychology & Psychiatry*. 45(4): 672–86.

Frost, L., & Bondy, A. S. (1994). *PECS: The Picture Exchange Communication System training manual*. Cherry Hill, NJ., Pyramid Educational Consultants.

Garvey, C. (1977). *Play*. London, Fontana.

Gerlach, E. K. (2003). *Autism Treatment Guide*. 3rd Edition. Eugene, Oregon, Four Leaf Press.

Gillberg, C. & Wing, L. (1999). 'Autism not an extremely rare disorder.' *Acta Psychiat. Scand.* 99(6): 399–406.

Gillberg, C. (1999). 'Neurodevelopmental process and psychological functioning in autism.' *Developmental Psychopathology*. 11(3): 567–87.

Gillberg, C. (2002). *A Guide to Asperger Syndrome*. Cambridge University Press.

Gillberg, C., Ehlers, S., Schaumann, H., Jakibsson, G., Dahlgren, S., Lindblom, R., Bagenholm, A., Tjuus, T. & Blinder, E. (1990). 'Autism Under Age 3 Years: a Clinical Study of 28 Cases Referred for Autistic Symptoms in Infancy.' *Journal of Child Psychology and Psychiatry* 31: 921–34.

Gillberg, I. C. & Gillberg, C (1989). 'Asperger Syndrome — Some epidemiological considerations: A research note.' *Journal of Child Psychology and Psychiatry* 30(4): 631–8.

Gilliam, J.E. (1995). *The Gilliam Autism Rating Scale.* Texas, ProEd.

Glenys, J. (2002). *Educational Provision for Children with Autism and Asperger Syndrome.* London, David Fulton Publishers.

Goldstein, H. & Wickstrom, S. (1986). 'Peer Intervention Effects on Communicative Interaction Among Handicapped and Nonhandicapped Preschoolers.' *Journal of Applied Behaviour Analysis* 19(2): 209–14.

Grados, M. A. & McCarthy, D. (2000). 'Stereotypies and Repetitive Behaviors in Autism.' *Autism: Clinical and Research Issues.* P. J. Accardo, Magnusen, C. & Capute, A. J. Baltimore, York Press.

Grandin, T. & Scariano, M. M. (1986). *Emergence Labelled Autistic.* Cornwall, Great Britain, DJ Costello.

Grandin, T. (1995). 'The learning style of people with autism: an autobiography.' *Teaching children with autism: Strategies to enhance communication and socialisation.* K. Quill. Albany, N.Y., Delmar Publishers.

Grandin, T. (1996). *Making the Transition from the World of School into the World of Work.* Centre for the Study of Autism. Online article: <http://www.autism.org//temple/transition/html>.

Grandin, T. (1996). *Thinking in Pictures.* New York, Vintage Books.

Gray, C. (1994). *Comic Strip Conversations.* Future Horizons, Texas.

Gray, C. (Ed.). (2000). 'Gray's Guide to Bullying.' *The Morning News.* 12(4), 13(1), 13(2): Jenison Public School, Jenison, MI.

Gray, C., & Garand, J. (1993). 'Social Stories: Improving responses of students with autism with accurate social information.' *Focus on Autistic Behaviour* 8(1): 1–10.

Gray, C., (Ed). (1993). *The Social Story Book.* Jenison, MI, Jenison Public Schools.

Grofer, L. (1996). 'Helping the child with autism to understanding transitions.' *Autism Tasmania News:* 8–9.

Hadden, M. (2003). *The Curious Incident of the Dog in the Night-time.* London, Jonathan Cape.

Happe, F. & Frith,U. (1996). 'The neuropsychology of autism.' *Brain.* 119(4): 1377–400.

Happe, F. (1993). 'Communicative competence and theory of mind in autism: a test of relevance theory.' *Cognition* 48(2): 101–19.

Happe, F. (1994). 'An advanced test of theory of mind: understanding a story character's thoughts and feelings by able autistic, mentally handicapped, and normal children and adults.' *Journal of Autism and Developmental Disorders.* 24(2): 129–54.

Happe, F. (1994). 'Wechsler IQ profile and theory of mind in autism: a research note.' *Journal of Child Psychology and Psychiatry.*

Happe, F. (1994). *Autism, an Introduction to Psychological Theory.* London, UCL Press.

Happe, F. (1995). 'The role of age and verbal ability in the theory of mind task performance of subjects with autism.' *Child Development* 66(3): 843–55.

Happe, F. (1999). 'Autism: cognitive deficit or cognitive style?' *Trends in Cognitive Science* 3(6):216–22.

Happe, F. (2003). 'Theory of mind and the self.' *Annual N.Y. Academic Science* Oct:1001: 134–44.

Happe,F. (1996). 'Studying weak central coherence at low levels: children with autism do not succumb to visual illusions. A research note.' *Journal Child Psychology Psychiatry.* 37(7): 873–7.

Harris, P. (1993). 'Pretending and planning.' *Understanding other minds — Perpectives from autism.* S. Baron-Cohen, H. Tager-Flusberg & D.J. Cohen (Editors). Oxford, Oxford University Press.

Harris, S., Handleman, J.S., Kristoff, B., Bass, L. & Gordan, R.. (1990). 'Changes in Language Development Among Autistic and Peer Children in Segregated and Integrated Preschool Settings.' *Journal of Autism and Developmental Disorders* 20: 23–32.

Hatch- Rasmussen, C. (1995). *Sensory Integration.* Beaverton, Oregon, Therapies Northwest.

Hauck, M., Fein, D., Waterhouse, L. & Feinstein, C. (1995). 'Social Interactions by Autistic Children to Adults and Other Children.' *Journal of Autism and Developmental Disorders* 25(6): 579–95.

Healy, J (1982). 'The Enigma of Hyperlexia.' *Reading Research Quarterly.* 3: 319–38.

Heilman, K.M. & Valenstein, E. (1993). *Clinical Neuropsychology.* 3rd ed. Oxford University Press, N.Y.

Hermelin, B. & O'Connor, N. (1970). *Psychological Experiments with Autistic Children.* London, Pergamon.

Hermelin, B. (1976). 'Coding and the sense modalities.' *Early Childhood Autism.* L. Wing. London, Pergamon.

Hesmondhalgh, M. & Breakey, C. (2001). *Access and Inclusion for Children with Autistic Spectrum Disorders.* London, Jessica Kingsley Publishers.

Hodgdon, L. A. (1995). *Visual Strategies for Improving Communication* Vol. 1. Michigan, Quirk Roberts Publishing.

Hodgdon, L. A. (1999). *Solving Behaviour Problems in Autism.* Michigan, Quirk Roberts Publishing.

Hopkins, J. M. & Lord, C. (1981). 'The social behaviour of autistic children with younger and same-age non-handicapped peers.' Papers and reports from international meetings of the National Society for Autistic Children. D. Parke (Ed.). Boston, M.A.

Horner, R. H., Carr, E. G., Strain, P. S., Todd, A. W. & Reed, H. K. (2002). 'Problem Behaviour Interventions For Young Children with Autism: A Research Synthesis.' *Journal of Autism and Developmental Disorders* 32(5): 423–46.

Horner, R. H., Dunlap, G., & Koegal, R. L. (Eds.). (1988). *Generalisation and Maintenance: Life-style Changes in Applied Settings.* Baltimore, Paul H. Brookes Publishing Co.

Horton, R. (2004). 'The lessons of MMR'. *The Lancet.* Mar. 6: 363(9411):747–9.

Howlin, P. (1997). 'Prognosis in Autism: Do Specialist Treatments Affect Long-Term Outcome?' *European Child and Adult Psychiatry* 6(2): 55–72.

Howlin, P., Baron-Cohen, S, & Hadwin, J. (2000). *Teaching Children with Autism to Mind-Read.* N.Y., Wiley.

Hoyson, M., & Jamieson, B. & Strain, P.S. (1984). 'Individualized Group Instruction of Normally Developing and Autistic-Like Children: A Description and Evaluation of the LEAP Curriculum Model.' *Journal of the Division of Early Childhood* 8: 157–71.

Huebner, R.A. (1992). Autistic disorder: a neuropsychological enigma. *American Journal of Occupational Therapy.* 46(6): 487–501.

Huebner, R.A. (2001). *Autism: A Sensorimotor Approach to Management.* Gaithersburg MD, Aspen Publishers.

Hughes, C. (1996). 'Brief Report: Planning problems in autism at the level of motor control.' *Journal of Autism and Developmental Disorders* 26: 99–107.

Hughes, C., Russell, J., Robbins, T. W. (1994). 'Evidence for executive dysfunction in autism.' *Neuropsychology* 32: 477–92.

International Molecular Genetic Study of Autism Consortium (IMGSAC). (1998). 'A full genome screen for autism with evidence for linkage to a region on chromosome 7q'. *Human Molecular Genetics.* 7: 571–8.

International Molecular Genetic Study of Autism Consortium (IMGSAC). (2001). 'A geneomewide screen for autism: strong evedence for linkage to chromosomes 2q, 7q, and 16p'. *American Journal for Human Genetics.* 69(3): 570–81.

Ives, M. & Monro, N. (2002). *Caring for a Child with Autism.* London, Jessica Kingsley Publishers.

Jackson, L. (2002). *A User Guide to the GF/CF Diet for Autism, Asperger Syndrome and AD/HD.* London, Jessica Kingsley Publisher.

Janzen, J. (1996). *Understanding the Nature of Autism.* Texas, Therapy Skill Builders.

Janzen, J. E. (1999). *Autism. Facts and Strategies for Parents.* USA, Therapy Skill Builders.

Jarrold, C., Boucher, J. & Smith, P. (1993). 'Symbolic Play in Autism: A Review.' *Journal of Autism and Developmental Disorders* 23(2): 281–307.

Jarrold, C., Boucher, J., & Smith, P. (1996). 'Generativity deficits in pretend play in autism.' *British Journal of Developmental Psychology* 14: 275–300.

Jarrold, C., Smith, P., Boucher, J. & Harris, P. (1994). 'Comprehension of Pretense in Children with Autism.' *Journal of Autism and Developmental Disorders* 24(4): 433–55.

Jordan, R. & Jones, G. (1999). *Meeting the Needs of Children with Autistic Spectrum Disorders.* London, David Fulton Publishers.

Jordan, R. & Libby, S. (1997). 'Developing and using play in the curriculum.' *Autism and Learning: a Guide to Good Practice.* S. Powell & R. Jordan (Editors). London, David Fulton Publishers.

Jordan, R. (1999). *Autistic Spectrum Disorders.* London, David Fulton Publishers.

Joseph, R. M. & Tager-Flusberg, H. (1997). 'An Investigation of Attention and Affect in Children with Autism and Down Syndrome.' *Journal of Autism and Developmental Disorders* 27(4): 385–98.

Kanner, L. & Eisenberg, L. (1956). '*Early infantile autism*, 1943–55.'

Kanner, L. (1943). 'Autistic disturbances of affective contact.' *Nervous Child* 2: 217–50.

Kasari, C. (2002). 'Assessing change in early intervention programs for children with autism'. *Journal of Autism and Developmental Disorders* 32(5):447–61.

Kaye, J. A., del Mar Melero-Montes, M. & Jick, H. (2001). 'Mumps, measles and rubella vaccine and the incidence of autism recorded by general practitioners: a time trend analysis.' *British Medical Journal* (322): 460–3.

Kientz, M. A., & Dunn, W. (1997). 'A comparison of the performance of children with and without autism on the sensory profile.' *American Journal of Occupational Therapy* 51: 530–7.

Koegal, R. L., Egel, A. L., & Dunlap, G. (1980). 'Learning characteristics of autistic children.' *Methods of Instruction with Severely Handicapped Students.* W. Sailor, B. Wilcox & L.J. Brown (Editors). Baltimore, MD, Paul H. Brookes Publishing Co.

Koegel, R. L. & Koegal, L. K. (1995). *Teaching Children with Autism.* Maryland, Paul H. Brookes Publishing.

Kranowitz, C. (1998). *The out-of-sync child: Recognising and coping with sensory integration dysfunction.* New York, Skylight Press.

Lane, S. & Royeen, C. (1991). 'Tactile processing and sensory defensiveness' In Fisher, Murray & Bundy (eds) *Sensory Integration Theory and Practice.* Philadelphia, F.A. Davis Co.

LaVigna, G. W. & Willis, T.J. (1991). Nonaversive behaviour modification. Minneapolis, Minnesota, Workshop presentation, Institute for Applied (5): 659–85. Behaviour Analysis.

Le Blanc, L.A., Coates, A.M., Daneshvar, S., Charlop-Christy, M.H., Morris, C. & Lancaster, B.M. (2003). 'Using video modeling and reinforcement to teach perspective-taking skills to children with autism'. *Journal of Applied Behaviour Analysis.* 36: 253–7.

Le Breton, M. (2001). *Diet Intervention and Autism.* London, Jessica Kingsley Publisher.

Le Page, M. & Ainsworth C. (2001). 'MMR Vaccine: A parent's dilemma'. *The New Scientist.* 3 Feb,2001. No 2276, p 8–9.

Lears, L. (1998). *Ian's Walk, A Story about Autism.* Illinois, Albert Whitman & Co.

Leslie, A. M. (1987). 'Pretense and representation: the origins of theory of mind.' *Psychological Review* 94(4): 412–26.

Lewis, V. & Boucher, J. (1995). 'Generativity in the Play of Young People with Autism.' *Journal of Autism and Developmental Disorders* 25(2): 105–21.

Libby, S., Powell, S., Messer, D. & Jordan, R. (1997). 'Imitation of Pretend Play Acts by Children with Autism and Down Syndrome.' *Journal of Autism and Developmental Disorders* 27(4): 366–83.

Libby, S., Powell, S., Messer, D., & Jordan, R. (1998). 'Spontaneous play in children with autism: a reappraisal.' *Journal of Autism and Developmental Disorders* 28(6): 487–97.

Linder, T.W. (1993). *Transdisciplinary Play-based Intervention.* Baltimore, Paul H. Brookes.

Lord, C. & Risi, S. (2000). *Diagnosis of Autism Spectrum Disorders in Young Children. Autism Spectrum Disorders. A Transactional Developmental Perspective.* A. M. Wetherby, & B.M. Prizant, (Editors). Baltimore, Paul H. Brookes. 9.

Lord, C., Rutter, M. & Le Couteur, A. (1994). 'Autism Diagnostic Interview Revised: a revised version of a diagnostic interview for caregivers of individuals with possible pervasive developmental disorders.' *Journal of Autism and Developmental Disorders*: 24.

Lovaas, I. O. &. Smith, T. (1988). *Intensive Behavioural Treatment for Young Autistic Children. Advances in Clinical Child Psychology.* B. B. Lahey and A. E. Kazdin. New York, Plenum Press. 2.

Lovaas, I. O. (1977). *The Autistic Child: Language Development Through Behaviour Modification.* Oxford, England, Irvington.

Lovaas, O. I. (1987). 'Behavioural Treatment and Normal Educational and Intellectual Functioning of Young Autistic Children.' *Jounral of Consulting and Clinical Psychology* 55: 3–9.

Loveland, K. A. & Landry, S.H. (1986). 'Joint Attention and Language in Autism and Developmental Language Delay.' *Journal of Autism and Developmental Disorders* 16(3): 335–49.

Lowdon, G. (1991). 'Some thoughts on the nature of perception in autism.' *Communication* 25(3).

Lucyshyn, J., Olson, D. & Horner, R. (1995). 'Building an ecology of support: A case study of one young woman with severe problem behaviours living in the community.' *Journal of the Association for Persons with Severe Handicaps* 20(1): 16–30.

Luria, A. R. (1966). *The Higher Cortical Functions in Man.* New York, Basic Books.

Mahoney, G. & Filer, J. (1996). 'How Responsive is Early Intervention to the Priorities and Needs of Families?' *Topics in Early Childhood Special Education* 16(4): 437–57.

Mahoney, G. & Wheeden, C.A. (1997). 'Parent-Child Interaction — The Foundation for Family-Centred Early Intervention Practice : A Response to Baird and Peterson.' *Topics in Early Childhood Special Education* 17(2): 165.

Mahoney, W., Szatmari, P., Maclean, J., Bryson, S., Bartolucci, G., Walter, S., Hoult, L., & Jones, M. (1998). 'Reliability and accuracy of differentiating pervasive developmental disorder subtypes.' *Journal of the American Academy of Child and Adolescent Psychiatry* 37: 278–85.

Mars, A. E., Mauk, J. E. & Dowrick, P. W. (1998). 'Symptoms of pervasive developmental disorders as observed in prediagnostic home videos of infants and toddlers.' *Journal of Pediatrics* 132: 500–4.

McAfee, J. (2002). *Navigating the Social World.* Arlington, Future Horizons.

McArthur, D. & Adamson, L.B. (1996). 'Joint Attention in Preverbal Children: Autism and Developmental Language Disorder.' *Journal of Autism and Developmental Disorders* 26(5): 481–96.

McBride, S. L. & Peterson, C. (1997). 'Home-Based Early Intervention with Families of Children with Disabilities: Who is Doing What?' *Topics in Early Childhood Special Education* 17(2): 209–33.

McEachin, J., Smith, T. & Lovaas, D. (1993). 'Long-Term Outcome for Children with Autism who Received Early Intensive Behavioural Treatment.' *American Journal on Mental Retardation* 97: 359–72.

McEvoy, R. E., Rogers, S. J. & Pennington, B. F. (1993). 'Executive function and social communication deficits in young autistic children.' *Journal of Child Psychology and Psychiatry.* 34(4): 563–78.

McGee, G. G., Feldman, R. S. & Morrier, M. J. (1997). 'Benchmarks of Social Treatment for Children with Autism.' *Journal of Autism and Developmental Disorders* 27(4): 353–63.

Medical Research Council. (Dec. 2001). *Review of Autism Research: Epidemiology and Causes.* Medical Research Council.

Mesibov, G. & Handley, S. (1998). 'Adolescents and adults with autism'. In D.J. Cohen & F.R. Volkmer (eds). *Handbook of Autism and Pervasive Developmental Disorders.* 2nd ed. N.Y. Wiley, pp 309–22.

Mesibov, G. B. (1997). 'Preschool Issues in Autism: Introduction.'

Meyer, R. N. (2001). *Asperger Syndrome Employment Workbook.* London, Jessica Kingsley Publishers.

Mirenda, P., & Erickson, K.A. (2000). *Augmentative Communication and Literacy. Autism Spectrum Disorders. A Transactional Developmental Perspective.* A. M. Wetherby, & Prizant, B.M. Baltimore (Editors), Paul H. Brookes.

Mirenda, P., & Mathy-Laikko, P. (1989). 'Augmentative and alternative communication applications for persons with severe congenital communication disorders: An introduction.' *Augmentative and Alternative Communication* 1: 143–50.

Mirenda, P., & Schuler, A., (1989). 'Augmenting communication for persons with autism: Issues and strategies.' *Topics in Language Disorders* 9: 24–43.

Moon, E. (2002). 'Speed of Dark.' Great Britain, Orbit Books.

Mundy, P. & Crowson, M. (1997). 'Joint Attention and Early Social Communication: Implications for Research on Intervention with Autism.' *Journal of Autism and Developmental Disorders* 27(6): 653–75.

Mundy, P. & Markus, J. (1997). 'On the nature of communication and language impairment in autism'. *Mental Retardation and Developmental Disabilities Research Review* 3(4): 343–9.

Mundy, P. & Sigman, M. (1989). 'Social attachments in autistic children.' *Journal of American Academy Child Adolescent Psychiatry* 28(1): 74–81.

Mundy, P., Sigman, M & Sherman, T. (1987). 'Nonverbal Communication and Play Correlates of Language Development in Autistic Children.' *Journal of Autism and Developmental Disorders* 17 (349–64).

Mundy, P., Sigman, M., Ungerer, J. & Sherman, T. (1986). 'Defining the Social Deficits of Autism: The Contribution of Non-Verbal Communication Measures.' *Journal of Child Psychology and Psychiatry* 27(5): 657–69.

Mundy, P., Sigman,M & Kasari, C. (1990). 'A Longitudinal Study of Joint Attention and Language Development in Autistic Children.' *Journal of Autism and Developmental Disorders* 20(1): 115–28.

Mundy,P. (1995). 'Joint attention and social emotional approach behaviour in children with autism.' *Development and Pschopathology* 7(1): 63–82.

Musselwhite, C. R., & Waterman, K. (1988). *Communication Programming for Persons with Severe Handicaps.* St. Louis, Little, Brown & Co.

Myles, B. S. & Southwick, J. (1999). *Asperger Syndrome and Difficult Moments.* Kansas, Autism Asperger Publishing Co.

Myles, B. S. (2003). 'Behavioural forms of stress management for individuals with Asperger's syndrome'. *Child Adolescent Psychiatric Clinic N. America* 12(1):123–41.

Myles, B. S., Dun, W. & Orr, S. (2002). 'Sensory processing issues associated with Asperger's syndrome: a preliminary investigation'. *Journal Occupational Therapy* 56(1): 97–102.

Myles, B. S., Tapscott Cook, K., Miller, N. E., Rinner, L., & Robbins, L. A. (2000). *Asperger Syndrome and Sensory Issues.* Kansas, Autism Asperger Publishing Co.

Myles, B., Bock, S. & Simpson, R. (2001). *The Asperger Syndrome Diagnostic Scale.* Kansas, Autism/Asperger Publishing Co.

Nansel, T. R., Overpeck, M., Pilla, R. S., Ruan, W. J., Simons-Morton, B., & Scheidt, P. (2001). 'Bullying behaviours among U.S. youth: Prevalence and association with psychosocial adjustment.' *Journal of the American Medical Association.* 285(16): 2094–100.

National Institute of Mental Health (NIMH). (2001). 'Facts about Anxiety Disorders'. Fact Sheet Publication No. OM-994152.

New Scientist: 'Vaccine autism link retracted'. 181: issue 2438. 13 March 2004, p 4.

O'Neill, J. L. (1999). *Through the Eyes of Aliens: A Book about Autistic People.* London, Jessica Kingsley Publishers.

O'Neill, M. & Jones, R. (1997). 'Sensory-Perceptual Abnormalities in Autism: A Case For More Research?' *Journal of Autism and Developmental Disorders* 27(3): 284–93.

Oliver, C., Murphy, G. H. & Corbett, J. A. (1987). 'Self injurious behaviour in people with mental handicaps: a total population study'. *Journal Mental Deficiencies Response.* 31(2): 147–62.

Olley, J. G. (1987). 'Classroom structure and autism.' *Handbook of Autism and Pervasivve Developmental Disorders.* D. J. C. A. M. Donnellan. New York, Wiley.

Olweus, D. *Bullying at school: What we Know and What we can Do*, Schwab Foundation.

Ornitz, E. M. (1970). 'Vestibular Dysfunction in schizophrenia and childhood autism.' *Comprehensive Psychiatry.*

Ornitz, E. M. (1973). 'The modulation of sensory input and motor output in autistic children.' *Psychopathology and Child Development.* S. Reichler. New York, Plenum.

Ornitz, E. M., Guthrie, D. & Farley, A. H. (1977). The early development of autistic children. *Journal of Autism Childhood Schizophrenia.* 7(3): 207–29.

Osborn, K., & Wilcox, B. (1992). *School to community transition: A Planning and Procedures Handbook for Parents and Teachers in La Porte County.* Bloomington, IN, Indiana University, Institute for the Study of Developmental Disabilities.

Osterling, J. & Dawson, G. (1994). 'Early Recognition of Children with Autism: A Study of First Birthday Home Videotapes.' *Journal of Autism and Developmental Disorders* 24(3): 247–58.

Ozonoff, S. (1995). 'Executive functions in autism.' *Learning and Cognition in Autism.* E. Schopler & G. Mesibov (Editors). New York, Plenum Publishers.

Ozonoff, S., Pennington, B.F. & Rogers, S.J. (1991). 'Executive function deficits in high functioning autistic individuals: relationship to theory of mind.' *Journal of Child Psychology and Psychiatry.* 32(7): 1081-105.

Patja, A., Davidkin, I., Kurki, T., Kallio, M. J., Valle, M., & Peltola, H. (2000). 'Serious adverse events after measles-mumps-rubella vaccination during a fourteen year prospective follow-up'. *Pediatric Infectious Disease Journal* 19(12): 1127–34.

Peterson, S. L., Bondy, A. S., Vincent, Y. & Finnegan, C. S. (1995). 'Effects of altering communicative input for students with autism and no speech: Two case studies.' *Augmentative and Alternative Communication* 11: 93–100.

Phillips, W., Gómez, J. C., Baron-Cohen, S., Laa, V. & Riviere, A. (1995). 'Treating People as Objects, Agents, or "Subjects": How Young Children With and Without Autism Make Requests.' *Journal of Child Psychology and Psychiatry* 36(8): 1383–98.

Piaget J. (1969/91). 'Advances in child and adolescent psychology'. In P. Light, S. Sheldon, & M. Woodhead (eds). *Learning to Think.* (p 5–15), London, Routledge.

Piaget, J. (1954). 'The development of time concepts in the child'. Procedures Annual Meeting of Americam Psychopathological Association discussion. p 45–55.

Piaget, J. (1962). Play, *Dreams and Imitation.* New York, W.W. Norton & Co.

Piaget, J. (1969) *The Mechanisms of Perception.* London, Routledge & Keegan.

Pierce, K., Glad, K. S. & Schreibman, L. (1997). 'Social Perception in Children with Autism: An Attentional Deficit?' *Journal of Autism and Developmental Disorders* 27(3): 265–82.

Porges, S. (2003). The Sound Connection 9(4): 1–2. *Quarterly Newsletter of the Society for Auditory Intervention Techniques.*

Potter, C. & Whittaker, C. (2001). *Enabling Communication.* London, Jessica Kingsley Publishers.

Powell, S. (Editor). (2000). *Helping Children with Autism to Learn.* London, David Fulton Publishers.

Powers, M. (1992). *Early intervention for children with autism. Autism: Identification, education and treatment.* D. E. Berkell (Editor). Hillsdale N. J., Lawrence Erlbaum Associates.

Pratt, C. (2002). *Transition: Preparing for a Lifetime,* BBB Autism Support Network. Article 39 The Indiana Resource Centre for Autism.

Prior, M. & Cummings, J. (2000). *Understanding Asperger's Syndrome.* Melbourne, Royal Children's Hospital.

Prior, M. (2003). 'Is there an increase in the prevalence of autism spectrum disorders?' *Journal of Paediatric Child Health.* 39(2): 81–2.

Prior, M.R. (1979). 'Cognitive abilities and disabilities in infantile autism: a review'. *Journal of Abnormal Child Psychology.* 7(4):357–80.

Prizant, B. & Rubin, E. (1999). 'Contemporary Issues in Interventions for Autism Spectrum Disorders: A Commentary.' *Journal of the Association for Persons with Severe Handicaps* 24(3): 199–208.

Prizant, B. & Rydell, P. J. (1984). 'Analysis of functions of delayed echolalia in autistic children'. *Journal of Speech Hearing Response.* 27(2):183–92.

Prizant, B. & Schuler, A. L. (1987). *Facilitating communication: Theoretical foundations. Handbook of Autism and Pervasive Developmental Disorders.* C. A. Donnellan (Editor). New York, Wiley.

Prizant, B. (1983). 'Language acquisition and communicative behaviour in autism: towards an understanding of the "whole' of it".' *Journal of Speech Hearing Disorders* 48(3): 296–307.

Prizant, B. M. & Wetherby, A. M. (1988). 'Providing Services to Children with Autism (Ages 0 to 2 Years) and Their Families.' *Topics in Language Disorders* 9(1): 1–23.

Prizant, B. M. (1996). 'Brief Report: Communication, Language, Social, and Emotional Development.' *Journal of Autism and Developmental Disorders* 26(2): 173.

Prizant, B."M. & Wetherby, A. M. (1987). Communicative intent: a framework for understanding social-communicative behaviour in autism. *Journal of American Academy of Child Adolescent Psychiatry* 26(4): 472–9.

Quill, K. A. (1997). 'Instructional considerations for young children with autism: the rationale for visually cued instruction.' *Journal for Autism and Developmental Disorders* 27(6): 697–714.

Quill, K. A. (2000). Do-Watch-Listen-Say. Baltimore, Paul H. Brookes.

Quill, K. A. (Editor). (1995). *Teaching Children with Autism: Strategies to Enhance Communication and Socialisation.* Albany, New York, Delmar Publishers.

Rand, B. *How to Understand People who are Different.* Online article <http://www.isn.net>.

Restall, G. & Magill-Evans, J. (1994). 'Play and preschool children with autism.' *The American Journal of Occupational Therapy* 48(2): 113–20.

Richer, J. & Coates, S. (eds.) (2001). *Autism. The Search for Coherence.* London, Jessica Kingsley Publishers.

Richman, S. *Raising a Child with Autism* . London, Jessica Kingsley Publishers.

Rimland, B. & Baker, S.M. (1996). 'Brief Report: Alternative Approaches to the Development of Effective Treatments for Autism.' *Journal of Autism and Developmental Disorders* 26(2): 237–41.

Rimland, B. & Edelson, S. M. (1995). 'Brief report: a pilot study of auditory integration training in autism'. *Journal of Autism and Developmental Disorders* 25(1): 61–70.

Roberts, J. M. A. (1988). 'What is echolalia?' Autism Association of N.S.W. Sydney.

Rogers, S. J. & DiLalla, D. (1991). 'A Comparative Study of the Effects of a Developmentally Based Preschool Curriculum on Young Children with Autism and Young Children with other Disorders of Behaviour and Development.' *Topics in Early Childhood Special Education* 11(2): 29–47.Rogers, S. J. & Lewis, H. C. (1989). 'An Effective Day Treatment Model for Young Children with Pervasive Developmental Disorders.' *Journal of Child and Adolescent Psychiatry* 28: 207–14.

Rogers, S. J. & Pennington, B. F. (1991). 'A theoretical approach to the deficits in infantile autism.' *Development and Psychopathology* 3: 137–62.

Rogers, S. J. (1996). 'Brief Report: Early Intervention in Autism.' *Journal of Autism and Developmental Disorders* 26(2): 243.

Rogers, S. J., Lewis, H. C. & Reis, K. (1987). 'An Effective Procedure for Training Early Special Education Teams to Implement a Model Program.' *Journal of the Division of Early Childhood* 11: 180–8.

Rojahn, J., Hammer, D. & Kroeger, T. L. (1996). 'Stereotypy'. In N. N.Singh (ed) *Prevention and Treatment of Severe Behaviour Problems: Models and Methods in Developmental Disabilities* (pp 199–216), Pacific Grove CA, Brooks/Cole.

Romski, M. A., & Sevcik, R. A. (1996). *Breaking the Speech Barrier: Language Development Through Augmented Means.* Baltimore, Paul H. Brookes Publishing Co.

Ruble, L. A. & Dalrymple, N. J. (1996). 'An Alternative View of Outcome in Autism.' *Focus on Autism and Other Developmental Disabilities* 11(1): 3–14.

Russell, J., Saltmarsh, R., & Hill, E. (1999). 'What do executive factors contribute to the failure on false belief tasks by children with autism.' *Journal of Child Psychology and Psychiatry* 40(6): 859–68.

Rutter, M. (1978). 'Diagnosis and Definition of Childhood Autism.' *Journal of Autism and Childhood Schizophrenia* 8: 139–61.

Rutter, M. (1985). The Treatment of autistic children. *Journal of Child Psychology and Psychiatry* 26(2): 193–214.

Rydell, P. J. & Mirenda, P. (1994). 'Effects of High and Low Constraint Utterances on the Production of Immediate and Delayed Echolalia in Young Children with Autism.' *Journal of Autism and Developmental Disorders* 719–35.

Saitoh, O. & Courchesne, E. (1998), 'Magnetic resonance imaging study of the brain in autism.' *Psychiatry Clinical Neuroscience* 52: 219–22.

Sattler, J. (1992). *Assessment of Children* (3rd ed rev), San Diego, Jerome M. Sattler.

School Therapy Services. (2002). *Learning Through the Senses.* Northern Territory, Territory Health Services.

Schopler, E., Reichler, R. J. & Rochen-Renner, B. (1993). *The Childhood Autism Rating Scale.* Western Psychological Services, Los Angelos.

Schopler,E. (1965). Early infantile autism and receptor processes. *Arch. Gen. Psychiatry* 13(4): 327–35.

Schopler,E. (1976). 'Toward reducing behaviour problems in autistic children.' *Journal of Autism and Childhood Schizophrenia* 6(1); 1–13.

Schreibman, L. (1996). 'Brief Report: The Case for Social and Behavioural Intervention Research.' *Journal of Autism and Developmental Disorders* 26(2): 247.

Schuler, A. L., Prizant, B. M. and Wetherby, A. M. (1997). 'Enhancing language and communication development: prelinguistic approaches.' *Handbook of Autism and Pervasive Developmental Disorders.* D. J. Cohen & F. R. Volkmar (Editors). New York, Wiley.

Schuler, A., & Baldwin, M. (1981). 'Nonspeech communication and childhood autism.' *Language, Speech and Hearing Services in the Schools* 12: 246–57.

Schwartz, I. S., Garfinkle, A. N., & Bauer, J. (1998). 'The picture exchange communication system: Communicative outcomes for young children with disabilities.' *Topics in Early Childhood Education* 18(3): 144–59.

Seal, B., & Bonvillian, J. (1997). 'Sign language and motor functioning in students with autistic disorder.' *Journal of Autism and Developmental Disorders* 27: 437–66.

Seibert, J. M. & Oller, D. K. (1981). 'Linguistic pragmatics and language intervention strategies'. *Journal Autism and Developmental Disorders* 11(1):75–88.

Seifer, R., Clark, G. N. & Sameroff, A. J. (1991). 'Positive Effects of Interaction Coaching on Infants with Developmental Disabilities and Their Mothers.' *American Journal on Mental Retardation* 96(1): 1–11.

Shah, A. & Frith, U. (1993). 'Why do autistic individuals show superior performance in the block design task?' *Journal of Child Psychology and Psychiatry* 34(8):1351–64.

Sherratt, D. (1999). 'The importance of play'. In G. Jones (ed) *Good Autism Practice.* London, David Fulton.

Sherratt, D. (1999). *The Development of Pretend Play in Children with Autism.* London, Teacher Training Agency.

Siegel, B. (2000). 'Behavioural and educational treatments for autism spectrum disorders.' *The Advocate* 33: 22–25.

Siegel, B., Anders, T. F. Ciaranello, R. D., Bienenstock, B. & Kraemer, H. C. (1986). 'Empirically Derived Subclassification of the Autistic Syndrome.' *Journal of Autism and Developmental Disorders* 16(3): 275–93.

Sigman, M., & Capps, L. (1997). *Children with Autism: A Developmental Perspective*. Cambridge MA, Harvard University Press.

Sigman, M., Mundy, P., Sherman, T. & Ungerer, J. (1986). 'Social Interactions of Autistic, Mentally Retarded and Normal Children and Their Caregivers.' *Journal of Child Psychology and Psychiatry* 27(5): 647–56.

Simmons, K. L. (1998). *Little Rainman*. Texas, Future Horizons.

Sinha, Y., Silove, N., Wheeler, D., & Williams, K. (2004). 'Auditory integration training and other sound therapies for autism spectrum disorders'. *Cochrane Database System Review* (1) CD003681.

Smith, M. D., Belcher, R. G., & Juhrs, P. D. (1995). *A Guide to Successful Employment for Individuals with Autism*. Baltimore, Paul H. Brookes.

Snyder, J., Brooker, M., Patrick, M.R., Snyder, A., Schrepferman, L., & Stoolmiller, M. (2003). 'Observed peer victimization during early elementary school: continuity, growth and relation to risk for child antisocial and depressive behaviour.' *Child Development* 74(6): 1881–98.

Spague, J. R. & Rian, V. (1993). 'Support systems for students with severe problem behaviours in Indiana: A descriptive analysis of school structure and student demographics'. Unpublished manuscript Indiana University, Bloomington.

Sparling, J. W. (1991). 'Brief Report: A Prospective Case Report of Infantile Autism from Pregnancy to Four Years.' *Journal of Autism and Developmental Disorders* 21(2): 229–36.

Sparrow, S. S., Balla, D. A. & Cicchetti, D. V. (1984). *Vineland Adaptive Behaviour Scales*. AGS Publishing, MN.

Stahmer, A. C. (1995). 'Teaching Symbolic Play Skills to Children with Autism Using Pivotal Response Training.' *Journal of Autism and Developmental Disorders* 25: 123–41.

Stahmer, A. C. (1999). 'Using pivotal response training to facilitate appropriate play in children with autistic spectrum disorders.' *Child Language Teaching and Therapy* 15(1): 29–40.

Stewart, R. (Spring 2000). 'Should We Insist on Eye Contact with People Who Have Autism Spectrum Disorders?' *Indiana Resource Center for Autism Reporter* 5(3): 7–12.

Stokes, T. F. & Baer, D. M. (1977). 'An implicit technology of generalisation.' *Journal of Applied Behaviour Analysis* 10: 349–69.

Stone, W. L.& Lemanek, K. L. (1990). 'Parental Report of Social Behaviours in Autistic Preschoolers.' *Journal of Autism and Developmental Disorders* 20: 513–22.

Stone, W. L., Ousley, O. Y., Yoder, P. J., Hogan, K. L., & Hepburn, S. L. (1997). 'Nonverbal Communication in Two-and-Three-Year-Old Children with Autism.' *Journal of Autism and Developmental Disorders* 27(6): 677–96.

Stratton, K. (2001). 'Immunization safety review: measles-mumps-rubella vaccine and autism.' Institute of Medicine. Washhington D.C., National Accademy Press.

Surian, L., Baron-Cohen, S, & Van der Lely, H. (1996). 'Are children with autism deaf to Gricean maxims?' *Cognitive-Neuropsychiatry* 1(1): 55–71.

Sussman, F. (1999). *More Than Words*. Ontario, The Hanen Program.

Szatmari, P. (1991). 'Asperger's Syndrome: Diagnosis, treatment and outcome.' *Psychiatric Clinics of North America* 14(1): 81–92.

Tager-Flusberg, H. (1985). The conceptual basis for referential word meaning in children with autism. *Child Development* 25(5): 1167–78.

Tager-Flusberg, H. (1996). 'Brief Report: Current Theory and Research on Language and Communication in Autism.' *Journal of Autism and Developmental Disorders* 26(2): 169–72.

Tager-Flusberg, H. (2004). 'Strategies for conducting research on language in autism.' *Journal of Autism and Developmental Disorders* 34(1): 75–80.

Taylor, B., Miller,E., Farrington, G. P., Petropoulos, M. C., Favout-Mayaud, I., Li, J., & Wright, P. A. (1999). 'Autism and measles, mumps and rubella vaccine: no epidemiological evidence for a causal association.' *Lancet* (353): 2026–29.

Teitelbaum, P. (1998). 'Movement analysis in infancy may be useful for the early diagnosis of autism.' Procedures from the National Academy of Science USA 95: 13982–7.

The Times. Edition 4M. Thurs 04 Mar 2004, p 4.

Thieman, K. S., & Goldstein, H. (2001). 'Social Stories, written text cues, and video feedback: Effects on social communication of children with autism.' *Journal of Applied Behaviour Analysis* 34: 425–46.

Thorp, D. M., Stahmer, A. C., & Schreibman, L. (1995). 'Effects of Sociodramatic Play Training on Children with Autism.' *Journal of Autism and Developmental Disorders* 25(3): 265–82.

Tonge, B. & Einfeld, S. (1999). 'Psychopathology and Intellectual Disability: the Australian child to Adult Longitudinal Study'. In L.M. Glidden (ed) *International Review of Research in Mental Retardation* Vol.26. Academic Press, Maryland.

Tonge, B. J. (2002). 'Autism autistic spectrum and the need for better definition.' *MJA* 176: 412–13.

Tonge, B., Brereton, A., Gray, T. & Einfeld, S. (1999). 'Behavioural disturbance in high functioning autism'. *Autism* 3(2): 117–30.

Trad, P.V., Bernstein, D., Shapiro, T., & Hertzig, M. (1993). 'Assessing the Relationship Between Affective Responsivity and Social Interaction in Children with Pervasive Developmental Disorder.' *Journal of Autism and Developmental Disorders* 23(2): 361–77.

Trevarthen, C., Aitken, K., Papoudi, D., & Robarts, J. (1996). *Children with Autism: Diagnosis and Interventions to Meet Their Needs*. London, Jessica Kingsley Publishers.

Ulliana, L. (2001). *Visual Strategies: Developing Visual Supports*. Autism Association of NSW, Sydney.

Ungerer, J.A. & Sigman, M. (1981). 'Symbolic play and language comprehension in autistic children'. *Journal American Academy Child Psychiatry* 20(2): 318–37.

Vermeulen, P. (2000). *I am Special. Introducing Children and Young People to their Autistic Spectrum Disorder*. London, Jessica Kingsley Publishers.

Vygotsky, L. S. (1964). *Thought and Language*. New York, John Wiley & Sons.

Vygotsky, L. S. (1967). 'Play and its role in the mental development of the child'. *Soviet Psychology* 12: 62–76.

Wakefield, A. J. (1998). 'Ileal-lymphoid-nodular hyperplasia, non-specific colitis and pervasive developmental disorder in children.' *Lancet* (351): 637–41.

Wakefield, A. J. (2002). 'Enterocolitis, autism and measles virus'. *Molecular Psychiatry* 7 Suppl 2: S44–6.

Waterhouse, S. (2000). *A Positive Approach to Autism.* London, Jessica Kingsley Publishers.

Weitzman, E. (1994). *Learning Language and Loving It.* Ontario, Hanen Center Publication.

Wellman, H.M. (1992). *The Child's Theory of Mind.* Cambridge MA., The MIT Press.

Wetherby, A. B., & Prizant, B. M. (2000). *Autism Spectrum Disorders: A Transactional Developmental Perspective.* Baltimore, Paul H.Brookes.

Wetherby, A. M. (1986). 'Ontogeny of communicative functions in autism'. *Journal Autism and Developmental Disorders.* 16(3) 295–316.

Whalen, C. & Schreibman, L. (2003). 'Joint Attention Training for Children with Autism Using Behaviour Modification Procedures.' *Journal of Child Psychology and Psychiatry* 44(3): 456–86.

Wheeler, M. & Pratt, C. (2001). 'When your Child is Diagnosed with an Autism Spectrum Disorder'. Indiana Resource Center for Autism. IRCA Online Publication. <http://www.iidc.indiana.edu.irca/family>.

Whiteley, P, Rogers, J. & Shattock, P. (1998). Clinical features associated with autism. *Autism* 2(4):415–42.

Whiteley, P. & Shattock, P. (2002). 'Biochemical aspects in autism spectrum disorders: updating the opioid-excess theory and presenting new opportunities for biomedical intervention.' *Expert Opinion Therapy Targets* 6(2): 175–83.

Whitely, P., Rogers, J., Savery, D. & Shattock, P. A. (1999). 'A gluten free diet as an intervention for autism and associated spectrum disorders.' *Autism* 3: 45–65.

WHO (1992). *International Classification of Diseases and Related Health Problems.* Geneva, Switzerland, WHO.

Wilbarger, P. & Wilbarger, J (1991). *Sensory Defensiveness in Children Aged 2–12: A Guide for Oarents and Other Caregivers.* Denver CO. Avanti Educational Programs.

Willey, L. H. (1999). *Pretending to be Normal.* London, Jessica Kingsley Publishers.

Willey, L. H. (2001). *Asperger Syndrome in the Family.* London, Jessica Kingsley Publishers.

Williams, D. (1992). *Nobody Nowhere.* London, Doubleday.

Williams, D. (1994). *Somebody Somewhere.* New York, Times Books.

Williams, D. (1996). *Autism. An Inside-Out Approach.* London, Jessica Kingsley Publishers.

Williams, D. (1998). *Autism and Sensing. The Unlost Instinct.* London, Jessica Kingsley Publishers.

Williams, E., Reddy, V. & Costall, A. (2001). 'Taking a closer look at functional play in children with autism.' *Journal of Autism and Developmental Disorders* 31(1): 67–77.

Williams, K. (2001). 'Understanding the Student with Asperger's Syndrome: Guidelines for Teachers.' *Intervention in School and Clinic* 36(5): 287–92.

Williamson, G. G., & Anzalone, M. E., (1997). 'Sensory Integration: A key component of the evaluation and treatment of young children with severe difficulties in relating and communicating.' *Zero to Three Bulletin* 17: 29–36.

Wing, L. & Gould, J. (1979). 'Severe Impairments of Social Interaction and Associated Abnormalities in Children: Epidemiology and Classification.' *Journal of Autism and Developmental Disorders* 9: 11–29.

Wing, L. (1976) 'Diagnosis, clinical description annd prognosis.' In L. Wing (ed.) *Early Childhood Autism* (pp 15–48), Oxford, Pergamon.

Wing, L. (1980). *Autistic Children, A Guide for Parents* Constable, London.

Wing, L. (1981). 'Language, social and cognitive impairments in autism and severe mental retardation.' *Journal of Autism and Developmental Disorders* 11(1): 31-44.

Wing, L. (1988). 'The continuum of autistic disorders'. In E. Schopler & G.M. Mesibov (eds.) *Diagnosis and Assessment in Autism.* (pp 91–110), N.Y. Plenum.

Wing, L. (1996). *The Autistic Spectrum: a Guide for Parents and Professionals.* Constable Publishers, U.K.

Wing, L. (1997). *The Autistic Spectrum.* London, Constable and Company Ltd.

Wing, L., & Attwood, A. (1987). 'Syndromes of autism and atypical development.' *Handbook of Autism and Pervasive Developmental Disorders.* D. Cohen & A. Donnellan (Editors). New York, John Wiley and Sons.

Wolfberg, P. J. & Schuler, A. L. (1993). 'Integrated Play Groups: A Model for Promoting the Social and Cognitive Dimensions of Play in Children with Autism.' *Journal of Autism and Developmental Disorders* 23(3): 467–89.

Wolfberg, P. J. (1999). *Play and Imagination in Children with Autism.* New York, Teachers College Press.

Wulff, B. (1985). 'The Symbolic and Object Play of Children with Autism: A Review.' *Journal of Autism and Developmental Disorders* 15: 139–48.

Yack, E., Aquilla, P., & Sutton, S. (2002). *Building Bridges Through Sensory Integration*, 2nd Ed. Las Vegas, Sensory Resources.

Yarnall, P. (2000). 'Current interventions in autism — a brief analysis.' *The Advocate* 33: 25–27.

Index